MW01283562

"Pain is complex, requiring a multifaceted approach to successfully understanding and designing effective interventions for pain care. As a psychologist and yoga therapist who has worked in the field of pain management for over four decades, I deeply appreciate *Yoga and Science in Pain Care* as a valuable addition to the field of pain management. This carefully crafted book offers us a vast and priceless array of theoretical and practical insights, interventions, and resources for enhancing our ability to fully understand, support, and provide effective pain care for individuals living with pain."

*—Richard C. Miller, PhD, Co-Founder, The International Association of Yoga Therapy and developer of iRest Meditation: Restorative Practices for Health, Resiliency, and Well-Being*

"The authors of *Yoga and Science in Pain Care* have elegantly illuminated theory, history, clinical expertise, and personal practice so that laymen, clinicians, and the yoga community can have a resource on every page of this text. Jump into any chapter and deepen the trust you have in your own experience of pain while gaining insight, hope and new coping strategies for yourself or your clients."

*—Jill Miller, author of* The Roll Mode *and creator of Yoga Tune Up®*

"*Yoga and Science in Pain Care* is an extraordinarily in-depth, multi-dimensional look at pain. Utilizing both the lenses of the state-of-the-art neurobiological understanding of pain and the broad therapeutic wisdom from the yoga tradition, this text is a necessary reference for anyone wanting to better understand the complexity of chronic pain and the conceptual models for skillfully addressing the suffering of this epidemic."

*—Kimberly Carson, MPH, C-IAYT, co-author of* Relax Into Yoga for Chronic Pain, *www.mindfulyogaworks.com*

"This insightful research and experience-based book explores yoga therapy as a treatment and living practice. The authors provide an integrated, in-depth understanding of how yoga therapy can be incorporated within a modern understanding of pain as an experience. The book encompasses perspectives from people living with pain, summarises research progress in the field, debates theories of pain and pain management, considers the many different yoga practices, describes pain biology, self-regulation and examines breath, body awareness, nutrition, emotions and responses to pain, and above all, integrates concern for practitioners and people with pain as humans sharing an intangible experience together. The authors write with precision and care to ensure novice and expert alike will learn more about how yoga therapy can provide a uniting and compassionate approach to helping people with pain learn to live well."

*—Bronwyn Lennox Thompson, PhD, MSc, DipOT, Postgraduate Academic Programme Leader, Pain and Pain Management, Orthopaedic Surgery and Musculoskeletal Medicine, University of Otago, Christchurch, NZ*

"*Yoga and Science in Pain Care* is a 'master text' that seamlessly integrates contemporary scientific understanding with the breadth of yogic body-mind principles. Written in a manner that will appeal to both those appreciating a level of scientific rigor and those more attuned to the broader, more holistic approach, this text should be part of the professional library for all yoga teachers and therapists. The list of editors and contributors is a 'who's who' of leaders in the field of therapeutic yoga."

—*Leigh Blashki, C-IAYT, Past-President, Yoga Australia,*
*Founder, Australian Institute of Yoga Therapy*

"*Yoga and Science in Pain Care* is a beautiful blending of creativity, hope, science, enthusiasm, and compassion. This is a must-have resource for clinicians and movement therapists of all types. The individual chapters are immediately useful, and taken as a whole it is a guide to helping people (or ourselves) live well with pain. I especially appreciate the joy of movement and positivity that are represented throughout the book. Keep this in your clinics and gift it to new healthcare professionals, it will save you time and help focus recovery."

—*Sandy Hilton, PT, DPT, MS, Entropy Physiotherapy,*
*Chicago, www.entropy-physio.com*

"*Yoga and Science in Pain Care* will help the world see that the yogic wisdom of the ages is converging with scientific revelations—that the only way toward sustainable transformation for those suffering with pain is to restore the whole person and facilitate change in all of its complexity."

—*Melissa Cady, D.O., Board-Certified in Anesthesiology and*
*Pain Medicine, author of Paindemic, www.painoutloud.com*

"I am confident you will learn as much as I did while reading this amazing timely collaborative book about unique approaches to yoga in the setting of chronic pain. This text is destined to become an instant classic and required reading in the field of yoga therapy, and its impact will no doubt be felt in many other fields working with persistent pain!"

—*Baxter Bell, MD, co-author of* Yoga for Healthy Aging

"*Yoga and Science in Pain Care* is a book that every yoga teacher and therapist should study. It offers current, real, and inspired wisdom on the effects of acute or chronic pain and how to manage it through yoga. It addresses the complex issues around pain, and how mind/body yoga techniques can change the responses of our nervous system toward pain. This book offers hope to those suffering from pain and those who treat them. These compassionate therapists have provided for us through stories, scientific research, and experience, a safe and invaluable pathway to the future of successful pain management."

—*Marion (Mugs) McConnell, author of* Letters from the Yoga Masters:
Teachings Revealed Through Correspondence from Paramhansa
Yogananda, Ramana Maharshi, Swami Sivananda and Others

# Yoga and Science
# in Pain Care

*of related interest*

**Yoga Therapy as a Creative Response to Pain**
*Matthew J. Taylor*
*Foreword by John Kepner*
ISBN 978 1 84819 356 7
eISBN 978 0 85701 315 6

**Yoga Therapy for Stroke**
A Handbook for Yoga Therapists and Healthcare Professionals
*Arlene A. Schmid and Marieke Van Puymbroeck*
*Forewords by Matthew J. Taylor and Linda Williams*
ISBN 978 1 84819 369 7
eISBN 978 0 85701 327 9

**Yoga for a Happy Back**
A Teacher's Guide to Spinal Health through Yoga Therapy
*Rachel Krentzman, PT, E-RYT*
*Foreword by Aadil Palkhivala*
ISBN 978 1 84819 271 3
eISBN 978 0 85701 253 1

**Yoga Therapy for Parkinson's Disease and Multiple Sclerosis**
*Jean Danford*
ISBN 978 1 84819 299 7
eISBN 978 0 85701 249 4

**Principles and Themes in Yoga Therapy**
An Introduction to Integrative Mind/Body Yoga Therapeutics
*James Foulkes*
*Foreword by Mikhail Kogan, MD*
*Illustrated by Simon Barkworth*
ISBN 978 1 84819 248 5
eISBN 978 0 85701 194 7

**Yoga Teaching Handbook**
A Practical Guide for Yoga Teachers and Trainees
*Edited by Sian O'Neill*
ISBN 978 1 84819 355 0
eISBN 978 0 85701 313 2

**Scoliosis, Yoga Therapy, and the Art of Letting Go**
*Rachel Krentzman, PT, E-RYT*
*Foreword by Matthew J. Taylor PT, PhD*
ISBN 978 1 84819 272 0
eISBN 978 0 85701 243 2

# YOGA and SCIENCE in PAIN CARE

## TREATING THE PERSON IN PAIN

Edited by NEIL PEARSON, SHELLY PROSKO and MARLYSA SULLIVAN

Foreword by Timothy McCall

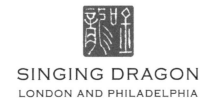

SINGING DRAGON
LONDON AND PHILADELPHIA

Quote on page 141 is reprinted from *The Miracle of Mindfulness* by Thich Nhat Hanh. Copyright
© 1975, 1976 by Thich Nhat Hanh. Preface and English translation Copyright © 1975, 1976,
1987 by Mobi Ho. Reprinted with permission from Beacon Press, Boston Massachusetts.
Figure 11.2 is reprinted from Farb, Anderson and Segal (2012)
with kind permission from the authors.
Figures 12.1 and 12.2 are reprinted from National Institute on Drug
Abuse (2015) with kind permission from NIDA.
Bullet list on pages 211–12 is reprinted from National Institute on
Drug Abuse (2018) with kind permission from NIDA.
Quote on page 260 is reprinted from *Man's Search for Meaning* by Viktor E.
Frankl. Copyright © 1959, 1962, 1984, 1992 by Viktor E. Frankl. Reprinted
with permission from Beacon Press, Boston Massachusetts.
Figure 15.3 is reprinted from Sullivan *et al.* 2018 with kind
permission from Innovision Health Media.

First published in 2019
by Jessica Kingsley Publishers
73 Collier Street
London N1 9BE, UK
and
400 Market Street, Suite 400
Philadelphia, PA 19106, USA

*www.jkp.com*

Copyright © Jessica Kingsley Publishers 2019
Foreword copyright © Timothy McCall 2019

All rights reserved. No part of this publication may be reproduced in any material form
(including photocopying, storing in any medium by electronic means or transmitting)
without the written permission of the copyright owner except in accordance with the
provisions of the law or under terms of a licence issued in the UK by the Copyright Licensing
Agency Ltd. www.cla.co.uk or in overseas territories by the relevant reproduction rights
organization, for details see www.ifrro.org. Applications for the copyright owner's written
permission to reproduce any part of this publication should be addressed to the publisher.

Warning: The doing of an unauthorized act in relation to a copyright work may
result in both a civil claim for damages and criminal prosecution.

**Library of Congress Cataloging in Publication Data**
A CIP catalog record for this book is available from the Library of Congress

**British Library Cataloguing in Publication Data**
A CIP catalogue record for this book is available from the British Library

ISBN 978 1 84819 397 0
eISBN 978 0 85701 354 5

Printed and bound in the United States

# Contents

# Foreword

Several years ago, I received an email with tragic news. My college friend Todd, brilliant, talented and one of the funniest people I've ever known, had committed suicide. He'd suffered from an extremely painful neurologic condition and apparently couldn't take it anymore. We'd lost touch years earlier, and I imagined that he had exhausted every treatment option offered to him without finding relief. I felt especially sad because I suspected that some of the tools I'd learned in yoga and yoga therapy—that he likely hadn't been exposed to—might well have made a difference. That emotion was only heightened when I discovered that Todd, who I'd met in Madison, Wisconsin, and I had been living in the same Northern California town.

More recently, in my own journey through metastatic head and neck cancer, I had a few months of severe pain due to tissue damage caused by chemoradiation. My radiation oncologist had prescribed opioids during my second week of treatment—a good choice I felt given the acute nature of my discomfort and my low risk of becoming addicted. Likely due to all the yogic, Ayurvedic and the other holistic healing approaches I was using, however, I didn't end up needing to take those narcotics until more than a month later, and easily weaned myself off as the pain diminished. In the meantime, the drugs had made a big difference in keeping me more comfortable.

Unfortunately, opioids are turning out to be more problematic for chronic pain. One reason is that when pain-relieving drugs are taken long term, they tend to lose effectiveness, a phenomenon known medically as tachyphylaxis. To get the same analgesic effect you need to steadily increase the dose—simultaneously increasing the side effects and the addiction potential. The unskillful use of narcotic pain relievers in chronic pain is widely considered a major contributor to the current opioid crisis.

What is needed urgently are non-drug measures for chronic pain, and yoga and its varied toolbox—including meditation, mindful awareness, mindful movement and breathing techniques aimed at lessening the reactivity of the nervous system as well as the mind—offer great promise. Better still, not only are yogic approaches not subject to tachyphylaxis, the opposite seems to be true. The longer and more steadily yoga tools are employed the more powerful they become. Slowly, like interest building in a compound savings account, the benefits accrue. The practice of yoga even offers the possibility of entirely transforming the patient's relationship to their pain, even in cases where it cannot be entirely relieved—something that no drug can do.

As this book skillfully documents, there is promising, though incomplete, scientific support, for the use of yogic approaches in chronic pain. Some cautious observers say more data are needed before we can recommend yoga to patients in pain. While no one disputes the desirability of further scientific investigation, given all that is at stake, such reticence may cause unfortunate side effects, both for society in general and for countless individuals, desperate like my late friend Todd, for whom yoga might offer some measure of relief.

Good doctors weigh the risks versus the benefits of any medical intervention. When this logic is applied to yoga for people with chronic pain, the equation is lopsided. Unlike drugs which kill tens of thousands of patients every year— even when used as prescribed—as far as we know there has never been a single death attributable to yoga therapy. Yoga, particularly the vigorous yoga taught in some classes, can cause injuries, but they appear to be rare in yoga therapy, which by definition is tailored to each client's unique constellation of aptitudes and limitations. Compared to conventional medical approaches, the cost of yoga therapy is low. Most people who try it seem to like it.

Finally, consider this: almost all studies of yoga are of short duration due to the chronic shortage of funding for such research. Studies lasting a few weeks or months will tend to underestimate the benefits of a practice, which builds in effectiveness slowly over time. Further, due to the requirements of evidence-based medicine, yoga studies are almost always of standardized treatment protocols, in which every person is prescribed the same exact same poses, breathing techniques, etc. These protocols lack the personalization that skilled yoga therapists insist boosts both the effectiveness and safety of the practices prescribed. Of course, this notion needs to be studied, but to the extent that it's true, the research to date will have once again systematically underestimated yoga therapy's true potential.

Modern medicine has spent billions of dollars in its efforts to understand and relieve chronic pain, with some notable successes, yet it lacks satisfactory solutions for many patients. What medicine has focused on much less, however, is the relief of suffering. Suffering can fuel the fire of chronic pain. Understanding the causes of suffering and how it can be lessened has been a central focus of yoga for thousands of years. The time is right to apply this wisdom to the millions of chronic pain sufferers whose need for it is pressing. *Yoga and Science in Pain Care*, scientifically savvy, informed by clinical experience and rich in yogic insight, shows us the way.

*Timothy McCall, MD*

# Acknowledgements

To all the people in pain with whom we have had the privilege to work, we extend tremendous gratitude. Our efforts are a reflection of what you have taught us. Your capacity to be open, vulnerable, courageous and curious has been inspirational in our lives and our work. We are grateful for your patience and trust, but also your willingness to tell us when we have failed to truly understand or offer the help you really need. We are blessed and honored to be on this healing path with each of you.

We are grateful to all of the authors who contributed to this book: Joletta Belton, Steffany Moonaz, Matthew J. Taylor, Matt Erb, Lori Rubenstein Fazzio, Tracey Sondik, Antonio Sausys and Michael Lee. Thank you for offering your brilliant gifts of time, energy, expertise and wisdom. Your important and valuable work to help reduce suffering in the world is extraordinary. We are honored to share this experience with you.

Thanks to all teachers who have come before us, lighting the way for this book and our work. Thanks also to our supportive bridge-building colleagues, including clinicians and researchers, who walk alongside us and continue on this path of integrating yoga into healthcare. Building these bridges with your courage, perseverance, dedication, creativity and commitment to enhance healthcare and pain care is inspiring and greatly appreciated.

We want to thank our publisher, Singing Dragon, for their guidance and support and making this enjoyable experience possible.

## Marlysa

In addition to the above, I want to express my gratitude to the amazing support system of friends, teachers and colleagues who have encouraged me in my work and life to continuously follow my heart and trust in my path.

Most of all to my husband, John Sullivan, for his understanding, patience, unconditional love and constant belief in me and my work. Our life together is a source of inspiration, discovery, exploration and enjoyment—I am continuously thankful for all of our journeys and conversations.

I want to also express my immense gratitude to the teachers and mentors who have helped encourage my curiosity, as well as showing me both acceptance and compassion in my learning process. To name a few of these teachers—Karen Davis Warren, for introducing me to the field of physical therapy from the beginning with a focus on holistic, collaborative and integrated care. To Leslie Taylor and Gordon Cummings, who inspired me to integrate the social/spiritual domains into physical therapy care. To incredible yoga teachers and therapists who have helped the ancient wisdom of yoga become a personal and professional journey for both myself and my clients—Julie Wilcox, Richard Miller, Priti Robyn Ross, Sue Hopkins, Matthew J. Taylor. To Stephen Porges, for the generous support in helping an idea become a well-defined theory in the paper on polyvagal theory and yoga. To incredible friends and colleagues Matt Erb and Laura Schmalzl, for all of your help, encouragement and inspiration in our writing endeavors—it has been an honor to get to know you both and to work with you.

To James Snow, who introduced me to the idea of eudaimonia and for all of your encouragement in my academic path. To Steffany Moonaz, for being a compassionate, supportive teacher of research and critical thinking—I am incredibly grateful for your patience and guidance in helping my "big ideas" find their way into a path of research and work. To Diane Finlayson, for all of our conversations and inspirations to encourage my creativity and growth in teaching and life. To all the Maryland University of Integrative Health faculty and students who have been of immense support, inspiration and encouragement in my teaching, research and writing.

To all the friends and colleagues who have helped me through the years and have shown me compassionate and heartfelt connection and friendship—to Holle Black, Corbett Jordan-Oldham, Jeffrey Shoaf, Tra Kirkpatrick, Kelli Bethel, Tracey Sondik, Tina Paul, Ann Swanson, Laurie Robertson, Veronica Lewinger, Amy Wheeler, Sherry Brourman, Melinda Atkins.

And to Shelly and Neil, for being on this path of writing and sharing in this experience—I am continuously grateful and inspired by the work you do and who you are. Thank you for being a part of this journey with me.

## Shelly

In addition to those thanked above, I would like to thank the teachers who have supported and guided me with compassion and patience and allowed me the freedom to explore, make mistakes and offer direction without rigidity while learning. There are too many to mention, but these teachers take many forms: my parents, family, friends, patients, creative bridge-builder colleagues, students, coaches, school teachers, yoga teachers, coworkers and the children in my life. You have been instrumental on this path and have influenced my work and writing in this book.

Neil Pearson, thank you for being a gracious, humble and generous teacher and mentor to me on this path of better understanding pain and people in pain and improving pain care. Your dedication and integrity are inspiring and contagious.

Special thanks to Helene Couvrette, Sherry Brourman, Chrys Kub, Christine Carr, Marlysa Sullivan, Matthew J. Taylor, Staffan Elgelid, Lori Rubenstein Fazzio, Rachel Krentzman, Diana Zotos-Florio, Baxter Bell, Joanne Gailius, Ron Naresh King, Liz Duncanson, Carolyn Vandyken, Stacey Lovo Grona, Tianna Meriage-Reiter, Rajam Roose, Cassi Kit, Anne Pitman, Linda Boryski, Matt Erb, Diana Perez, John Kepner, Nydia Tijerina Darby, Joe Tatta, Antony Lo, Kim Deschamps, Amy Wheeler, Jaimie Perkunas, Ann Parkinson, Dustienne Miller, Ann Green, Maggie Bergeron, Eryn Kirkwood, Eoin Finn and Paula Clayton. I appreciate the way in which each of you has shown your love, support and faith in me and my work.

Thanks to the good people behind the academic institutions that provided me with the luxury of exceptional education: University of Saskatchewan, E.D. Feehan and St. Dominic in Saskatoon, Saskatchewan, Canada.

I want to acknowledge all people who have made it possible for yoga to be with us today and all those who continue to believe in the therapeutic value of yoga and are dedicated to finding accessible ways to use it and teach it in order to help those in pain.

Thank you to Marlysa and Neil for being loving and supportive friends, colleagues and co-editors on this journey. It has been an honor and pleasure to work together towards this shared vision we all have of integrating yoga, science and pain care. I admire your creativity and wisdom and have learned from your kindness, curiosity, professionalism and patience. Thank you for the opportunity to collaborate and create. Thanks to Lisa Pearson for contributing your insights and wisdom with such grace to Chapter 14, Compassion in Pain Care.

Thank you Chris Ulmer, my husband, for lovingly encouraging me to take the path less traveled so I could share my work in a way that would be of better service and for believing in me and supporting me regardless of the path I chose. Your unwavering trust and support continues to carry me on this journey. I am grateful for our precious connection and am inspired and influenced by your curiosity and passion for finding ways to better serve humanity and help create thriving, flourishing and equitable communities. I admire and continually learn from your warm heart, humility and ability to see others' perspectives.

And thanks to my mom, dad and sister, Kim, for consistently leading by example and being such loving and compassionate role models. You have each shaped and influenced this work of helping people in pain.

## Neil

Additional thanks from me start with those who have strived to fill in the answers in pain care—when what we learned in school was not sufficient to understand pain, the experiences of people in pain or how to provide effective physical therapy addressing the complex and multifaceted suffering of the person seeking out my expertise. Many of these clinicians, authors and researchers have developed or are now involved in sustainable organizations such as NOIGroup, Pain BC, the Canadian Physiotherapy Pain Science Division and the International Spine and Pain Institute, are involved in yearly conferences such as the San Diego Pain Summit, the Montreal International Symposium on Therapeutic Yoga, the conferences of the International Association of Yoga Therapists and the International Association for the Study of Pain and are involved in educational and community-building social media groups. Like Lorimer Moseley and David Butler, for whom I am deeply grateful, from many of these individuals we learn through their role-modelling that it is one's heart and soul more than knowledge and expertise that are the answers for effective pain care. Thank you to Cheryl Van Demark for her assistance with pain and biology editing in Chapter 4.

Unending gratitude to my parents—your love and support are immeasurable positive forces in who I am.

Within yoga, I am humbled by all those who have passed down these wonderful paths and techniques, allowing all of us to find more peace. I am blessed as I continue to learn from teachers and students how to integrate yoga and pain care. To Mugs (Marion) McConnell and Dr. Ananda Bhavanani, who have inspired me, filled my mind and been incredible role-models, I offer the most heartfelt gratitude. And to Shelly and Marlysa, I am grateful to be partners with you in this project.

To Lisa, Swami Swarupananda, my love, my wife, you have shown me how to link my knowledge and expertise, all that I have learned from those mentioned above, into compassionate and loving language moving me forward as I hoped in my evolution as a physical therapist and as a teacher of pain care.

# Preface

NEIL PEARSON, SHELLY PROSKO, MARLYSA SULLIVAN

The three of us share a passion for helping people in pain. Combined, we have decades of experience in both working with clients in pain and providing education to healthcare professionals on how to help people in pain through yoga. Separately, we had each thought about and been approached to write on this topic. As we thought about what a book would look like on this topic of yoga, science and pain care, it was apparent that this project would be best served through collaboration. A book about pain should mirror the complexity and multifaceted nature of the subject.

Just as pain can only be understood from holistic and integrated perspectives, our intention was to create a book that could reflect the multifaceted nature of pain and the human experience. With the complexity of the topic, and to ensure we offered a variety of perspectives to prevent our own biases from dominating the project, we decided to invite esteemed colleagues to share their knowledge, experience and wisdom. As a group effort, we felt this book could provide a more expansive and in-depth understanding while capturing the essence of important aspects of pain and pain care.

We each contemplated our own gifts, focus and perspectives on pain care as well as that of inspiring colleagues. This book is an attempt to demonstrate this collective dialogue through exploring various perspectives on pain care. We sought to include essential and relevant topics that would cover an understanding of pain itself, the lived experience of pain and fundamental topics for pain management and pain care.

We hope this book meets your needs. A growing number of people are seeking yoga when they have pain and a growing number of rehabilitation professionals are integrating yoga into their work. As well, health professionals are seeking support and guidance on how to incorporate a biopsychosocial-spiritual (BPSS) approach into their treatments. This book will help alleviate the system-wide lack of available resources, specifically on a BPSS approach to helping individuals with persistent pain.

Yoga therapy is an emerging complementary and integrative healthcare field with recent accreditation, credentialing and certification processes. Since 2007, research (systematic reviews and meta analyses) and the American Medical Association have supported the use of yoga for people with chronic pain. In 2017, the American College of Physicians, also on the basis of research evidence, recommended yoga as one of the non-pharmacologic, non-invasive clinical treatment options for patients with chronic low back pain. Other systematic reviews have supported the effectiveness of yoga for people with fibromyalgia, osteoarthritis, rheumatoid arthritis, neck pain and irritable bowel syndrome. Yet, there is a lack of comprehensive resources for yoga teachers and therapists to learn about pain and for health professionals to learn about yoga and pain. Combined with the astonishing prevalence of chronic pain worldwide and the opioid crisis, we believe our book will be of service, hopefully inspiring other authors and clinicians.

This book is intended to be used in course study for yoga therapist programs, medical and rehabilitation universities/colleges, mind-body institutions and schools that have mind-body programs. It is a book of theory, and not meant as a thorough training on pain or yoga therapy. It is also not meant as a practical guide to all that is required to provide effective pain care. It is our hope that this book reaches and serves:

- all healthcare professionals who work with people in pain and want to better understand pain and the value of integrating yoga and mind-body practices into clinical practice

- yoga professionals (teachers and therapists) who want to better understand pain, pain science and aspects of the science behind yoga and are interested in enhancing their practice and working with the persistent pain population

- mind-body contemplative practitioners and researchers who want to better understand pain and how yoga as a mind-body practice works as an aspect of pain care

- yoga practitioners, integrative health consumers and people suffering from pain, particularly those keen to learn more about pain biology and yoga, and who want an in-depth read with practical knowledge in this field.

The three of us would like to share a bit about our own history behind how we became interested in this path of integrating yoga into pain care.

**Marlysa**: A driving inspiration in my work has been exploring how our beliefs—about ourselves and the world around us—shape and influence our health and wellbeing. Through college I studied medical anthropology, and religion, before deciding on a clinical path through physical therapy. As a physical therapist I became intrigued by the variability and complexity of each patient's experience of pain and illness. I sought ways to address and incorporate the psychological, spiritual/existential aspects of a person's experience into physical therapy care. The study of yoga and yoga therapy provided me with a both personal and professional path for this exploration and a practical means for its application. The integration of yoga into physical therapy, and my work as a yoga therapist, have helped me find ways to help others explore their pain, or illness, and the beliefs (about themselves, relationships, spiritual and existential) that impact their healing journey.

**Neil**: Curiosity and hope have been the driving forces in my journey. From noticing that patients' experiences of pain did not match what I learned in school, to wondering what changed when people living in pain began to improve, to watching some individuals learning to thrive without much change in the pain and others relying more on contemplative practices than what we offered as health professionals, I was continually informed that multiple perspectives on pain management were required. The identification of common factors within contemplative practices and the science of pain and the lived experience of pain assist us in the evolution of guiding more people to less suffering.

**Shelly**: My journey of the integration of yoga in pain care started with my personal experience of yoga. The physical, emotional, mental, social and spiritual benefits related to my personal yoga practice drove me to explore (and continually explore) how yoga can be integrated into physiotherapy to enhance patient care and outcomes, particularly for those patients who were struggling to find relief and ways to return to their most meaningful activities. Early on in my clinical practice, the necessity of taking a whole-person-valued approach was evident. I quickly learned I was not treating conditions or addressing body parts; I was helping a *human being* who was experiencing pain or living with an injury or condition, within the context of their environment. In my ongoing studies and exploration of yoga therapy, I have found that it offers an incredibly inclusive, accessible, practical and compassionate biopsychosocial-spiritual framework from which we can work while staying within our scope of practice as physiotherapists that is also in line with evidence-informed best practices and a contemporary understanding of the science surrounding pain. This integration of yoga and science in pain care has helped me be more understanding, compassionate, effective and creative in the way I guide and walk beside fellow humans who are suffering to help them find a way to live life with more ease.

Our vision is for this book to improve care for people living in pain, whether acute or chronic pain. We believe that health professionals and yoga therapists can enhance care through deeper understanding of pain, science and evidence-informed interventions. We also believe that professionals can enhance their work through integrating yoga concepts, practices and philosophies. As such, this book is meant to bridge yoga, pain science and evidence-informed rehabilitation in working with people in pain and will inform those committed to helping people with this largely undertreated issue that causes so much suffering in the world.

# Introduction

NEIL PEARSON, SHELLY PROSKO, MARLYSA SULLIVAN

Our final decision for the title of this book, *Yoga and Science in Pain Care: Treating the Person in Pain,* required considerable deliberation. We chose our language very intentionally:

**Yoga and science**: Both of these terms were essential, as we wanted the title and the contents to capture the attention of health professionals and yoga therapists. Our main goal is to enhance the outcomes of people living in pain when they seek help from yoga or health professionals. The title reflects the importance of an equal understanding of yoga and current science as relevant to helping the person in pain. Yoga therapists will be informed in how they can use knowledge from science and health professionals informed in how they can use knowledge from yoga to help people in pain.

**Pain care**: We chose the term *pain care* because we prefer this over *pain management*. Pain care intends to suggest that helping people in pain is not only a medical issue, but also a health and wellbeing issue. It also intends to express that effective care does not always succeed with focusing on *managing* the *pain*. Effective pain care is about assisting and *caring* for the *person* when pain persists, and there are situations in which the pain can be changed rather than managed.

**Treating the person in pain**: We considered using the phrase "*assisting* the person in pain" rather than "*treating* the person in pain," but we wanted to ensure we captured the attention of healthcare professionals who are accustomed to using the term "treating." At times, we are providing treatment "to" the person in pain. We also pondered "treating the *patient* in pain" but wanted to avoid always referring to people living with pain as *patients*. This decision does not intend to ignore the power differential between the person in pain and the practitioner, or the responsibilities of the treating practitioner. At all times, the practitioner must remember the dynamics of the therapeutic situation and know that the best outcomes arise from knowing when to be the expert, when to be the student and when to collaborate and brainstorm. We deliberately avoided titles that included "yoga *for* chronic pain" or "yoga and science *for* treating chronic pain," as we are not focusing on using yoga for pain or for a condition, rather we are using yoga and science to better understand, address and assist *individual human beings* who are living with and suffering from conditions and pain.

Throughout the book, you will note that we use the terms *chronic pain* and *persistent pain* interchangeably. At times, we use the term *chronic pain* since this is used as a diagnosis required for treatment to be received and can be seen by some as a validation that they have a real problem. However, *chronic pain* can also signify to the patient that the pain will never get better and likely continue to worsen. The term *persistent pain* signifies that there is hope of recovering function, ease of motion and/or quality of life, and that pain itself can potentially change. However, our experiences have taught us that using the term "persistent pain" can be invalidating to some patients. Consequently, we intentionally use both terms in this book.

Each chapter represents a vast subject. The contents are meant as a synthesis of relevant and essential information. For more information on each topic, we encourage you to refer to the resources and references included in each chapter, seek further study and continue to inquire. This is an evolving field.

Interpret what you read as the authors' attempts to include a current understanding. As soon as the book is published, aspects of it will already be outdated in such an evolving area of research and practice.

As you read each chapter, consider that the content is intended to offer an opportunity to consider the lived experience of pain and pain science from a yoga perspective, and to consider yoga therapy from a science perspective. We believe that yoga can benefit from integrating pain science and evidence-informed best practices, and that traditional pain management and rehabilitation can benefit from the integration of yoga practices and philosophy.

## Chapter 1: Lived Experience of Pain

We deliberately begin with a window into living with pain from the perspective of Joletta Belton, an advocate for people in pain. Pain is experienced as an individual, yet there are vast commonalities across individuals. Many of these are highlighted within Belton's chapter. This chapter includes a compassionate plea to healthcare professionals to not give up on people in pain, to have hope, to be inspired. It reminds us that there are *endless possibilities* to help people in pain. As you read this chapter, remember that listening to and offering an individual the opportunity to disclose their story is one of the, if not the most, effective pain care techniques we have. Just as we should start therapeutic interventions by listening to the individual's story, learning more about pain begins with considering how pain impacts life.

## Chapter 2: Current Research in Yoga and Pain

Chapter 2 presents the trajectory of yoga research, the state of the research on yoga for pain and why yoga therapy research matters. Moonaz also discusses general trends, limitations and future directions of yoga research. Pain care has three primary goals—improving ease of movement and function, enhancing quality of life and decreasing pain. Multiple meta-analyses and systematic reviews show positive functional outcomes when people with chronic pain engage in yoga. Many people in pain, and many professionals want to know, "will my pain change when I practice yoga?" As such, and at the risk of creating the impression that the author and editors believe that changing pain is the only valid goal of pain care or yoga, this chapter focuses on research into the uncertainty of whether pain itself will change when one practices yoga.

## Chapter 3: The Current State(s) and Theor(y)ies on Pain Management (sic)

Chapter 3 introduces the history and the context of understanding pain from different perspectives, cultures and time. Helping people in pain requires taking the time to consider our own beliefs about pain from multiple perspectives, as well as gaining improved ability to consider the understanding of pain from a patient's perspective. Taylor points out how we must let go of dogma and simple linear views of pain, of people in pain and of pain care, if we are to evolve and help more people. This chapter is worth reading multiple times, and even to continually consider as you read the other chapters. We all have biases we have yet to discover. Exploring them introspectively will even assist helping patients past similar linear dogmatic barriers to recovery.

## Chapter 4: Yoga and Yoga Therapy

Here we provide a background on yoga and yoga therapy and how we are defining certain key principles for the book. This chapter offers an understanding of different paths and aspects of yoga. Our hope is to explain the parts in such a way that also shows that yoga is only well understood as a complete and integrated practice. We pull ideas and practices apart for the purpose of explanation, but the practice is intended to be used as part of a cohesive system situated within a wisdom tradition.

The best way to understand yoga is to experience it by becoming a practitioner of it. We know that some practitioners, just like patients, learn best with a cognitive foundation. We encourage the reader to move beyond reading about yoga, and beyond the individual techniques of yoga, to experiencing the effects of a regular "classic" yoga practice.

As our journey through the book progresses, we will travel from the grosser levels of experience such as the body to more subtle levels of experience such as the mind, emotions, compassion, social relationships and spirituality. Each author presents their understanding, expertise and work.

## Chapter 5: Pain Biology and Sensitization

Chapter 5 details the current understandings of pain biology including the complexity of defining and understanding pain from a physiological perspective. This understanding is one of the foundations of success in the work we do assisting people in pain. Consider this chapter as a summary and as incomplete. Our understanding of human biology is vast and ever-changing. Strangely, this knowledge adds to uncertainty as much as to new understanding. Every system of the organism impacts our experiences, and we can observe how experiences impact the person, their systems, organs, tissues, cells, etc... and even epigenetics. There are also diverse views of the importance of different aspects of biology, both on the experiences of pain and effective pain care. All this requires acquisition of knowledge and tolerance of uncertainty far beyond this chapter.

## Chapter 6: Polyvagal Theory and the Gunas: A Model for Autonomic Regulation in Pain

Chapter 6 offers a deep dive into the autonomic nervous system and its relationship to pain. Polyvagal theory and its relationship to yoga philosophical theories offers a foundation for the applications of the practices that can influence the pain experience. The relationship of autonomic regulation to physiological, emotional, behavioral states; pain; and their connection to yoga is explored through this chapter. This chapter offers a fresh perspective in pain care in that the context within which we provide pain care, or the "how" pain care is provided, may be of far greater importance than has yet been considered in health professional training.

## Chapter 7: Integrating Pain Science Education, Movement and Yoga

Chapter 7 describes the importance of pain education in facilitating change and transformation and yoga as a form of such education. Knowledge is often the foundation from which change arises. Research shows the benefits of providing verbal and written education to people in pain, especially when combined with movement therapy. Knowledge is powerful, yet this chapter emphasizes a shift in perspective to one in which movement and yoga practices are viewed as not only movement and contemplative practices, but also educational agents. This perspective shift has the potential to enhance outcomes of pain care and to innovate research methodologies.

## Chapter 8: Breathing and Pranayama in Pain Care

Chapter 8 moves us into the more subtle realm and power of breath, its relationship to pain and its potential for affecting the many aspects of physiological, psychological and emotional states and in transformation. This chapter not only provides an understanding of breath that will help health professionals explain the importance of breath in pain care, but also offers skeptics a new understanding of people who report it as the most impactful aspect of their therapy and provides an understanding of the views of yoga therapists who see it as foundational to effective pain care.

## Chapter 9: Body Awareness, Bhavana and Pratyahara

Chapter 9 discusses the topic of body awareness from both biomedical and yoga perspectives and how yoga can facilitate a process through which the person can draw their attention inward and cultivate insight and healthier relationships with body, mind and the experience of pain. This chapter offers the opportunity to discuss an important new understanding of people in pain and of effective pain care. Disruptions of body awareness and body image seem far more common and far more impactful on pain care than previously considered. Yoga provides multiple practices that address body awareness, as Rubenstein Fazzio discusses in this chapter.

## Chapter 10: Ingredients for Pain Care: Nutrition and Yoga

Chapter 10 moves into the topic of nutrition and understanding the connections between nutrition and pain and how to approach this topic from a yoga perspective. This chapter discusses the link between pain, stress, inflammation and the immune system and the important connections between the gut and brain. The application of these topics to yoga philosophy and lifestyle is offered through experiential activities.

## Chapter 11: Transforming Psycho-Emotional Pain

Chapter 11 dives deeper into understanding the psycho-emotional experience of pain and how yoga can be used as a transformative process as an aspect of pain care. Lee thoroughly differentiates between the symptom management approach and transformational approach of yoga therapy. The delineation between physical pain and psycho-emotional pain is only of value if we maintain a hold on the understanding of integration. We discuss them as separate, knowing that the human is not.

## Chapter 12: Pain, Addiction, and Yoga

Chapter 12 explores addiction and its intersection with pain. This is particularly important in the climate of the opioid crisis and the increased public awareness on addiction and the movement towards identifying viable and effective nonpharmacological interventions for pain. Sondik discusses the philosophical context and practices of yoga in connection to these topics. We hope that a greater understanding of addiction will increase compassion towards the people living in pain and decrease one of the most powerful stigmas around pain.

## Chapter 13: Pain, A Loss to be Grieved

In Chapter 13, Sausys writes about loss, grief and pain, their relationships and similarities and how they affect one another. Specific ideas and practices of yoga to work with loss, grief and pain through this lens are offered. Grief counselling may be the most neglected aspect of pain care within Western pain-management programs. We lose so much when pain persists. Given the power of grief, and that anything able to drive the hypervigilance of the individual and the nervous systems can maintain pain, understanding grief and pain is vital.

The final chapters, 14 and 15, move into the topics of compassion, connection, social relationships and the spiritual/existential realms of human existence as they relate to pain care.

## Chapter 14: Compassion in Pain Care

Chapter 14 explores in-depth interpretations of compassion and the science surrounding compassion. It focuses on the value and importance of compassion in pain care, which consists of compassion for the patient by the health practitioner and self-compassion in both the patient and the practitioner. The context for compassion and its relationships to core yoga philosophical principles and practices are described and ways of cultivating compassion in pain care are outlined. Without compassion for the patient, we cannot form an effective therapeutic alliance/relationship. And without practicing self-compassion, it is difficult to continue helping people with this complex phenomenon of changing pain.

## Chapter 15: Connection, Meaningful Relationship, and Purpose in Life: Social and Existential Concerns in Pain Care

Our final chapter on this journey explores the social and spiritual/existential domains of experience and how they both affect and are affected by the pain experience and influence physical and mental health. This chapter hopes to shed light on this important topic from both current scientific and philosophical perspectives, as well as bridging this information with the yoga tradition. Through the cultivation of connection (personal, interpersonal and existential/spiritual) and purpose/meaning, yoga provides a practical philosophical path that can be of benefit to the person in pain. This information is often mentioned within health professional education and yoga therapy training; however, we believe much more attention to these domains is required. Again, context including how care is provided and the actions/behaviors of the therapist are as important as the "things" or "techniques" we use as "pain care" for the people we serve.

Our hope is that you will read this book to gain a deeper appreciation and understanding of pain, people in pain and how to help people living in pain. Accumulating more information, clinical skills and techniques is important, but a deeper understanding and ongoing exploration of the complexity of pain is required. Use this book as a first step. Take time to learn more. Then take more time to consider what you have learned.

We also hope that this book will help bring together yoga therapists and health professionals. There is value in blending science and yoga therapy in pain care—for the person in pain, for the health professional and for the yoga professional.

Maybe this book will even impact research. Sometimes clinicians seeing certain patterns in patients or in treatment are motivated to research a new theory. Sometimes budding researchers learn of new connections they had not considered or that were previously outside their typical area of expertise. Pain and pain care are expansive topics that will benefit from looking at commonalities across related fields, while people in pain will benefit from sharing and integrating the knowledge and practice between healthcare and yoga.

## Chapter 1

# Lived Experience of Pain

JOLETTA BELTON

When we live with pain for a long time, it changes who we are. It changes how we see the world and how we relate to that world.

It changes everything. It is hard.

We often don't have very good answers for why we're in pain or what to do about it. That makes it even harder. Things just don't make sense. I know; I've been there. I have lived with unexplained, debilitating pain that ended my career, threatened my relationships, and turned my world upside down. Pain that kept me housebound and isolated, lost in hopelessness and despair. Pain that reverberated through my entire being, rippling out to every corner of my life. Pain that affected every aspect of my existence yet was invisible.

There were beacons of light amidst the darkness, though, and they led me forward. Led me back to an active, meaningful, purposeful life. The beacons came in many forms, the first of which was discovering pain science and exploring how I could use what I learned to take an active role in my own recovery. It was the key that opened the door onto everything else. To introspection and reflection, which played a necessary role in changing my experience. To the active strategies that helped me get back to living well and with ease, such as movement, mindfulness, creativity, and connecting with the people, places, and experiences that mattered to me.

My life changed. I changed. The journey was long, but it was mine, is still mine. I've learned a lot along the way. I'm grateful to still be learning as I go.

## My pain story

My pain first started with a twinge in my hip as I stepped off the fire engine on a routine call. Something I'd done literally thousands of times but, this one time, I missed a step. It was just a twinge. A twinge I thought would resolve fairly quickly. It didn't. The twinge morphed into ongoing, unrelenting, intractable pain and I went from being a strong, capable, athletic firefighter one moment— at the height of my career and the peak of my strength and physical fitness—

to frail, weak, and broken by pain the next. It all started with a twinge. A missed step that led me down a wholly unexpected path of career-ending, life-altering, self-altering pain.

It didn't make any sense.

My pain was worse when I sat, so I didn't sit. For over two years I stood or laid down everywhere. It's hard to live a normal life under such circumstances. Hard to live any sort of life, as I'm sure you can imagine. I didn't socialize. I withdrew from family and friends. No more going out for coffee or a drink, no dinners out, no movies, no driving to the store, no lounging on the couch. My world became very, very small. Within that small, pained world I'd ruminate over the past and the person I could no longer be and worry that my future would be nothing but pain, nothing but suffering. The present terrified me. The pain was scary and all-consuming. It colored everything and painted a bleak future. I wanted nothing to do with it. I wanted it to be gone. I wanted someone, something— anyone, anything—to fix me.

## Not knowing

In those early years I didn't think about pain as a complex experience. I didn't know that many factors contribute to pain and its persistence or that many of those same factors can contribute to recovery. I thought pain could only mean injury and damage—that to recover from pain meant the injury needed to heal, the damage to be fixed. When my pain persisted, I naturally thought I was still damaged—still injured, still broken, and in need of fixing. So, I searched for the fix. From medications to physical therapy to injections to surgery to alternative medicine. With each new doctor, new therapist, new treatment I went in with high hopes that *this* would be the thing that fixed me, then plunged into the depths of despair when it didn't. I felt like a failure, every single time. It was an exhausting, demoralizing roller coaster ride of emotions, of highs and lows, of unfulfilled promises and diminishing hope.

I recognize now that the biggest problem back then wasn't the pain so much as not understanding what the pain meant and not knowing what to do about it. Not knowing there was anything I *could* do about it. My life, my very existence, was on hold until the damage was repaired, the injury healed. Only then could I get back to living, back to myself, I thought. Yet, after years of manual therapies, injections that didn't work, and a surgery that fixed my anatomy but didn't fix me, I still had pain. I had still failed. I had lost my career, and with it my identity, my sense of who I was, my life as I had known it. I felt worthless, purposeless, hopeless…just less.

## The personal toll

I'm not alone in this. We become diminished, unknown even to ourselves, when we experience ongoing, unrelenting pain that makes no sense. Pain that is too often dismissed and invalidated by others, by friends and family, by medical professionals. There is shame and guilt, feeling as though we are a burden to our partners and families, our friends and coworkers, even our healthcare providers. We withdraw from our loved ones, from work and play, from society in general. We become more and more isolated, less and less understood. There's anger, grief, frustration, and the seeming unfairness of it all. We can't think, can't sleep, can't dream, can't express what we are going through. Pain becomes everything. We become pain.

Unrelenting pain can do that to a person. It has a way of taking over our lives. Pain that doesn't let up makes us experience our bodies, our worlds, in a wholly different way. While living my day-to-day life before pain I never had reason to think much about my body or the sensations within it. I never thought much about how I moved; I just moved. There was no reason to pay attention to it. With worsening pain, though, came an all-encompassing attention to my hip, to where it hurt. Nothing else mattered. Over time it was as though the entirety of my being became my hip and the pain that had taken up residence there. Pain that consumed my thoughts, demanded all of my attention, sapped all of my resources, and robbed me of my ability to think clearly, to engage with my friends and family, to live my life how I wanted to. How I expected to.

I didn't like who I'd become during those worst years of my pain. I was no longer fun, no longer funny. No longer present in the presence of others, always focused on the pain. I was short of temper, unable to have a conversation, incapable of making the simplest decisions. I could no longer *do* things. I was no longer active, no longer an athlete, no longer a firefighter. No longer me.

Pain was the enemy. All it did was take. It took my career, identity, friends, hobbies, and financial security. My joy, my laughter, my hope. My body had betrayed me; it'd become a hostile environment I wanted desperately to escape but couldn't escape. Pain had become my world, my universe, my life. Who could blame me, though? Who could blame any of us who start to focus solely on the pain when we don't know what it means and we don't know what to do about it?

## A new understanding

But pain was not the enemy, my body not a traitor. There was no need to escape. There was a different way forward; it just took me some years to happen upon it. The way was paved for me when I learned about pain science. I finally saw the possibility of my world expanding again. I had hope, realistic hope, that things could change, that they would change. Understanding more about pain biology allowed me to better make sense of *my* pain. By reconceptualizing what the pain meant and didn't mean, I could redefine success, I could re-find myself. I was empowered to live my life again, to become more flexible in body and mind. I no longer had to wait for pain to be gone to get back to the things that mattered to me—the people, places, and experiences that provided me with purpose and filled my life with meaning.

Slowly, bit by bit, the change I had hoped for for so long became a reality.

## Making sense of pain

This new understanding of pain took some time for me to wrap my head around. That the pain wasn't a direct reflection of what was happening in my hip—that it wasn't just an issue in my tissues—was a revolutionary way of thinking. It was so different to what I'd believed for so long: that if there was pain there *had* to be injury, there *had* to be damage where the pain was felt. There is rarely a single, linear cause when it comes to pain, though, especially pain that lasts a long time.

Rather, pain is a biopsychosocial, consciously lived experience that is influenced by, and in turn influences, every aspect of our being, every aspect of our lives. From our genes to our immune, endocrine, and nervous systems, to our beliefs, thoughts, and perceptions, to our movements, emotions, and behaviors. All of which happen within the wider world of our families, social systems, cultures, and society. Pain is not so simple as degenerated joints, poor posture, or dysfunctional biomechanics. It is not just about weaknesses, instability, or asymmetries, as many of us have been told for so long. Pain is much more complex than that.

I felt validated. I wasn't just a difficult case, not just a failure. I had no reason to be ashamed, I wasn't to blame. My pain was real, with very real biological processes underlying it. My pain was not all in my head. Not made up. Not exaggerated or fabricated. I wasn't damaged goods, wasn't some broken, dysfunctional, weak person. After years of being told conflicting things, after so many failed treatments, my pain finally started to make some sense. My perspective started to shift. My outlook started to change.

## Empowerment

While it was a bit daunting to discover that pain involves complex interactions between the biological, psychological, and social factors in our lives, it was also empowering. I believed, for the first time in a long time, that there was something I could do. That I had some control. I no longer thought of pain as some external force acting upon me, nor some enemy attacking from within. Rather, pain was something that was a part of me. A part of my human experience, just as it is a part of many people's human experiences. It was a hard realization to come to, yet also a relief. I no longer had to fight the pain and could begin to work *with* it instead.

By understanding that pain is predictive and protective by nature, as you'll learn in later chapters of this book, and not a damage meter, I could get back to living again, even if pain was still present. I didn't have to wait anymore. That was empowering.

## Acceptance

Making sense of my pain allowed me to develop a different relationship with it and to come to a new understanding of myself. For so long, I'd wanted to go back to my life before pain, to who I was before pain. I was stuck in ruminations about the past and what was and what would no longer be and in worry about the future, anxious and fearful about what was to come. It was affecting my pain and wasn't allowing me to move forward. I came to realize that accepting my pain, accepting all that had led up to it no matter how unfair it seemed, didn't mean accepting it as my future fate, too. Acceptance was not about giving up or resigning myself to a life of unchanging pain and endless suffering, it was quite the opposite. It was about hope. It was about making space for pain so there was room for everything else. For all the things that really mattered. By accepting all that had changed, including me, I was finally able to move on from who I'd been and move toward what was possible.

## Reflection and introspection

What was possible? Could viewing my pain through a different lens change things? I wondered if I could I bring a new perspective to my thoughts, emotions, fears, and worries. To my beliefs and expectations. Rather than continually yearning for things to be different, which kept me mired in despair and hopelessness, acceptance gave me the space to become more introspective and reflective about what might be contributing to my experience and what I could do to change it. Taking notice of what was affecting my pain, rather than just taking notice of the pain, was transformative. I felt empowered to take steps that would minimize the things that sent my protective systems into overdrive and maximize the things that made my life better. I had some control over what my life could be again.

It wasn't easy, by any means, but neither was the unforgiving pain. At least along this new path pain was no longer at the center of things. I was. My life was.

## My path forward

My path forward included many things that were all interconnected and interrelated, just as all of the biological, psychological, and social influences on our pain, on our lives, are inextricably interconnected and interrelated. It involved contemplating the biopsychosocial nature of pain and what it meant for my unique experiences, and how I could use what I discovered to make changes. It was about going inward, facing my fears, my pain, my suffering rather than always trying to escape them. It was asking myself some difficult questions, going into dark corners that were scary and uncomfortable, which was difficult, is still difficult. However, I discovered that being *with* my feelings, rather than fighting against them, shined light on a path out of the darkness. It came down to learning more about myself, getting curious and exploring who I was as a person—what was my story and what did I want it to be?—and rewriting it as I went along.

What did I value and find meaningful, and why? What could I do to engage with those things more often? I needed to go outward, too, to find resources that could help me connect the dots and come to new understandings. I needed trusted guides—coaches who could gently challenge my beliefs about my pain and my capabilities and could help me discover all that was possible, walking with me as those possibilities became reality.

## *Self-care*

This introspection and reflection also led me to the see the value of self-care. During the worst years of my pain, I felt guilty taking time to take care of myself. It felt selfish. I found it much easier to care for others, even at the expense of my own wellbeing. It took some time for me to recognize that I was of value, that I was worthy of care. That I deserved kindness and compassion, just the same as anyone who is struggling with pain or is suffering. That we are all deserving of kindness and compassion—of care.

Self-care means different things to different people, because we all have unique needs and goals, likes and dislikes. For me it has been about reconnecting with the things in life I value most. The people, places, and experiences that give me purpose and fill my life with meaning. It's learning and reflecting, breathing and moving, meditation and mindfulness. It's playing outside, challenging myself in new ways. It's expressing myself in new ways and being creative. It's connecting with the things that matter to me over and over and over again. A form of training of sorts. And as with any training, with anything we practice consistently, it leads to real biological change, real functional, and real structural changes in our brains and bodies. We are bioplastic beings, after all, changing and adapting with new and repeated activities, until our very last breath.

So, self-care isn't selfish; it's healthcare. It's empowerment. It leads to real, measurable, physiological changes. That's really cool. Not only did understanding the biology of pain validate my experiences and confirm that my pain was very real, it also showed me a meaningful, accessible path forward by using bioplasticity to my advantage.

## Re-engaging with the world

My first step in taking care of myself led me back into nature. It seemed an easy and accessible place to start. I had withdrawn from nature, like everything else, in my pain, despite it being where I have always found solace, where I have always found peace, calm, and healing. It took knowing that I wasn't doing harm to myself with each painful step to get me to take that step back into nature. To reconnect with the great outdoors, with the trees, the earth, the sky, the moon, and the stars. To once again feel the wind through my hair, the sun on my face. To commune with the flora and fauna.

Being out in nature, I felt as though a great weight was lifted, a heaviness on my soul I hadn't known was there. I felt lighter, filled with hope. I also felt pleasantly surprised: the world was still out there in all its glory, in all its awesomeness, despite my absence from it for so long. There was still beauty and wonder. Still the magic of sunlight filtering through tree branches, the majesty of evening sunsets that fill the sky with color. It had been there all along, I had just stopped noticing it, stopped looking for it. For so long all I had noticed, all I had looked for, was pain.

Nature became a healing, soothing, welcoming place once again. Somewhere I could go to breathe and just be without fear of judgment or failure. Without worrying that I was doing this pain thing wrong. It was freeing. I wanted to capture it—for those times I might forget again—so I started taking pictures, literally seeing the world through a new lens. A world full of colors and vibrancy, sound and sensations. Full of life. I could *feel* it again. The joy of a blue sky dotted with white wispy clouds, the simple wonder of a dewy blade of grass, the awesomeness of a wave crashing upon the shore or a mountaintop shrouded in mist.

When I sought beauty, it was there. It was a revelation.

It wasn't just my view of the world that had changed, so, too, had my view of myself. Where before I'd only seen barriers and limitations, only what I'd lost and could no longer do, I suddenly saw possibility. What I could do, what I could be. I started moving through the world differently, feeling more at ease, more natural, more able, as I bent and stooped, crawled and scrambled to get a clearer shot, a better view. A different perspective.

The world was still a beautiful, wondrous place, and I belonged in it. I was a part of it.


## Breathing

Out in nature, I could just breathe again. I could get out of my hip, out of my head, and into the world. Into the present, no longer stuck in yearning for the past or worrying about the future. And the present was OK, it was no longer terrifying. I was OK. I discovered that I could ground myself in the present moment at anytime, anywhere, with my breath. It sounds so simple, we all know how to breathe, yet bringing awareness to the breath is different. It was akin to becoming aware of the world around me again after so many years of being aware only of pain.

The breath became a training tool to ground myself in the here and now when my thoughts and feelings had a mind of their own, trying to carry me off to the land of worry and dread. The breath also became a useful way for me to detect when my protective systems were ramping up, which would precede a provocation of pain or a flare-up. If I found myself holding my breath or that my breaths were short and quick, I could breathe more slowly, more deeply, and work on relaxing in order to calm my protective systems down. While the concept was simple, the practice was difficult. Perhaps unsurprisingly, protection was not so easy to "let go" of. It was a bit scary to relax after protecting myself from pain for so long. It took training and consistency, but eventually it became easier.

## Moving

My protective responses not only affected my breath, but my movement, too. My muscles would tense up, my joints would become stiff, my movement braced and rigid. Being rigid and stiff affected the way I moved, the way I walked, the way I sat. The way I existed in the world. The tenser and more guarded I was, the more pain there was, so I started moving less. The less I moved, the more painful movement became. Fear of more pain, of more damage, made me move even less. A vicious cycle. Over time I developed rigid and inflexible rules surrounding my posture and movement, without even realizing it. I planned every motion from sitting to standing, lying down to lifting groceries. It became more and more difficult, impossible even, to move with ease.

It wasn't always that way, I wasn't always so careful, so protective. Early on in my pain experience, I hit exercise and physical therapy hard, thinking that improving my strength and stability would improve my pain, as I'd been told. When my pain became progressively worse rather than improving, the worsening pain became progressively worrying. The more I worried, the less I moved, going from one extreme to the other. From boom to bust. I went through these cycles a few times over the course of various treatments. I had needed the middle ground between the extremes of pushing through pain and doing hardly anything at all for the pain.

Once I discovered that I wasn't doing more harm to myself with each painful movement, understanding that movement was safe, that it was beneficial, this allowed me to find the "just right" amount of effort. Over time my fears and worries lessened and my confidence in my hip, in myself, increased. I was able to more consistently calm my protective systems down through breathing and relaxing, which allowed me to move with more ease. I began to notice habits, postures, and movements that provoked my pain and took steps to change them up. I explored movement more freely, with curiosity and flexibility, rather than with rigid rules.

That was important because how I moved affected how I saw myself, too. Moving is about so much more than muscles, joints, and anatomy. When my movement became limited, my sense of self became limited, too. So, too, what I believed I was capable of doing. Being able to move with ease allowed me to relate to my body, myself, my world, differently. I could stay engaged with my life and demonstrate that hey, I'm safe, this is OK. I'm OK. I'm safe.

I was no longer just a painful hip, I was a whole person again. My hip, which had often felt "other" during the worst years of my pain, became reintegrated back into the whole of my being. My hip, my body, was no longer the thing that betrayed me, harboring the enemy. I trusted it again. I trusted my body, myself. I had confidence. I felt strong and adaptable and resilient. I felt like myself.

## Mindfulness

Being out in nature, breathing, and moving with ease were all a part of a more mindful approach. Over time I was able to become more present, more curious and exploratory, and less reactive and judgmental. Eventually, my accidental engagement with mindfulness led to a more purposeful pursuit: meditation. It was something I had tried for years with no success, but in those early attempts I had a goal of pain reduction in mind. It didn't work. When I pursued meditation with a goal of just meditating in mind, it became an instrumental part of my day. Having a formal practice helped me cultivate the ability to take a step back and see the whole picture, of which pain was but a part. To put things in perspective. To respond differently. To see that there was more to my life, more to me, more to my story, than pain.

Through my meditation practice I also came to realize how hard I had been on myself over the years. How much I blamed myself for my pain and for not getting better. Perfectionism is a lifelong pattern of mine: I've always been one to beat myself up when things didn't go as planned. Being able to love myself, to care for myself, to be kind and compassionate with myself, has perhaps been the greatest lesson I have learned. I needed a lot of practice. I needed to keep coming back to it, over and over again. I am grateful for that lesson, though, as it has helped me so much with pain and in life. It wouldn't have happened without all the rest of it, though. And all the rest of it wouldn't have happened without mindfulness. It is all connected.

## It all matters

I'm often asked what has helped the most over the years. What led me from debilitating pain where I couldn't sit, couldn't think, couldn't function for the pain, to being able to live the life I want to without pain being so much of a problem? It's such a difficult question to answer because it's no one thing; it was everything. It's hard to put into words just what that means, but I'll try. It was:

- feeling heard and believed, supported and empowered

- feeling understood, as well as understanding and making sense of my pain

- acceptance and a willingness to get back to living, even if pain was still present

- reconnecting with nature and myself, breathing, meditating, being more mindful

- reconnecting with family and friends and maintaining those connections

- engaging in enjoyed activities like reading, writing, cooking, hiking, snowboarding, camping, travel, photography, watching movies, and spending time with my boys

- moving with more ease and less worry, more play and fewer rules

- being of service to others through volunteering and starting a non-profit

- being kind and compassionate with myself and others, being grateful, loving and being loved.

It was all of that, and so much more. It was everything. It was all interconnected and interrelated. Each part, each interaction between parts, mattered. It all affected me; it all changed me. Down to my very cells, it changed me.

## It is not an easy path

When we live with pain, it changes who we are as people. It changes how we see the world and how we relate to that world. We protect ourselves through isolation and withdrawal, through guarding and tension, through altered thoughts, beliefs, and movements. We disconnect from the people, places, and activities that are meaningful to us.

It is hard.

That doesn't even begin to hit upon the truth, though. Living with pain is so much more than hard. So much more than difficult. Yet living with pain can also be a great teacher. It forced me to simplify my life, to determine what was really meaningful to me. And when I made space for pain, there was room for all that was meaningful. There was room for beauty, laughter, love, and purpose. For joy as well as sorrow. For the entire spectrum, the entire depth, of being human. There were setbacks and flare-ups, and they were hard, too. With each flare-up

I reminded myself, or was reminded by others, that I'd always gotten through it, that I knew what to do, that I didn't have to do it all on my own.

That I am strong, adaptable, resilient. Capable. That I can do this. And I keep coming back to that over and over again.

## Conclusion

I've shared my story here because I want you to know how difficult it is to live with pain. How dark, demoralizing, and distressing it is. How life- and self-altering it is. And I want you to know it takes hard work to get out of those dark places, too. I want you to know that change is possible, but it's not easy. It takes time and persistence, compassion and courage. My hope is that my story bolsters your own compassion and courage, your kindness and patience, your hope, when you are working with people in pain. And I hope it gives you hope, realistic hope, for the future of pain care. There is so much that you can do to help people living with pain.

We need to feel safe—physically, emotionally, cognitively. You can provide safety. We need to know we are strong, adaptable, resilient, and capable. You can tell us that. Even better, you can show us. We need to be heard, believed, and validated. You can hear us. Listen as much as you educate. Learn from us, just as we will learn from you. We need to be understood and we also need to understand. You can help us make sense of things.

Discover who we are as people. Who we were before pain, who we are now, who we want to be. Find out what is meaningful to us. Help us engage with the things that matter to us. Combine your expertise with ours. Use our values and goals as the compass to help us map our paths forward and use your skills, education, and training to help us navigate along the way. Empower us to live well, whether pain is present or not. Help us foster our patience. Encourage our persistence. Emphasize our strengths, our resilience, our adaptability. Our courage. Recognize our efforts and celebrate our successes, knowing that no success is too small. Guide us back to the valued, meaningful, purposeful lives we want to live. You can do all that.

There is hope, such realistic hope, for everyone living with pain. There is so much that is possible, so much that can be done, no matter how long someone has lived with pain, no matter how many limitations they may have. Bring that hope forward to all of the people you work with. Be convincing so that they will be convinced. There is such hope that pain can change, that lives can change. You can help make that change happen.

There are many paths forward; there are endless possibilities. You can show us the way.

*Chapter 2*

# Current Research in Yoga and Pain

Steffany Moonaz

## Background

### *Why research matters to yoga therapy*

It is sometimes thought that modern scientific evidence is not relevant to an ancient practice such as yoga. After all, yoga has been practiced for thousands of years. Some might suggest that its teachings are of Divine origin and therefore beyond the scrutiny that the scientific method espouses. However, it is a core concept within yoga to become a witness to one's own experience and the surrounding world. Detached curiosity is very much aligned with both yoga and science.

Evidence-informed practice is critical for optimal care in the applied field of yoga therapy. Along with skills/knowledge and the individual client's priorities/preferences, we should be compelled to avail ourselves of the best available evidence in clinical decision making. An understanding of the modern literature is not only useful for informing yoga therapy practice, but can also provide a common language for collaborative care and can improve the clarity with which we explain and describe our work to clients, students, and others. Lastly, the strength of the evidence ultimately informs recommendations, referrals, and policy decisions related to access and availability of yoga for underserved populations who are desperately seeking viable solutions for ongoing pain management.

Pain reduction is most certainly not the original intention of yoga. However, in the process of working toward a state of union, many changes may occur on the levels of mind, body, and spirit, including a reduction in pain-related outcomes and other sequelae of life with a chronic pain condition. People may come to yoga to change their pain, but stay to change their lives, which may ultimately change their pain.

## Current trajectory of yoga research

Science is an iterative process. Each step builds on the step prior. Each research study makes a small contribution to a growing body of evidence, much like adding a single puzzle piece until a pattern begins to emerge. Relative to other fields, the yoga research literature is small but rapidly expanding. In fact, there has been exponential growth in both the quantity and quality of yoga research in the past decade alone. That being said, we are still quite far from a readiness to study the nuanced questions that will guide best practices in yoga therapy.

Early yoga research in the West tended to be unfunded passion projects completed by interested researchers working primarily in other areas. Such studies were necessarily small and often lacked strong scientific rigor. These pilot studies began to demonstrate that a yoga intervention could be generally feasible, acceptable, and relatively safe. Given the connotations of yoga at the time, this alone was important. Small trials also bring challenges to light that can be addressed prior to the investment of substantial time and funds. As yoga research expanded, randomized clinical trials began to compare yoga with a control group, which can begin to demonstrate the effects of yoga practice for outcomes such as pain intensity, pain interference, pain coping, and more. As these studies collect, they can be gathered by likeness and combined through systematic reviews and meta-analyses, which determine an overall effect that might not be apparent when looking at a single study alone.

Currently, there is very little evidence to suggest which yoga practices are most effective at which times, for which individuals, with which conditions. Additionally, while there is much conjecture about how or why yoga is effective for pain, evidence is limited regarding the specific mechanisms. Lastly, published manuscripts may not describe the yoga intervention or the study methods in sufficient detail for critical examination, future replication, or reasonable comparison. Improving the clarity of reporting as the yoga research expands will also improve the possibility for more evidence-informed practice among yoga therapists.

## Diversity of study designs

The randomized controlled trial (RCT) is often held up as the ideal research design. It is certainly true that many aspects of a RCT help to minimize bias and isolate variables for comparison. But the RCT was primarily developed for studying pharmacological approaches that could be more easily standardized and masked than yoga practice. Research on mind-body practices such as yoga requires more creative study designs. Pragmatic research, observational studies, qualitative and mixed methods approaches, and comparative effectiveness research will help to answer different questions beyond what we can learn from RCTs.

## Research reported in this chapter

The evidence discussed in this chapter comes from RCTs, pilot studies, qualitative research, and literature reviews. I have included more varied types of research than would be found in a typical systematic review, yet also included results of such reviews. This is not an exhaustive discussion of the evidence on yoga for pain, but it provides an indication of the current state of the evidence. Much more research on practices and mechanisms related to yoga is also important for informing yoga therapy practice. Research on the effects of exercise for pain is relevant, as is the evidence for meditation and mindfulness practices from outside of the yoga tradition. Research that studies sleep patterns and respiration is relevant to yoga, as is the evidence relating meaning and purpose to the experience of pain. These exciting and important areas of research should all continue to inform the way we think about yoga and its role in pain management. In this chapter, however, the focus is specifically on the direct relationship between yoga and pain.

## The evidence

### Neck pain

The literature on yoga for neck pain, while somewhat sparse, has been well characterized. A 2017 meta-analysis of three studies on 188 patients with chronic neck pain revealed robust, short-term, clinically meaningful effects for pain intensity when comparing yoga with usual care.[1] In fact, the full range of the 95 percent confidence interval for mean difference on this outcome represented a meaningful difference between groups; in other words, even a conservative estimate of the results suggests an important improvement associated with yoga. Effects on pain-related disability and mood were also large, and these effects were consistent for both exercise-based and meditative-based yoga programs.

While much of the research on yoga for pain involves Hatha yoga interventions with physical postures and breath integration, included in the above meta-analysis was a RCT involving 60 patients with chronic neck pain comparing physiotherapy followed by an audio-CD guided yogic relaxation with mantra repetition to physiotherapy followed by supine rest.[2] The yoga group rested supine and listened to the mantra first, followed by audible repetition, with the instruction to feel the sound resonance throughout the body. After ten days, the yoga group had significantly better pain and neck movements compared to the control group. Improvements were significantly greater for neck disability and anxiety, although both groups improved for all variables.

The authors of this small meta-analysis concluded that while the physical practices of yoga can bring the benefits of muscle stretching and strengthening, mindful movement, and intentional breath work, the meditative practices of yoga may also increase body awareness, resulting in changes to postural patterning and habitual muscle tension. The optimal combination and relative contributions of various yoga practices for affecting neck pain has yet to be examined.

In addition to the quantitative literature, 18 participants in a RCT of Iyengar yoga for chronic neck pain were recruited for a qualitative study[3] in which they were asked to complete a drawing of their neck and shoulders before and after the nine-week intervention, based on their subjective perceptions, and then were interviewed about their body perceptions, emotional status, coping skills, and changes to any of these. Changes to the line drawings of the neck and shoulders were dramatic and their interviews reflected renewed body awareness, greater control over their health, increased acceptance of their pain and disability, more use of active coping strategies, and enhanced participation in life activities. As with other studies, some reported reduced reliance on pain medications. One participant stated, "I know for example that this half forward bend, that is now like a painkiller for me…" (p.540). Another reported an "awareness that you can change a lot yourself" (p.539). Overall, shifts in experience were reported on a physical, cognitive, emotional, behavioral, and social level, reflecting a whole-person response to the yoga intervention.

Overall, the evidence on yoga for neck pain is small but promising. While both movement and meditative practices seem to be effective, the relative efficacy and specific mechanisms have yet to be explored. Additionally, the movement practices included above are all Iyengar-based and the benefits may not be generalizable to community-based or non-Iyengar yoga programs.

## Low back pain

The yoga literature on chronic low back pain (cLBP) is perhaps the most robust of all pain conditions. While summary research has been conducted, a few select studies are reported here, as their study designs reflect the type of creative research designs needed in the field. Dr. Robert Saper and his lab beautifully designed and executed a non-inferiority study comparing yoga, physical therapy (PT), and an educational control in a low-income, racially diverse sample with moderate to severe cLBP.[4] (Classes were held once weekly due to prior research demonstrating similar improvements in pain and function for groups receiving yoga either once or twice per week.[5]) Classes included relaxation, breath work, yoga philosophy, and postures, accompanied by world music. Classes were taught by one to three teachers with no more than four to five students per teacher for any class. Thirty minutes of daily home practice was encouraged.

Unlike a comparative effectiveness study, which is designed to demonstrate which intervention is more effective, non-inferiority studies are powered to show whether two interventions are comparable. In this case, the study was designed to determine whether yoga is at least as effective as the established treatment of physical therapy. (Greater statistical power via a larger sample size would be necessary to determine whether one of these is more effective than the other.) The results demonstrated that yoga was non-inferior to physical therapy with regard to improved pain, and the similarity carried across most secondary outcomes also.

Additionally, both groups were less likely to use pain medication than the education control and the improvements were sustained at one year for both active groups, regardless of whether they were assigned to home practice only or ongoing live sessions. There was also no demonstrable difference in adverse events between yoga and PT, most of which were mild and self-limited. Interestingly, the PT group had a greater loss to follow-up.

The non-inferiority study above was preceded by a RCT[6] that also compared yoga to stretching and an educational book that was used in both studies. In this study, yoga was more effective than the educational group but similar to the stretching group—the latter of which included much more stretching than what would generally be found in publicly available stretching classes. More than half of active participants improved by at least 50 percent for both primary outcomes (back-related functional status and bothersomeness of pain) compared to 23 percent for education (p<0.001). Those assigned to yoga were more likely to attend at least one class, suggesting an acceptance of yoga for those with cLBP. Additionally, home practice was substantially higher for yoga than stretching, with 59 percent and 40 percent respectively reporting home practice on at least three days in the prior week. Yoga participants also reported that they would definitely recommend the class to others at higher rates than stretching (85% versus 54%). Similar to the non-inferiority study, the active groups reported twice the incidence of reduced medication compared to the education group at both follow-ups.

Nineteen participants from the dosing trial mentioned above[7] were recruited for individual semi-structured interviews to understand the impact of yoga on back pain qualitatively.[8] Participants reported that yoga served as a pain management strategy while also improving mood, stress management, relaxation, and self-efficacy for pain-related self-care. Mindfulness of emotions and greater acceptance of pain were noted as helpful outcomes of yoga practice. Some reported that yoga reduced or eliminated the need for pain medication, and breathing practices were harnessed as a coping strategy for pain, stress, and sleep. Noticing a connection between mind and body was felt to foster greater regulation of the pain experience, and the social support of both classmates and friends/family was said to improve adherence to class attendance and home practice. Yoga was not seen as a permanent cure but a long-term strategy for pain management.

The literature on yoga for cLBP overall suggests strong evidence for a modest to moderate benefit,[9] with most RCTs indicating reduced pain and disability, safety, and acceptability.[10] Practice guidelines from the American College of Physicians and the American Pain Society based on best evidence also suggest that yoga should be considered for individuals unresponsive to conventional treatment.[11] This evidence demonstrates that yoga is feasible, acceptable, and effective across demographics and in populations with a lower general uptake of yoga practice. Clear and publicly available protocols make it possible to replicate such programs more broadly.

## Arthritis and related conditions

Arthritis is an umbrella term that captures over 100 unique diagnoses and is the leading cause of disability in the US. These various conditions are sometimes included in trials for their similar features or studied individually for greater specificity. The most common form of arthritis is osteoarthritis (OA), which is often thought of as a biomechanical condition but is now known to also have a component of systemic inflammation. The knee is the most common joint affected with OA and several studies have explored the effects of yoga on knee OA, which were recently summarized by Kan *et al.*[12] Using the Western Ontario and McMaster Universities OA Index Scale (WOMAC), Kolasinski *et al.*[13] found significantly improved pain after eight weeks of asana, while Cheung *et al.* reported significant between-group differences at eight weeks.[14] They also found a significant difference in pain comparing four weeks to eight weeks and from four weeks to twenty weeks. By visual analog scale (VAS), Ebnezar *et al.*[15] noted significant differences in pain both within and between groups after a three-month intervention that combined a comprehensive yoga practice (asana, pranayama, meditation, lectures, counseling, relaxation, and subtle exercises) with PT compared to therapeutic exercise combined with PT. Nambi and Shah saw a greater reduction in pain among asana participants than controls after eight weeks, while change scores (difference over time) were significantly better for yoga compared to controls.[16] Another small RCT[17] saw no significant difference in pain between yoga (asana, pranayama, and meditation) and control (home-based activities), but within-group difference was significant for yoga and not for controls. Aside from the study from Ebnezar *et al.*, the sample sizes are quite small, all but one failed to blind assessors to treatment group, and adverse events reporting was inconsistent. This work would benefit from larger, more rigorous trials and meta-analysis when possible.

In contrast with OA, rheumatoid arthritis (RA) is an autoimmune condition with substantial systemic inflammation as a central feature. A systematic review[18] was conducted to summarize the literature on yoga for both RA and spondyloarthropathies, which are forms of inflammatory arthritis that primarily affect the spine. They found that yoga seems effective in decreasing pain and inflammation while increasing quality of life. Bosch et al.[19] reported improved disability scores, pain perception, and depression after ten weeks of Hatha yoga for nine post-menopausal RA patients compared to controls. A RCT[20] with a much larger sample size (40 in each group) for a seven-week program including daily yoga and lifestyle changes showed a significant improvement for the yoga group in both pain and inflammatory markers. A smaller group of young persons with RA in a study by Evans et al. noted significantly greater improvements for pain disability, acceptance of chronic pain, and self-efficacy regarding pain after six weeks of Iyengar yoga compared to controls, while disease activity and pain scores did not change significantly.[21] A recent pilot study of an eight-week yoga program used pain as a secondary outcome and reported its improvement, along with better sleep,[22] though no significant between-group differences. While these small studies make it difficult to generalize to large populations, mind-body practices can move the body toward parasympathetic engagement[23] and therefore potentially reduce the effects of stress on disease processes such as RA. There is also evidence that pain perception and quality of life could be fostered in part by the release of endorphins associated with yoga practice.[24]

Ward et al. summarized the research on yoga for a variety of musculoskeletal conditions.[25] They included RA, OA, cLBP, and fibromyalgia (FM), which is further discussed in a later section of this chapter. Across a total of 17 studies, including eight with good methodological quality, yoga improved pain in OA, RA, and mild–moderate cLBP. A moderate effect was demonstrated in meta-analysis of good-quality studies for both functional outcomes and pain outcomes. For those reporting pain outcomes, all favored the yoga intervention and only one found no statistical difference in pain between yoga and passive control.[26] It is also noteworthy that a 24-week intervention for cLBP showed no difference at week 12, but a significant improvement in favor of yoga at 24 weeks, suggesting that dose may be important.[27] The current evidence suggests that yoga is safe and acceptable with potential benefits in pain and function for a variety of musculoskeletal conditions. However, it should be noted that yoga interventions were very heterogeneous in style, duration, and frequency, and many studies failed to report whether any adverse events occurred. Additionally, the more rigorous studies tended not to report sufficient detail for study replication, echoing an ongoing need for greater transparency in yoga research reporting.

In our work reviewing the literature in arthritis and rheumatic conditions, we found no evidence of disease worsening or increased joint pain, and some improvement in disease activity, including a reduction in tender and swollen joints. Improvements were consistently demonstrated for disease symptoms, including pain, function, mood, energy, and self-efficacy.[28] And in a review of yoga for rheumatic diseases (FM, OA, RA, and carpal tunnel syndrome) by Cramer *et al.*, yoga was associated with improvements in both pain and disability for FM, OA, and RA, although methodological quality was deemed to be generally low.[29] A later review also found an effect of yoga for carpal tunnel syndrome.[30]

In our RCT conducted at Johns Hopkins University,[31] we found significant improvements in pain for participants with RA or OA after eight weeks of yoga (asana, pranayama, relaxation, meditation, chanting, philosophy) compared to waitlist control, as well as improvements in other domains of health-related quality of life (physical roles, general health, vitality, mental health), physical fitness (flexibility, mobility), and psychological outcomes (depression, positive affect). Patient-reported outcomes (PROs) were assessed again after nine months and found to be largely sustained. In particular, pain had improved 25 percent for those participating in yoga and the change remained significant after nine months. While adherence is often discussed as a challenge, most who began the yoga intervention attended at least 12 out of 16 classes and 79 percent completed the intervention. Study withdrawal was not associated with any measured disease characteristics, but was associated with minority race, most commonly due to life events or scheduling.

The yoga intervention from the study above was replicated in a feasibility pilot for underserved minority patients from the Community Health Clinic at the National Institute of Arthritis and Musculoskeletal and Skin Diseases (NIAMS) at the National Institutes of Health.[32] This was of particular interest since minority race was the only significant predictor of attrition in the diverse study sample discussed above. Similarly, most participants who began the intervention completed it, as attrition was highest prior to the first class. Additionally, all who completed the intervention were still practicing yoga three months after the intervention period. While this was primarily a feasibility study, statistically significant improvements were measured for health-related behaviors, as measured with the Health-Promoting Lifestyle Profile II (HPLP-II). Selected physical measures also improved, including balance, functional reach, and disability of the arm/shoulder/hand (DASH), as well as improved self-efficacy. Because the measure used to assess pain (PROMIS-29) does not currently evaluate minimally clinically important differences, change over time was not statistically analyzed; however, both pain interference and pain intensity shifted in the desired direction, along with sleep disturbance and satisfaction with social roles. A larger RCT with a comparison of pain-related outcomes would be necessary to confirm these preliminary findings.

The above was a mixed-methods feasibility study and qualitative data were reported separately.[33] Participants were asked to keep personal journals and exit interviews were conducted. Additionally, study staff maintained field notes and observational data during the interviews and from contact with the participants at or between yoga classes. During interviews, 94 percent of participants viewed yoga as a way to care for their arthritis symptoms. Most were satisfied with the classes, agreed that the classes should be bilingual, and would recommend yoga to a friend with arthritis. Themes that emerged from their journals included both mental/emotional (gratitude, calm, stress, relaxation) and physical (flexibility, pain, sleep, energy) benefits from yoga practice. Support from props, written instructions, and family members were facilitators of home practice. As with other studies, insufficient time and space were barriers to practice, as well as illness, lack of motivation, and arthritis flares. Challenges to class attendance included transportation issues, such as distance, directional navigation, and cost of public transit. These factors should be taken into consideration when designing future studies and when endeavoring to make yoga more accessible to diverse populations.

While there are a growing number of clinical trials on yoga for various forms of arthritis, the studies are generally small, may be uncontrolled, and have inconsistent methodological rigor. Most studies report improvements in pain after completion of a yoga program, regardless of frequency or duration. However, several studies report within-group differences but not between-group differences. This may be due to non-specific effects related to research participation, baseline differences between groups, or insufficient power to detect differences. Periodic meta-analyses are needed to better synthesize the growing evidence. Nonetheless, yoga seems feasible and acceptable among diverse groups with different forms of arthritis. It also appears to be a relatively safe option for remaining active and managing stress, both of which are recommended for general arthritis management.

## Neurological pain

While FM is often included in the category of musculoskeletal conditions or arthritis as above, it is now known to involve dysregulation of the descending pain pathways and is therefore included here as a neurological condition. A systematic review and meta-analysis examining the effects of meditative movement therapies (Qigong, Tai Chi, and yoga) for FM[34] found that in subgroup analysis, only yoga was associated with significant changes in pain, fatigue, depression, and health-related quality of life at the end of treatment. None of the included yoga studies reported outcomes data beyond the end of treatment to explore longer-term effects. All therapies had high acceptance compared with medication treatment, and no serious adverse events were reported.

A systematic review of yoga for headaches[35] found that only one was a RCT, originating in India.[36] The program studied in this RCT included asana, pranayama, and kriya (nasal water cleansing) performed five days per week for three months. It found significant differences between groups for headache intensity, headache frequency, and symptom medication use, as well as both depression and anxiety scores. A RCT published after that review compared Rajyoga meditation to inactive control for individuals in outpatient psychiatric care for chronic tension headaches.[37] Meditation sessions were offered on alternate days for two weeks and participants were instructed to meditate for 20 minutes in the morning and evening. Significant improvements were seen in meditators for headache severity, frequency, and duration (all via VAS), a headache index (frequency × severity), depression, and anxiety (Hamilton scales). However, significant improvements were also seen in non-meditators who were receiving similar psychiatric care. While both groups improved significantly, improvements were much larger in the intervention group (87–93% improvement versus 23–38% improvement) but no direct comparison was reported between groups at posttest.

Research on yoga for multiple sclerosis (MS) usually focuses on outcomes such as fatigue, mood, cognition, and/or physical fitness. Some studies have also assessed changes in pain and pain management for this population. A RCT involving 60 Iranian women with MS measured pain and quality of life (QOL) with a six-point and ten-point scale, respectively.[38] The yoga intervention included mental focus, breath control, and slow movements, twice per week for 60–90 minutes. Both pain and QOL improved significantly in the yoga group but not in the inactive control group. However, no comparison was reported between groups at either time point. It is worth noting that the yoga group had poorer ratings for both items at baseline, and while significant improvements were made, they may not have sufficiently surpassed control group values for a statistical between-group difference. A four-month, single-arm Ananda yoga intervention,[39] while primarily focused on physical measures, also measured pain-related aspects of QOL using the Health Status Questionnaire (SF-36) and Pain Effects Scale (PES) for 22 study completers. The mental health components of the SF-36 showed significant changes before and after the intervention, while the physical health components, which include pain, were not significantly different. Additionally, other QOL measures improved but not the PES.

Chronic fatigue syndrome (CFS) is a systemic chronic condition with unknown etiology that has been classified as a neurological condition by the World Health Organization (WHO). The symptoms of CFS, including chronic pain, seem to stem largely from a variety of chronic neurological disturbances, impacting a variety of body systems.[40] A 2014 RCT included 30 persons (15 per group) with CFS who were previously unresponsive to conventional care.[41] While fatigue and vigor were the primary outcomes, within-group changes in pain were also assessed using the SF-8 and found to be significantly improved for yoga participants. Qualitative findings were also reported, although detailed methodology about its collection and analysis was not. Five participants reported pain relief during yoga, including two who also had FM. Participants mentioned that "as their practice proceeded, they were able to become detached from the pain, and they noticed that the severity of the pain decreased during a yoga session" (p.6). Seven participants also mentioned reduced muscular tension during yoga.

Evidence for the efficacy of yoga in neurological pain conditions is limited. Studies often assess pain as a secondary outcome, which means that sufficient statistical power may be lacking, and many trials in such conditions fail to include an assessment of pain in favor of other condition-related outcomes. Additionally, comparison between the intervention and control groups is sometimes excluded or not significant. Several studies utilized meditative yoga practices while others included movement, and it is not clear what the relative differences may be between these approaches. There are potential mechanisms by which both movement and meditation may help to change pain processing pathways and, given the dearth of effective pain management strategies for some of these conditions, further research is sorely needed in this area.

### Abdominal pain

A systematic review[42] reported on the literature regarding yoga for irritable bowel syndrome (IBS). It reported that twice-weekly Iyengar yoga for six weeks[43] was associated with significant improvements in "worst pain," which was maintained at two months follow-up, but there were no significant group differences for pain at posttest when compared to usual care waitlist. In the Evans study, 44 percent of adolescents experienced a reduction of 1–1.73 points on a numeric rating scale (NRS) and 46 percent experienced a reduction of at least 1.74 points on the NRS for abdominal pain, reflecting a clinically significant difference. A pilot study comparing yoga to a walking program[44] also reported within-group improvements in abdominal pain after eight weeks of twice-weekly Iyengar yoga, as well as improved visceral sensitivity and severity of somatic symptoms. A third study collected pain data for a 12-week Hatha yoga intervention (asana, pranayama, concentration, relaxation), but it was not assessed because of baseline differences between groups, although IBS symptom severity and IBS-related QOL improved.[45] The authors of the review conclude that yoga seems promising and safe for IBS, but no recommendations can be made due to heterogeneity of studies. However, practice need not be discouraged for those with IBS, especially when they feel it is beneficial for health, QOL, and IBS-related co-morbidities.

Nested within a RCT assessing the effects of twice-weekly yoga for eight weeks was a qualitative study exploring the experience of yoga for 15 women with pain-associated endometriosis.[46] All participants reported that yoga reduced pelvic pain, which was reflected in the quantitative findings of the full RCT with 40 participants.[47] It is worth noting that the interventionist, who was also the first author for both studies, conducted all interviews and analyzed data for thematic content, with cross-check by the second author. Interviewees reported awareness of mind-body integration, which assisted in pain management. Specifically, pranayama (breathing) techniques were cited as key to managing pain, as the breath work fostered introspection and therefore pain relief, especially when awareness allowed them to anticipate increases in pain and use pranayama preventatively. Participants also noted a decrease in their use of both pain and psychiatric medication through decreased dose and increased time between doses. Being able to share their stories and experiences helped them to reframe their beliefs about their condition and fostered social support within the group.

Very few studies have been conducted assessing the efficacy of yogic practices for the management of abdominal pain. While robust evidence may be lacking, yoga may serve as an adjuvant approach, in conjunction with conventional pain management and disease-modifying strategies. In addition to more common Hatha approaches, the roles of pranayama, social support, and belief reframing through yoga might be of interest to explore further.

### Special populations

Older adults and military populations (both veterans and active duty) are populations with high levels of reported pain and insufficient pain management.[48] As yoga is adapted to the unique needs of these populations, it may become an increasingly viable option for complementary care. Two review articles report on the role of yoga for seniors[49] and military[50] populations and their findings are summarized here.

As Bruckenthal *et al.* report in their review on older adults, use of yoga and other mind-body approaches among middle-aged and older adults is approximately 6–9 percent, rating it as one of the most common integrative health strategies (behind nutritional supplements and chiropractor or osteopathic manipulation).[51] Seventy-three percent of older adults use complementary and integrative health (CIH) approaches specifically to manage pain or a pain condition, and mind-body therapies are used most often in this regard. While it has been suggested that the direct evidence for yoga's impact on persistent pain in older adults is limited, growing evidence supports changes in the brain that are associated with chronic pain. Additionally, small studies of older adults with chronic stroke, joint pain, and OA have demonstrated reduced pain associated with yoga classes.[52] Unfortunately, CIH approaches are discussed in provider–patient encounters only 33 percent of the time, and only in 25 percent of encounters is the discussion initiated by the provider.[53] Approaches such as yoga that foster self-efficacy and can be practiced in group settings with the added element of social engagement and support may be particularly appropriate for older adults.

As for military populations, Miller *et al.* note that over 65 percent of veterans report pain, including almost 10 percent experiencing severe pain, according to data from the National Health Interview Survey.[54] Additionally, 44 percent of active duty service members report chronic pain.[55] While opioids are often used to manage chronic pain, the effects may not be sustained and the treatments are often misused, with 15–20 percent of active duty veterans reporting opioid misuse,[56] which includes a doubling from 2002 to 2005 and a tripling from 2005 to 2008. Most studies exploring the effects of yoga for pain in veterans are weakened by single-group design or non-randomized groups.[57] Nonetheless, these studies do indicate a change in pain outcomes warranting further study with rigorous designs. In a RCT of yoga for veterans with low back pain, pain intensity was reduced for the yoga group compared to controls, while pain was also reduced at six months follow-up.[58] This area is of particular importance since half of all veterans report back pain specifically.[59] Treatment of chronic pain in veteran and military populations is further complicated due to the high co-morbidity of post-traumatic stress disorder (PTSD). A recent literature review[60] found no studies including only active duty service members and suggested that a more complex, trauma-informed yoga approach might be appropriate for addressing both chronic pain and PTSD, given not only their co-occurrence, but also their reinforcing of each other.

## Summary

Summarizing the comprehensive quantitative literature (controlled clinical trials) on yoga for pain across populations, an excellent meta-analysis was conducted in 2012,[61] which warrants updating to include more recent literature. The authors point out that chronic pain is not simply a physical condition but includes physical, psychological, and social aspects, while both psychological and social factors also influence chronic pain. In their meta-analysis of yoga for people with pain, all studies reported a positive effect in favor of yoga, with a moderate overall effect. When exploring those studies that used a VAS to assess pain, a significant group difference was found. Effect sizes for back pain and RA were better compared to other pain conditions. A funnel plot also suggested no asymmetry that would indicate publication bias. They conclude that four studies described strong effects for pain intensity/frequency, six studies reported moderate effects, while two showed weak effects. Additionally, reporting of pain-related disability included strong effects for five studies, moderate effects for four studies, and weak effects for three studies. All were in favor of the yoga intervention over comparison groups. Overall, the strongest evidence of a potential benefit from yoga practice appeared to be for improving pain (Standard Mean Difference -0.74; 95% Confidence Interval -0.97, -0.42), with similar effects evident for both pain-related disability and mood. As may be expected, longer trials were associated with suboptimal adherence, as with most exercise interventions.

As with the subsequent literature reflected in the body of this chapter, yoga appears to be consistently associated with reduced pain, as well as other outcomes of concern to chronic pain populations, such as disability, mood, and QOL. It is important to note that the reverse is very unlikely: yoga does not seem to exacerbate pain in chronic pain populations. This alone is noteworthy, since yoga may confer other benefits for these populations, such as increased physical fitness and reduced stress. If the evidence is not yet sufficiently robust to say with certainty that yoga decreases pain, we can more confidently say that yoga tends to not increase pain, and therefore need not be discouraged so long as it is practiced appropriately.

It is important to note that a lack of evidence is not evidence of lack. For some pain conditions, the evidence is limited simply because there have been very few studies in that area, or the studies have not been of sufficient vigor. It is still quite possible that mild, moderate, or even strong evidence for a reduction in pain or other related outcomes will emerge as the research evolves.

## General trends and limitations

To date, the vast majority of yoga research, on pain and otherwise, is comprised of small pilot studies, both controlled and uncontrolled. As these studies collect over time, the possibility of conducting systematic reviews and meta-analysis emerges, which can give us a better sense of the current collective evidence. Unfortunately, systematic reviews often limit the included studies to RCTs, which restricts the segment of evidence included, and meta-analyses require common outcome measures and robust research reporting, which does not necessarily reflect the existing yoga literature. Some large and rigorous trials have been conducted, and these show very promising findings, especially for pain outcomes and QOL. Most RCTs, however, compare yoga to usual care, waitlist, or inactive control. Especially because it is generally not possible to mask group assignment for the participants, there is high risk of non-specific effects differentiating the two groups.

Pilot studies are generally conducted to assess safety, feasibility, and acceptability. Overall, the existing literature suggests that yoga has all three, when developed in consideration of the needs and limitations for a specific population. While reported adverse events are few and minor, too many studies lack consistent reporting of adverse events, and since we cannot assume that lack of reporting means that no adverse events (AEs) occurred, strong conclusions about safety cannot yet be made. Participation rates and qualitative data reflect a general receptivity to yoga across clinical and demographic populations.

## Future directions

Larger and more rigorous RCTs are needed for most pain conditions in order to bolster the strength of the evidence. Systematic reviews should consider reporting findings from controlled and uncontrolled trials in order to provide a more comprehensive view of the evidence. Consistent and thorough research reporting is needed in order to facilitate more inclusive meta-analyses. AEs need to be reported for all clinical trials, including a report of no AEs or no AEs related to the intervention when appropriate. Active control groups should be considered to reduce the confounding of non-specific effects and to isolate specific components of yoga that are not shared with other self-care strategies. Pragmatic studies can help to differentiate yoga's efficacy from its effectiveness in real-world settings that are commercially available to chronic pain populations. Because of known racial and socioeconomic disparities in both pain and disability regardless of diagnosis, it is imperative that studies explore the effectiveness of self-care and non-pharmacological strategies for improving pain and function in diverse samples. Lastly, comparisons between various yoga practices and styles will help to improve evidence-informed yoga therapy and to establish best practices driven by all three components of evidence-informed practice (knowledge and experience, client preferences/values, and best available evidence).

## Chapter 3

# The Current State(s) and Theor(y)ies on Pain Management (sic)

## Matthew J. Taylor

What went wrong with the messy chapter title? It turns out the original title for this chapter using both "state" and "theory" in the singular isn't accurate, and we might ask, is "management" still appropriate for how we providers relate to pain? More importantly, the old title nicely captured the primary challenges rehabilitation professionals face today: despite our best efforts, to include Western medicine, there isn't a single, monolithic state or theory on the human experience of pain, and consequently no matching theory that provides a singular management practice for addressing those suffering. And, there's a pretty good chance there won't ever be a single state or theory, let alone some definitive, specific case "control/management" for pain either. And, that's OK.

Why is it OK? How did we arrive at these multiple states and theories with all the powerful technology and information explosion? Does having plural states and theories limit us or free us? What does this plurality portend for the future of pain understanding and the care to address pain?

I know, those questions are a hard-right turn after the last chapter exploring what we "know" about yoga and pain. But these questions also more comfortably hold the very real, lived experience of pain recounted in Chapter 1. Because of that, in this chapter we will explore the above questions and offer a robust framework for optimizing the remainder of this book. If done well, we will also be able to more easily adjust our future understandings around pain, as well as the related pain management practices as they continue to evolve. We will begin with a very brief history of pain and present states, followed by a summation of some the challenges we face today, and then finish by discussing the promising possibilities that lie before us by including yoga and the role it can play as it evolves as well. The good news is that it is my contention that we are at an exciting threshold, so let's explore where we've been and how to best step across this threshold into the future.

## How did we arrive at these multiple states and theories with all the powerful technology and information explosion?

In order to better understand our place in this history of pain and care for those in pain, it is helpful to first zoom out in a wide perspective across human evolution. The space constraints of this chapter prohibit a detailed, historical timeline rich in context. Fortunately, that doesn't mean we can't offer a functional understanding of the history that supports this textbook. The arc of the evolution of pain science and theory mirrors that of human consciousness. Just as our pain theories continue to evolve across time, so too has human consciousness, both as a species across the millennia, but also as a developmental arc within each of us as individuals in our lifetime à la Piaget.[1] These arcs are spectrums representing various aspects available for human experiencing and are not intended to describe fixed realities or some stable state. This will become clearer below when Table 3.1 is described. Conveniently, these arcs make nice bridgework for linking our conventional rehabilitation perspectives with yoga. For those new to yoga, it is an inquiry via lived experience that explores consciousness. Therefore, Table 3.1 illustrates how our consciousness level is reflected in our pain theories, setting a foundation for why yoga is a natural thread to connect the two. Understanding the assumptions and beliefs that underlie and guide our rehabilitation practice is of course a key component of clinical mastery. Consider the following summary outline of the arc of human consciousness and then we will overlay our arc of pain understanding.

There are many descriptions of human consciousness evolution with numerous overlaps between them. Table 3.1 is an amalgamation of the most common descriptions that ranges in an arc from magical to rational/reductionist/ materialism to postmodern/constructivism to integral.[2] Today we can find practitioners who practice along the entire arc and frequently move back and forth, often without realizing they are shifting, and at other times intentionally doing so to match the patient or audience. In Table 3.1, below each level of consciousness there is description of it, and beneath that, an example or two from the pain theories that exist representing those state(s) and their respective philosophical underpinnings.

Note, both postmodern and integral reject the singular idea of a single state of what we know and therefore are comfortable with a plurality of *states* and *theories*. Those levels also ask and acknowledge the importance of defining "Who is the 'we'?" in any inquiry to include the "us" as rehabilitation professionals of Western orientation compiling this text. This is evident as we see the discussions in the yoga community around appropriation of yoga (i.e. our nearly-all-Northern-European-descent contributing authors list) and even the possibility of an unintended medical colonialism of yoga as a commodity. One assumption we make is that the word "science" [Latin *scientia,* knowledge; noun; a branch of knowledge or study dealing with a body of facts or truths systematically arranged and showing the operation of general laws[3]] is synonymous with the present-day scientific method. This bias limits our discernment and appreciation for other sciences, especially if they are not European in origin.[4] This is an important topic emerging from the latter levels of consciousness. Readers unfamiliar with these concerns are invited to read Ganeri,[5] and you have also just experienced the utility of Table 3.1 in discovering how the levels affect our view of reality.

Table 3.1 Consciousness and pain theories

| Level of consciousness | Magical | Rational/ reductionist/ materialism | Postmodern/ constructivism | Integral |
|---|---|---|---|---|
| Description | Fanciful, no rigorous empirical examination, childlike wonder, pre-enlightenment. | Post-enlightenment, scientific method, predictability representing a singular reality determined by analysis of part; objectivity. Dichotomous, either/or answers. | Realities are constructed and varied, to include the scientific method as one. The role of the participant/ observer is critical in the construction. Paradoxical, both/and answers. | Relationship based; "everything is connected"; inclusive of prior levels, but not without ordering/ valuing. |
| Pain theory | Spirits, potions, humors, spells, retribution from the gods. | See specificity, intensity and pattern pain theories (page 57). | Dynamic systems theory, complexity and chaos theory; pain as distributed, self-organizing, representational and emergent. | The intention of a robust biopsychosocial model that includes individual, community, societal structures and environment in pain experiences. |

As with the field of consciousness, the history of pain theories is a subject as long as human history in our attempt to explain pain's existence and in seeking to ease it. Several modern theoretical frameworks have been proposed to explain the physiological basis of pain and are summarized below, although none of the theories completely accounts for all aspects of pain. In an effort to illustrate that history, I will offer a chronological list as a "glimpse" across that arc. As you read each item, consider where it fits in the arc on the table. Once you determine that, give it your best postmodern consideration: "Are there aspects that may be part of our most current theories or could reflect a lower or higher level of consciousness?" You might be surprised to see the sharp boundaries between theories as "rational" perspective begin to blur in an "integral" fabric of connection when adopted from that level of consciousness. Hopefully that's the case.

Some treatment pain theories have become part of our belief systems. Once a theory is a "belief," it becomes very difficult to challenge and question. Hopefully we can soften our grip on our beloved beliefs given that we now know pain thresholds vary from person to person and often *from culture to culture*. As our theories evolve, we also appreciate that not only is pain and suffering subjective, but so too are researchers holding onto their beliefs. It is therefore important to review the history of pain theories to understand that what we know (believe?) as truths can, have, and will change with research. And that's uncomfortable.

## Some history

- In traditional Chinese medicine (TCM), the term for pain appeared for the first time in the ancient medical text *Huang Di Nei Jing* more than 3000 years ago.[6] In this canon, "pain was believed to be a result of imbalance between *yin* and *yang*. Predominance of *yin* results in '*han*' (cold), causing damage to the '*xing*' (form of a substance) which is now known as tissue injury or damage, and leads to swelling, while predominance of *yang* results in '*re*' (hyperthermia or heat) which causes damage to the '*qi*', namely pneuma (previously referred to as '*chi*', the concept of energy circulating in the hypothetical 12 channels), and leads to pain" (p.343). Early nociceptive and inflammatory pain theory, perhaps? It is certainly describing a related systems view to include a complex network of flow of energy and information contrary to a simple local tissue damage description.

- In what is now India, the panca maya kosha model described from around the 6th century BCE in the *Taittiriya Upanishad* consists of five interwoven sheaths of human experience (body, breath, emotions, thinking, and spiritual) that when out of balance lead to suffering.[7] The early *Upanishads* (ancient yoga texts) viewed "humans' repeated drama of birth, life, and death to the yogin (one who practices yoga) as only pain (duhkha)" (p.174).[8] Also, Jainism's attitude is that mere physical existence is the source of suffering and painful limitation (p.203), and that "pain is transmitted by giving even the slightest pain to others is to be avoided and one should strive to be helpful at all times" (from the Jain *Yoga Drishti Samuccaya*, #150, p.206). Later, the *Bhagavad Gita*, 200 BCE, rightly identifies the instability of mind as the chief cause of suffering and that the root of the mental instability is desire (higher-order processing; default network dominance?).

- Buddhism's First Noble Truth: Life is suffering. Shared by Buddhism, Hinduism, and Jainism: "Because everything is impermanent and does not afford us lasting happiness, our life is, in the last analysis, shot through with sorrow and pain."[9] A bad tune from the orchestra that outputs pain tunes à la Butler and Moseley?[10]

- A lone example from the myriad of ancient and indigenous theories around the world: some Native American healers believed pain was all in one's head, literally, and they used pain pipes to "suck" the pain right out of a patient's head. Early editing of patient narratives about pain via a form of pain education?

- In the Western countries, the description of pain appeared for the first time in Homer's epics, *The Iliad* and *The Odyssey*, from around the 8th century BCE in ancient Greece. Homer (8th century BCE) described pain as "arrows shot by Gods." Aristotle (384–322 BCE) stated that pain was due to evil spirits and that the gods entered the body during injury.[11]

- The word "pain" itself derives from the Latin word "poena," which means "punishment or penalty." The Greeks named their goddess of revenge Poine, for inflicting pain upon mortals who angered the gods, and the Romans described the very spirit of punishment as "Poena." Many cultures and societies had developed their own theories regarding pain, including causations from deities, energy fields, the moon, and the stars. "Treatments" included attempted rituals, sacrifices, and other offerings to ward off the possibility of pain-related illness. See Moseley and Butler's chapter on metaphor for the significance in pain experiences.[12]

- Avicenna (980–1037), a renowned Muslim philosopher and physician, proposed for the first time that pain is an independent sensation that is dissociated from touch or temperature, in his work *Canon of Medicine and Poem of Medicine*.[13] The brain was not believed to have any direct influence and for years the liver or heart was thought to be the center for pain control, until the Renaissance (14th–17th centuries), when systematic autopsies were carried out by Andreas Vesalius, the founder of modern human anatomy.[14]

- Then, in the 17th century, the functions of the brain were further described by René Descartes and Thomas Willis. Descartes, a French writer and "Father of Modern Philosophy," provided a famous hypothetical drawing that showed the transmission of pain information via the peripheral nerves and the spinal cord to the ventricles of the brain and the pineal organ where the conscious perception of a painful stimulus was proposed to be produced. Thomas Willis, recognized as the discoverer of the "circle of Willis," was a pioneer of brain anatomy and in *Cerebri Anatome* (1664), he provided strong evidence supporting the roles of the brain in how pain is experienced (including the cerebral cortex), an ongoing theme today.[15]

Many important discoveries have since taken place that led to the following major theories that were proposed more recently. Note the rational, analytic process of reduction to the parts and their function in their effort to understand the whole. Attribution for what follows in the list to Physiopedia[16] (2018) and Chen (2011).

- Specificity theory (mid-1800s) attributed pain experience to specialized sense organs (nociceptors) that have thresholds at or near noxious levels, increasing activity with stronger noxious stimuli. These special peripheral afferent neurons have selective connections to particular spinal and brainstem projection neurons. The theory holds that specific pain receptors transmit signals to a "pain center" in the brain that produces the perception of pain. This theory considers pain as an independent sensation with specialized peripheral nociceptors, which respond to damage and send signals through nerve fibers to target specific areas in the brain. When these pain signals get to the pain centers, the individual then experiences pain. Match the parts to function and get a specific, predictable result.

- The intensity theory (later 1800s), which was first conceptualized in the 4th century BCE by Plato and revisited numerous times, suggests that peripheral sense organs are not differentiated into low- and high-threshold types. It proposes that afferent fibers transduce innocuous stimuli (for example, skin pressure) by generating a certain level of activity, whereas noxious stimuli are signaled by a greater level of discharge. It was concluded that there must be some form of summation that occurs for the subthreshold stimuli to become painful. Weak activation indicates innocuous stimuli; strong activation indicates painful (noxious) events. A linear relationship that adds up to a predictable result.

- Strong's theory (1895), not always included in historical lists, states that pain was an experience based on both the noxious stimulus and the psychic reaction or displeasure provoked by the sensation. Early suggestions of complexities ahead.

- The pattern theory (1920s) proposes that sense organs have a wide range of responses. Individual afferent neurons respond differently to stimuli of varied intensity. A composite pattern of the mode and location of activity is generated from a particular body region. Central projection neurons monitor and code the nature and place of stimulation by the pattern.

Non-painful or painful experiences are the result of differences in the patterns sent through the nervous system. Some early systems suggestions and more complex in its orientation and relationships.

- The Fourth Theory of Pain (by Hardy, Wolff, and Goodell, in the 1940s) stated that pain was composed of two parts: the perception of pain and the reaction one has toward it. The reaction was described as a complex physiopsychological process involving cognition, past experiences, culture, and various psychological factors that influence pain perception. See Strong (above) 50 years earlier. Losing our straight lines and control of the rational level of consciousness.

- According to Melzack and Wall's gate control theory (1965), pain stimulation is carried by small, slow fibers that enter the dorsal horn of the spinal cord; then T-cells transmit the impulses from the spinal cord up to the brain. These fibers can either inhibit the communication of stimulation or allow stimulation to be communicated into the central nervous system. For instance, large fibers can prohibit the impulses from the small fibers from ever communicating with the brain. In this way, the large fibers act as a "gate" that can open or close the system to pain stimulation. The gate can also at times be overwhelmed by a large number of small activated fibers and not be able to gate/block the pain. This theory was a precursor to an avalanche of complex findings in the late 20th century and early 21st century. Even by 1983, when I had the honor of attending a seminar by Ronald Melzack, I recall him describing how the theory had already been overwhelmed by new discoveries.

- The neuromatrix model of pain (1990–2013) was an attempt by Melzack to include all the theories and concepts of pain found in current research into a single model. The model attempts to illustrate the many complex relationships involved in pain perception, housed within the larger medical model of a biopsychosocial perspective first described by Engel in 1977.[17]

- Today, we observe that the clear, reductive lines between the multiple disciplines have blurred as the scientific method continues to reveal with greater clarity the complexity of living systems and behavior. Long laundry lists of predisposing, precipitating, and perpetuating factors for pain have been detailed, to include chronic low back pain alone now having over 200 prognostic factors[18] and ongoing confusion over the purpose and use of clinical prediction rules by clinicians.[19] The language of complexity and systems theory is now part of the most current pain science to include emergence, emergent properties, self-organizing, distributed networks, extended and embodied cognition, etc. All of these interwoven relationships hearken back to the *Taittiriya Upanishad*'s teaching on koshas noted earlier that described the complex contributors to illness and suffering. Which is magical and which postmodern/integral?

Even just this short summary leaves us with multiple *states* of both *theories* and *management practices*. It seems chronic pain ought to be viewed as the product of multiple dynamic factors that develop synergistically in combination with certain genetic, biomedical, psychological, behavioral, and environmental vulnerabilities. Unfortunately, it is safe to summarize that the dominant description of pain and management strategies early in the 21st century, and still most prevalent today, is incorrectly that pain is the result of a simple signaling system. Switched on—pain is experienced. Tissue damage healed, repaired, medicated, manipulated, or cut out, switch is off—and no pain. How can this be in light of the arc just described? This question and many others make up our present-day dilemma reviewed below.

## What challenges do we face today?

The various challenges rehabilitation professionals face in supporting people in pain can be understood in the context of Table 3.1. Ideally all of our theories and praxis would be situated in the column to the far right. Obviously, neither theories nor praxis are, so a brief review of some of the shortfalls will help orient us for our task at hand of creating a best possible future in pain care rehabilitation.

### *Healthcare providers and yoga professionals stuck in the parts/fixing model*

Despite the pain science suggesting otherwise, most providers still teach and practice from a bad parts/fix-it model. So, too, do most complementary and alternative medicine (CAM) providers including yoga professionals, even though it is the antithesis of an integral, non-dual philosophy. Name a part or pathology, and there's a "Yoga for…" DVD or workshop. We mirror the worldview that we live in where part of the dominant focus is on "fixing" the problem, "killing" the pain, or teaching people to "live with it." There's an ongoing reinforcement of mechanistic dualistic views of pain, pain management, and people in pain within both systems that is demonstrated in the segregation of medical, psychological, and spiritual (dare we use the word in rehabilitation?) perspectives. All of us trying to put Humpty together again and yet our institutions and practice settings result in pain management services awkwardly being "interdisciplinary"[20] and not reimbursed by insurers. Interdisciplinary is not synonymous with integral because it represents where each "silo" of a discipline contributes their respective care from their viewpoint. This often results in "awkward" input for their consumer, who is trying to understand and adhere to conflicting strategies, as well as billing nightmares, turf battles between disciplines, and no overarching guidance for resolving these challenges. Ironically, even some of those exposed to pain science that includes complexity and emergent aspects of pain slip into a mechanistic model, becoming "brain-centric," lacking an inclusive, integral practice approach to exercise and movement such as Malfliet et al.[21] This challenge bears some description and its own subsection.

### Providers already exposed to current pain science teaching and treating from a linear, rationalism perspective

Just being exposed to information and data doesn't shift a person with a rationalism consciousness to a postmodern or integral capacity. As a result, the acquisition of more "stuff," "pain theory de jour," which is a brain-centric, materialist emphasis with some additional tacked-on systems (immune, endocrine, circulatory, etc.), leaves the clinicians scrambling to find "tools" to singularly address each of those "parts" of a mechanistic understanding. Malfliet et al.[22] utilize operant conditioning models of instructing the patient that their pain isn't accurate and not to stop exercising. Well, that's a small, inaccurately applied "part" of pain education that produces a cold, stark treatment process that fails to address the "person" in front of them with all of the related and confounding complexities. A "simple" example is anyone with an adverse childhood experience of abuse or trauma. An unskilled, simplistic operant approach is just more trauma. What is required is transformational learning[23] where first the provider and then those they teach are given a safe environment to explore the assumptions underlying their current understanding and beliefs, then, in continued safety, are offered controlled opportunities to not just get facts, but have embodied experiences that they can safely attend to, reflect, and then edit both their narrative and movement/behavioral options in the future that yield practical application in their lives matching their goals and priorities. The result is a shift in the operating model in which the individual not only knows "new stuff," but also perceives and behaves differently as a result. In other words, shifts to the right in Table 3.1. When we undergo this type of process, we change our views of pain, our views of people in pain, and, subsequently, our pain management strategies. Again, yoga fits nicely into a part of the process, as it is a transformational learning system. The full practice of yoga offers skills and practices to consider our views, as well as integrate them into daily life as they change, and will be described further in the chapters that follow.

## *Omission of current pain science within pre-licensure rehabilitation curriculum and pre-credentialing, foundational yoga professional training*

The reasons for this large gap between existing emerging science and inclusion in either group's trainings are complex and many. Time constraints, teaching to the tests, faculty bias, research funding priorities, disciplinary turf battles are but a few. Elgelid[24] provides a deeper examination of the systems effects limiting innovation in rehabilitation academia, but we (the contributing authors) also already see it occurring in yoga trainings and professional associations as well.

## *Impact of national policy and funding for pain management and opioid addiction*

Levels of consciousness aren't limited to individual humans; organizations, institutions, and governments are described as having them too.[25] We see this play out in the way systems at those levels have medicalized pain management. That is, simplifying pain to a "thing" that is treated from a medical model limits our understanding and the possibilities for more effectively managing this complex phenomenon. An expanded, integral perspective would seek to incorporate the structures, policies, and societal norms that contribute to the pain crisis. Such things as: access to healthcare; food quality and nutrition; environmental controls; labor practices; pharmaceutical marketing, development, and costs; development and funding for community resources and self-management that often go unfunded or undeveloped by the larger systems' consciousness. A robust integral perspective would highlight and fund aspects of pain management that can be addressed in public health arenas that include prevention and addressing known "conditions of life" that increase chronic pain risks; these services don't require higher-paid healthcare services downstream and can be delivered in a more timely fashion rather than missing the critical early windows of intervention. As an example, in the US, the highest-level health policy agency (Agency for Healthcare Research and Quality) has just conducted a review intended to inform policy makers and set future funding. The review limited itself to single-intervention randomized controlled trials (RCTs) to address this complex problem. Note where that places this critical process in Table 3.1: directly in the center of the rational level of understanding: one thing to fix another thing. This process demonstrates four things:

- wrong methods
- wrong questions

- a conclusion that fails to yield insight or direction in authorizing an integrative response to the crisis

- a level of consciousness searching for a "silver bullet" single solution to a systems-generated catastrophe of unimaginable complexity.

Can you sense the harm such a lower level of consciousness by a governmental agency exacts on the very people it is charged with protecting?

### *The defending of turf between disciplines, cultural variances, and good old-fashioned hubris*

The human tendency to rigorously defend a belief extends all the way into the postmodern level (where they defend the "rightness" of multiple/plural perspectives as superior to the singular perspectives of earlier levels). Only at the integral level are people able to acknowledge and value plurality, *but* not in some wishy-washy, postmodern, "they are all equally valuable" frame. At the integral level values and priorities are adopted and applied when making decisions and setting policy and practice guidelines. The challenge is that very few of us are yet at this level of consciousness, and those who do reach it often move back and forth between levels (for example, "I'm good with emergence of pain, but don't make me get rid of my spine model with the red herniated disc wall"). As mentioned earlier, this includes our tendency to discount or exclude cultural perspectives that would have been relegated to the magical level 30 years ago. For instance, the early pioneers that began inquiring into meditation practices were often shunned, or discounted at best, for wasting their time and demeaning their respective professions. In hindsight, we can now appreciate that without their efforts, our neuroscience today would be far less developed and this book certainly wouldn't be going to press. The ancient Greeks warned of hubris (inflated, blinding pride). Can we personally and professionally set aside any hubris to both preserve and explore those pain theories and management practices that fall outside our habitual view? Adopting such plurality and diversity may be our biggest challenge and it is very much worth surrendering our hubris to achieve such freedom of sustaining metaperspectives.

### Does having plural states and theories limit us or free us?

What's worth keeping as we cross the threshold of moving between levels of consciousness and continuing to rigorously evolve our theories and practices? The challenges above point to what needs to be threshed out as chaff, if we can extend the "threshold" metaphor. What then is the kernel we want to find and cultivate? The short answer is: we don't know for sure; but it is tied to our personal embodied practice. The longer answer follows below.

It is worth repeating that by the definitions in Table 3.1, moving from a purely rationalist perspective to a postmodern and even integral view does not discount or eliminate the rational, but it does require a flexibility of perspective to include the concept of emergence that is not easy to attain.[26] Readers seeking a deeper inquiry into a science-based integral view of life should see Capra and Luisi.[27] One shouldn't then be surprised to see there is a connection between our collective and individual evolution of consciousness and the known creativity traits that facilitate our ability to hold multiple states and theories with their respective limitations and strengths. Frank Barron[28] in his seminal creativity research described traits creative individuals tend to exhibit:

- an independence of judgment rather than conformity

- a tolerance for ambiguity rather than a need for certainty

- a preference for complex thinking rather than polarized, simplistic, oppositional thinking

- androgynous behaviors with clarity on gender attributes and roles rather than a masculine preference

- a preference for complexity of outlook and a tolerance for asymmetry rather than symmetric, constrained possibilities.

What skills are required to cultivate these traits? The good news is that by continuing to read the rest of this book and then developing a broader, personal yoga practice you will cultivate those traits as sound developmental steps toward that goal.[29] And a personal practice is key to disrupting and evolving larger systems to include our professions and the societies where we practice.[30]

Given that perspective, it would seem that accepting plural states and theories would free us to create as we continue our practice development. The complexity of the pain and of the associated opioid crisis is certainly going to require creativity. There is nothing in human history to look back at to solve these situations. Our ability to generate new possibilities will be dependent on us being aware of what level of consciousness we are operating on along the way. Recognizing that we move between levels, we need to be patient with others and ourselves when we slip back into turf protection or old treatment/teaching patterns. Underscoring how challenging this new level of integral consciousness is, Moseley and Butler[31] go into significant detail about how difficult it is to just grasp the concept of emergence to both understand and teach in pain science education. Emergence is a single principle out of the many required in an integral view. This might be a good time to flip back to Table 3.1, pull out some paper, and reflect/journal to yourself where you find yourself on the table right now. During your last treatment session or teaching assignment? Where you spend most of your day? Where you would like to be a majority of the time?

Seriously, do it. If you don't know where you are, how are you ever going to get to where you want to be? Just like motor control, no? If the patient isn't sure where they are in space and can't accurately perceive changes in position across time, how can they learn a new movement strategy and perform it with skill?

For those who are new to this consciousness-levels discussion, it may be beneficial to use an example to reinforce the concept. Piaget's description of conservation of volume in the development of logical thinking from pre-operational to concrete operational is often used. This takes place between ages 7 and 11 where the younger child initially can't understand that if you pour a fixed amount of water in a tall, narrow glass and then into a short, squat glass, the volume remains the same (is conserved).[32] What is germane to our discussion, too, is that once the child moves into concrete operational thinking, they vehemently deny they ever couldn't understand it, even if shown videos of themselves claiming volume differences earlier. That implausibility is often seen in this arc of consciousness too, from the very rational lawyer donning the lucky golf shirt to the frustration of the postmodernist that the editor can only consider definitive black or white conclusions. My point being, we need to be patient with ourselves and each other as we move through time, evolving at different times and levels.

This need for patience is no more evident than when what is old brings forward the new and the new imagines it is new only to discover it is describing the old (e.g. try overlaying Melzack's neuromatrix model on the yoga indriyas concept from the Kashmiri Shaivism period after 850 CE).[33] Borrowing from Walsh's wisdom definition[34] can serve us well as we move across this threshold of pluralities from the old rational level. Wisdom is being researched and yoga is part of that long and evolving tradition. In his recent review of the literature, Walsh defines wisdom as, "deep accurate insight and understanding of oneself and the central existential issues of life, plus skillful benevolent responsiveness" (p.282). As we explore and observe our own and our collective experiences within our respective rehabilitation professions, can we work together in addressing the central existential issue of pain and suffering without creating more pain and suffering? This question finally brings us back to my use of (sic) in the title after "management." Management is a residual concept from the mechanistic, industrial era of parts. When applied to pain, it suggests control by someone and, in reality, unfortunately often ends in some form, at least from the consumer's perspective, of "learn to live with it." Adopting an integral perspective will include our reconciliation of the power imbalance of the "who" is the primary determinant and the process as an embodied, *skillful*, and evolving *benevolent responsiveness* to life circumstance.

There will be many new possible ways of serving our patients if we adopt systems and emergent theory, as well as applied creativity in rehabilitation, and the art and science of therapeutic relationship from the biopsychosocial model. We conclude this chapter by describing some of those "possibles."[35]

## What does this plurality portend for the future and what is the value of including yoga in that future?

This is where I set you up to be wildly excited about reading the remaining authors' chapters. We have appreciated the history of pain care and acknowledged the many challenges that exist in this new era, as well as where we are in terms of our own theories, perspective, and practice. Here I want to share an assistive framework as we step into the new terrain of integral pain study and practice. Navigating new theories and sustaining an integral perspective isn't easy even for the most seasoned of us. So, hang onto the following as hard or as long as you need to. There's no hurry to let it go and hopefully it will relieve future suffering for yourself (Patanjali Yoga Sutra 2.16)![36]

How do we bring yoga into pain rehabilitation? You are fortunate because the authors are sharing what they have learned so far. How will it look in the future? This is where we might need an assistive device of sorts because this integral level embraces uncertainty and, by definition, can't glimpse the emergent process ahead. And that's OK, again.

What I have found helpful is to maintain a couple of simple aphorisms (called sutras in yoga) about this integral level and participating in creative action specifically. For those who want to dive deeper, see Stuart A. Kauffman's work.[37] Dr. Kauffman is an MD, theoretical biologist, complex systems researcher, and former MacArthur "Genius" Fellow when he was serving as Professor of Biochemistry and Biophysics at the University of Pennsylvania. These aphorisms based on his text are for the rest of us.

As an integral therapist creating a future pain science and practice, it helps to remember the following.

- *The* solution doesn't exist and can't because the future isn't prestatable/predictable.

- The emergence of new possibles from complex systems is not prestatable, and these possibles enable but do not cause or predict the next possibles.

- The difference between Kauffman's causal versus enable is part of wisdom when describing living phenomena like human behavior and pain experience. Causal is the linear, predictable/prestatable quest of the rational consciousness, while in an integral, emergent worldview, new conditions (possibles) enable the emergence of new actuals but do not in fact cause them.

- Working together with patients to enable new possibles versus "doing to" is much less violent (yoga ahimsa/non-violence).

- Our individual practice being open to new possibles and recognizing new actuals is necessary in our personal and collective arc of conscious evolution and sound wisdom development.[38]

- Just as economies by their complexity are not prestatable, so too with healthcare and pain support practices, nevertheless we stay engaged and participate.

- Staying only in our silo of specialization in a complex era guarantees both *superficial* and *inaccurate insights* and sets us up for *unskillful* and *non-benevolent responses*. Not wise.

- "I don't know" and "Both/And or Yes, and…" are powerful answers at the integral level, followed by "Let's see what we can discover though…" as we all learn how to be with pain and suffering.

Yoga, as a wisdom tradition that plumbs the deepest inquiries into complex human experience, is a natural fit for this near era. Yoga, of course, is far more than the stereotypical acrobatics of the popular commodification of yoga. It too is continuing to evolve and is not some shell of a fixed, past practice. The discoveries you will make ahead while reading this book will foster many new possibles for you in understanding not just pain and suffering, but yourself as well. Remember, the first step in wisdom is *of oneself*. Hopefully, with this broader integral view, you can now at least glimpse a new horizon of possibles for all of us. Your continuing engagement and participation in this book will generate new possibles that will enable Kauffman's better future *actuals* to ease pain and suffering.

## Conclusion

One final frame of perspective, from 1977, lest we think this call to an integral level is new stuff:

> The proposed biopsychosocial model provides a blueprint for research, a framework for teaching, and a design for action in the real world of healthcare. Whether it is useful or not remains to be seen… In a free society, outcome (sic) will depend upon those who have the courage to try new paths and the *wisdom* to provide the necessary support.[39] (emphasis mine)

There's never been a more exciting time to be in rehabilitation. The new possibilities that yoga enables are incredible as you will soon learn. The next chapters are on the history of yoga therapy, the pain science that interfaces well with yoga, and what needs to be explored further. If we go with a sense of appreciating that these chapters are just a snapshot in the unfolding of our understanding on a larger scale, we can effectively take our place with wisdom in the ongoing arc of emergence of pain science and the care for those experiencing pain. Have fun!

*Chapter 4*

# Yoga and Yoga Therapy

Neil Pearson, Shelly Prosko, Marlysa Sullivan

## What is yoga?

Yoga is an ever-evolving practical philosophy intended to assist the individual in uncovering the causes of suffering and its alleviation. This wisdom tradition includes a philosophical perspective and worldview, as well as a systematic methodology of practices. An exploration of the context and history from which yoga developed including the texts that contain essential teachings, philosophies and practices is vital to our understanding of yoga.

These foundational texts point to the many ways yoga can be understood as both a state of "unity," "equanimity" or "liberation from suffering" and a set of practices leading toward that state.[1]

Table 4.1 offers some definitions from core texts. The first definition is from the *Katha Upanishad*, which is suggested to have been composed around the 3rd century BCE.[2] Next, the definitions from the *Mahabharata*, and the *Bhagavad Gita* contained therein, are presented in Table 4.1. These texts are said to have been finished between the 1st and 3rd century CE.[3] Lastly, the definition from the *Patanjali Yoga Sutras*, which is thought to have been solidified around the 4th century CE, will be provided.[4] At times, we have included the same verse from different translations of the texts. This is meant to illuminate the broad and wide-ranging meaning of yoga that will be utilized throughout this chapter and book.

These various definitions and translations demonstrate the nuanced and numerous ways yoga can be defined and understood. It is important to recognize that yoga is not a static nor fixed ideology, philosophy or practice. Rather it is a multifaceted and experiential process through which the individual realizes states such as: stillness; unity; equanimity; evenness of mind; unbinding or separation from pain or suffering; emergence of compassion; breaking free from negative states such as delusion or anger; cessation of the turnings of thought; disentangling from the misidentification with thought to one's true nature; the capacity to act skillfully in the face of life's occurrences.

Throughout all of these possible understandings is a common thread. At its foundation, yoga is a philosophy and practice meant to assist the practitioner in the alleviation, or liberation, from suffering. Yoga also describes a systematic methodology of practices for this attainment. Through this practice, the individual can realize a state of underlying connection or unity from which equanimity and qualities such as compassion emerge.

Table 4.1 Definitions of yoga

| *Katha Upanishad* | 3.11: "They say yoga is this complete stillness in which one enters the unitive state, never to become separate again, if one is not established in this state, the sense of unity will come and go."[5] |
|---|---|
| *Bhagavad Gita* | 2.48: "Yoga is said to be equanimity"[6] or "evenness of mind is yoga."[7]<br><br>2.50: "Yoga is Skill in Action."[8]<br><br>6.23: "Know that which is called yoga to be separation (viyoga) from contact (samyoga) with suffering…"[9]<br><br>"Let this dissolution of union with pain* be known as yoga; this yoga is to be practiced with determination and with an undismayed mind."[10]<br><br>"Since he knows that discipline** means unbinding the bonds of suffering, he should practice discipline resolutely, without despair dulling his reason."[11] |
| *Mahabharata* | "…the arguments of yoga are based on evidence…enjoin purity, compassion and observances…through yoga one can rid oneself of passion, delusion, affection, desire, and anger, and attain release; Yoga confers the power to break these bonds."[12] |
| *Patanjali Yoga Sutras* | 1.2–4: "Yoga is the cessation of the turnings of thought. When thought ceases, the spirit stands in its true identity as observer to the world. Otherwise, the observer identifies with the turnings of thought."[13] |

*The word "duhkha" is translated as "pain" in this version—we will offer more explanation on this term below.

** The word "yoga" is translated as "discipline" in this version.

## Understanding suffering

If yoga assists the individual in the alleviation of suffering—what is meant by suffering?

The word "duhkha" is used to refer to suffering in many of these texts. Some definitions of its meaning are:

- distress; dissatisfactoriness[14]

- dissatisfaction; uncomfortable, unpleasant, difficulty, pain, sorrow, suffering[15]

- suffering; pain.[16]

Another definition was offered during a lecture by a teacher who broke down the components of the word into its parts. She described the meaning as being akin to a wheel that was misplaced, imbalanced or off its axle. Duhkha can be understood as the discomfort or suffering that arises when things are not in alignment or are in a state of disharmony.

## Path of yoga: dharma and right action

If duhkha is about the discomfort or suffering of disharmony—how does one understand harmony and the alleviation of suffering?

The word "dharma" helps us to understand this concept of harmony. Dharma is another complex and nuanced term that can be understood as that which supports and sustains the individual and the environment around them.[17] Dharma includes a way of living that benefits oneself and the environment around them such that "skillful action" (one of the aforementioned definitions of yoga itself) can be undertaken. This skillful action in alignment with dharma supports the person in the alleviation of duhkha (suffering, disharmony).

Moreover, a definition of yoga is that of unity and connection through which states such as equanimity arise. This equanimity and connection to oneself and the environment can help provide the individual with the insight needed to discriminate between those actions that would be in alignment with dharma (for the betterment of the person and the environment) from those which would perpetuate duhkha (disharmony or suffering). As such, dharma provides an overarching framework from which to situate the application of the practices and philosophies of yoga for the promotion of right action in life leading to the mitigation of suffering.

The exploration of dharma includes an examination of the ways in which one's thoughts, emotions and behaviors support harmony with oneself and the environment around them. This exploration also helps to uncover the relationships to the body, mind and environment that lead to duhkha—a misalignment, disharmony or suffering.

Dharma helps the person determine the ways of relating and interacting with the body, mind and environment to foster cohesion and states such as equanimity. Therefore, this concept is at the heart of understanding yoga as a practical philosophy informing an approach to life. Ultimately, the person learns to cultivate the relationships with oneself, others and the environment in support of both oneself and the greater good.

As the adage says, there are many paths to the top of the mountain—there are also many paths and practices of yoga. Each of these can be utilized to foster the right and skillful action for the betterment and sustenance of oneself and the environment around them for the alleviation of suffering. These paths and practices will be described briefly in this chapter and in more detail throughout the book, however a prime example is the yamas and niyamas (detailed below). These ethical virtues can be utilized by the person to inquire into the right action in alignment with dharma to support the individual and those around them and towards the alleviation of suffering. Each practice and path of yoga holds this idea of supporting the person in finding a way of interacting with life such that suffering is alleviated and qualities such as equanimity, unity and connection are recognized and emerge.

In this way, yoga is understood as a practical application of philosophy for life. It is not simply something to be contemplated in a vacuum of experience. Yoga is fulfilled through right action in alignment with dharma. When the person understands this, their suffering is alleviated and unity or equanimity realized.

## Why does suffering occur?

Samkhya is a philosophical foundation that informs the yoga tradition and whose teachings are found within the *Bhagavad Gita*, *Mahabharata* and the *Patanjali Yoga Sutras*.[18] Samkhya describes two aspects of our experience. One aspect is that which is constantly changing and includes the ever-changing fluctuations of the body, mind and environment. This is termed "prakriti" and includes:

- the body with its ever-changing experiences such as age, bodily systems with their constant movement, illness, pain or disability

- the mind with the fluctuations and storehouse of thoughts, emotions, beliefs and habits

- the environment from which arises constant change in life occurrences and situations.

The ever-changing prakriti is differentiated from the unchanging aspect of our experience.

Purusha is defined as the observer to the fluctuations of the body, mind and environment. This unchanging observer experiences and perceives all of what arises in the body, mind and environment—yet remains separate from them.

In Samkhya and in yoga suffering, disharmony and misalignment arise when we misidentify as the fluctuations of the body, mind and environment—with prakriti. When we remember that we are experiencing prakriti—but are not these changeable aspects of experience—suffering can be alleviated. The reorientation of identity with the unchanging aspect of purusha supports the recognition of the unwavering equanimity, connection and unity within.[19]

Prakriti is broken down into three main constituents from which the myriad and changeable components of the body, mind and environment arise. These are termed the gunas. Everything of prakriti (body, mind and environment) is said to be made up of these gunas in different proportions.

The gunas are defined as follows.[20]

- **Raja guna**: Constituent of activation from which emerges a spectrum of mobilization, creativity to agitation, anxiety or anger.

- **Tama guna**: Constituent of solidity from which emerges a spectrum of form, mass to inertia, dullness, obscuration.

- **Sattva guna**: Constituent of clarity from which emerges illumination, lightness. While most of sattva is given positive qualities, one can become "addicted" to these qualities of joy in unhealthy forms of detachment.

## What is yoga therapy?

A yoga professional or healthcare provider can use yoga (practices and philosophy) within a therapeutic context. This may be described as therapeutic yoga or yoga therapy. However, the International Association of Yoga Therapists,[21] founded in 1989, has now developed a formal definition of yoga therapy along with standards of practice and accredited yoga therapy programs to train people to use yoga therapeutically. The term *yoga therapy* is defined by the International Association of Yoga Therapists: "Yoga therapy is the process of empowering individuals to progress toward improved health and wellbeing through the application of the teachings and practices of Yoga."[22]

For a more in-depth understanding of the definition, Taylor provides a perspective where he thoroughly breaks down this definition, emphasizing the operative words of *process, empowering, progress towards* and *application*.[23] In summary, yoga therapy does not consist of a prescriptive "fix-it" approach or protocol to helping people in pain. It is a *process* that promotes awareness and curiosity in the individual, so they can be open to changing beliefs and behaviors that would be better aligned with their values, goals and, as discussed above, their dharma, in order to alleviate suffering. Indeed, yoga therapy provides a process that is *empowering* for people in pain. The yoga therapist is not the "healer," rather, we are the facilitators of recovery and one's own internal processes that help the person in pain *progress towards* improved health and wellbeing, or eudaimonia, as Sullivan discusses in Chapter 15. Yoga therapists discern how to use yoga practices and philosophy appropriately, from the many paths and models described below, to provide a safe space for people in pain so that they can fully embody their experiences, create change and transform their pain so they can live with more ease and resilience and experience a steadfast joy. Yoga therapy is a transformational approach and not a symptom management approach like our current medical model, as Lee discusses in Chapter 11.

## Paths of yoga

There is more than one path or style of yoga. The *Upanishads*, ancient Sanskrit texts that discuss central concepts and philosophies of Hinduism, include reference to numerous styles of yoga, each intended to assist the yoga aspirant in liberation, discovering the meaning of atman (soul) and decreasing suffering. Here we offer descriptions of seven styles of yoga: Jnana, Bhakti, Karma, Hatha, Raja, Kriya and Tantra.

### *Jnana yoga*

Jnana in Sanskrit means knowledge, and Jnana yoga is both the path to self-realization through knowledge and the result of self-realization. This is different than intellect and deductive knowledge. Through the processes of listening, contemplating and meditating, through inquiry and curiosity, the mind is used to seek the truth beyond the mind. This is the process of Jnana yoga. When truth is realized, Jnana is the result.

Jnana requires that one believes nothing, at least in the realm of concepts, dogma and ideas. Facts are not disregarded, but belief is questioned. Certainty is not as important as curiosity and inquiry. Belief in nothing, and emptying the mind of preconceived and unexplored concepts, is extremely difficult. It is also not in alignment with the training most health professionals receive. We are expected to know, with certainty.

Jnana yoga is stated to involve intuitive flashes more than deductive and linear thinking. In this way it is similar to artistic creations, music and some aspects of scientific discovery. Each defies logic. The individual suddenly saw something as yet unseen or created something as yet unconsidered. For most, the intuition came after long periods of obsession with a certain question or problem. For the Jnana yogi, this may have been "What is my purpose in the world?" and for the scientist this might someday be "How can we reconnect a severed spinal cord?"

The Jnana yoga practitioner must know and feel in his or her heart that intellectual thought is limited. It can take time and experiences to realize that deep understanding and meaningful answers are not always attained through thought and discussion alone. Our lives, and especially pain, are much more complex and difficult to predict than what is dictated by logic. We know this. The Jnana yogi chooses to dive completely into this understanding.

Within Jnana yoga there are four pillars. A deep desire to decrease suffering, discernment, detachment and six virtues are these pillars. Within the pillars of virtue are the ability to remain calm, control over reactions to external stimuli, abandonment of anything not related to one's dharma, perseverance through suffering, faith in one's path and complete concentration/focus.

## Bhakti yoga

Bhakti in Sanskrit means to serve, adore, love and be devoted. Like other styles, Bhakti yoga is both the path and the result of the path. The Bhakti aspirant finds liberation through love, and so becomes love itself.

The Bhakti yogi is devoted to the divine in whatever form chosen. It is the devotion that is essential. Without devotion one cannot practice Bhakti yoga. The devotion can be to an individual, to one's god, to a purpose in life or to a cause. Many read of Bhakti festivals, which include opportunities to practice devotion in many forms, often including chanting and music.

The practices of Bhakti include compassion, japa (meditation on a mantra or repetition of a divine name), chanting, appreciation of wonder, inspiration, stillness and acknowledging sense of purpose. When devotion is strong enough, these practices take us past belief and past suffering. Some describe Bhakti as the expression of joy beyond words.

The practice of Bhakti also involves intense concentration. All one's energy is focused towards or drawn towards one direction. The intention is to take one away from identification with the body-mind, intellect and ego. Even though each of these is admired in modern times and useful in gaining knowledge, each can limit us in our path to less suffering.

## Karma yoga

Karma is the yoga of action, in which one acts without expecting a reward. The practice of Karma yoga is giving.

Karma is often thought to be about cause and effect. Yet it can be understood as almost the opposite. One acts not because of what one would gain or what would not be lost because of the action. Rather, one acts because it is right action, in service of others. Similar to Bhakti yoga, devotion is an aspect of Karma yoga— the devotion to giving to others, the world and the universe.

The actions of the Karma yoga practitioner are unselfish. They provide opportunities to increase awareness of our attachment to the "fruits" of our actions. These acts quiet and purify the mind. By being selfless, ego is lost, suffering decreases and the practitioner discovers the meaning of atman.

## Hatha yoga

In Sanskrit, ha means sun and tha means moon. Hatha is harmony between sun and moon aspects of one's being; between body and mind. The balance of these two is the basic aim of Hatha yoga.

Hatha yoga can be considered as the first part of Raja yoga. Without practicing Hatha yoga, Raja becomes very difficult for most. The practices of Hatha yoga include asana, pranayama, mudras and bandhas and techniques aimed at cleansing the body (shatkarmas). The mantras and mudras are both intended to induce deeper physiological, mental and psychic changes than would occur with the asana and pranayama alone.

The intention of Hatha yoga performed with these components is to bring about health and prepare the yoga practitioner for Raja or other styles of yoga. Through its practices, Hatha yoga is said to impact resistance to infection, absence of disease, mental and physical endurance, flexibility of body and mind, mental peace and perfect coordination and condition of internal organs, muscle and nerves in the body and their control by the brain and spinal nerves. The discipline of Hatha yoga allows the individual to not be hampered by the body during spiritual practices.

### Raja yoga

Raja yoga is the royal path. It is at times called classic yoga, and at other times Patanjali's yoga. This is the path of introspection. One attempts to explore different realms of the mind—subconscious, conscious, unconscious and beyond—through the eight limbs of Raja yoga. With disciplined practice one becomes increasingly aware of and in touch with the many and varied aspects of consciousness and being.

The eight limbs of Raja yoga are yamas, niyamas, asana, pranayama, pratyahara, dharana, dhyana and samadhi, as described below with examples of how they are relevant to pain care:

*Yamas*—five ethical considerations to guide interactions with others and the world.

- **Non-violence—kindness (ahimsa):** Both the person in pain and the therapist can practice kindness and compassion towards self and not be self-critical or harming in the words or tone used towards self when mistakes are made or actions performed of which we are not proud. In Chapter 1, Belton outlines the importance of kindness and compassion towards herself and others, and to love and be loved, on her journey to transforming her pain experience. Prosko talks about the components of compassion and kindness and the benefits in pain care at length in Chapter 14.

- **Truthfulness—to self and others, in actions and thoughts (satya):** As therapists, we can guide the patient to explore their view of reality and truth of the situation or moment. For example, perhaps the person is resisting the fact that they are in pain. If they deny and ignore the pain and are not honest or truthful with themselves that "this does indeed hurt," that can impact the process of changing the pain. It is important that the therapist finds ways to guide people to explore and discover their own truth and not place our own beliefs onto people.

- **Not stealing—material things, ideas or time from others (asteya)**: As therapists in the medical model, it is often our own discomfort in sitting with the person in pain's story and pain experience that can get in the way of the transformational process. Acknowledging and allowing the person in pain to have their experience, and providing them with the space by simply listening without trying to jump to "fix," can be seen as asteya, or not "robbing" or "stealing" the experience from the person.

- **Moderation—chastity and fidelity; some practice celibacy (brahmacharya)**: This also is often interpreted as not squandering our energy or making the best use of our energy and ourselves. Moderation can be seen as the "middle path" where there is a balance between "not too much" and "not too little." An example is using just the right amount of effort when recovering movement: excessive effort can create more resistance and rigidity, but too little effort may not produce the movement or stability required for the task. As the therapist, we need to ensure we empower patients to take an active approach in their pain care without leaving them unsupported and overwhelmed, but we need to give an appropriate amount of support without coddling or enabling the patient into a passive role. This can also apply to the home programs or homework we give people. Moderation is key.

- **Not coveting—non-attachment to or non-hoarding of ideas, beliefs or things and knowing we have enough and are enough (aparigraha)**: As therapists, it is important we stay open to challenging our own ideas and concepts about pain and our understanding of the human, so we stay open to expanding our options available to improve our capacity to help people in pain. We may not always know why practices help when they help, so it would be arrogant to continue to attach to old beliefs as new information is available. The person in pain can also practice not comparing themselves to a time where they thought they were "better" or "more productive" or contributing more to society. Coveting these ideas feeds into beliefs of being broken, not being whole or complete or "enough," and prevents progress on the path to change.

*Niyamas*—five considerations for how we view and treat our self.

- **Austerity and cleanliness—simplifying and uncluttering/cleaning body and mind (saucha)**: Impurity of thought, body or actions can impact any person's journey towards health and wellbeing, including people in pain and those who work with them. Making choices in line with our values and dharma, instead of allowing extraneous and unhelpful thoughts or behaviors to clutter our space, can also help the process. Additionally, the therapist can learn to cultivate purity of awareness and gain insight into how we can simplify helping the person in pain. We do not need to make things more complicated; this in fact may not serve the person we are trying to help. Pain and humans are complex; however, both simplicity and complexity can simultaneously exist.

- **Contentment—acceptance (santosha):** Not accepting the truth of reality can be a source of suffering. If we can compassionately guide people in pain to experience and understand this concept of the freedom behind accepting the moment as it is, they can then progress towards change and have a better chance at transforming the pain experience. As therapists, we can accept our role as facilitators and not "healers" or being the almighty savior. We can accept that we do not have all the answers and sometimes cannot help the person in pain in the way we desire or imagine.

- **Self-discipline—willpower and discipline (tapas):** Hard work and effort are also required in order to gain the skills of awareness and self-regulation and create change. People in pain also need to put in consistent and persistent, albeit adaptable, effort during this process. It is also the responsibility of the therapist to have the discipline and put in the hard work to become better at understanding pain and the human, better at being vulnerable and comfortable with uncertainty and more flexible to be willing to be open, learn, challenge our own beliefs and even change our language and way of thinking. We need discipline and effort to do this.

- **Self-study—learning from life experiences and exploring conditioned responses (svadhyaya):** It is valuable for the person in pain to practice the process of introspection and self-inquiry in order to gain insight into any habits or conditioned responses that contribute to their suffering. Consequently, this will support the insight and inner motivation required to create the desired change. A practical example of this would be to guide the patient to explore their thoughts, emotions and reactions during a movement that typically increases pain. The therapist can use a variety of techniques and motivational questioning to help the individual with this process.

- **Having faith—letting go, surrendering and trusting (ishvara pranidhana):** If we understand and accept that we do not have control over everything, we can ease into letting go and surrendering while trusting the process and the body's inherent wisdom to adapt and thrive. This niyama can highlight the person's spirituality. There is value in the therapist understanding the patient's underlying belief system. For example, being aware of whether or not the patient believes they are connected to and have support from a higher source can be useful information in order to guide our language and approach during the therapeutic interaction.

The yamas and niyamas can be integrated into pain care in numerous ways and are woven throughout the process. They are meant to be practiced and observed by both the person in pain and the therapist. They can inform the patient's goals, our language used and the specific practices, techniques or explorations we choose to offer the patient.

*Asana*—the physical postures of yoga vary between styles of yoga. In some styles, the postures are used primarily to keep the body healthy so that it can tolerate the sitting posture of meditation. In other styles, postures are held for long times (Yin) and, in others, movements are more flowing (Vinyasa). In Iyengar and Ashtanga yoga, body alignment during the asana practice is considered critical to attain the benefits of asana and yoga and to protect from injury. In Kundalini yoga, body alignment is of little concern, as the postures focus on prana rather than the anatomy and structure.

In yoga therapy, asana are used to restore ease of movement, flexibility, strength, balance and agility. Yet they are equally important for their psycho-emotional impact and effects on body awareness, body image and self-efficacy. In Chapter 7, Pearson further outlines the value of movement in pain care and how it can also be used as "pain education" or a way for the person in pain to better understand the pain experience.

*Pranayama*—the practices of pranayama involve consciously controlling breathing, with the goal of influencing prana (vital energy). In yoga therapy we use these same techniques to impact respiratory system physiology, but also to influence the autonomic nervous system, central nervous system, immune system and motor system. Prana is similar to Qi in traditional Chinese medicine. Good health requires free, unblocked movement of prana. In yoga philosophy, there are 72,000 pranic channels in the body. There is no known anatomical correlate of these found in the human body. Either they have not yet been identified or these channels may in fact not have a physical structure. Prana may not need specific structures through which to flow. In Chapter 8, Prosko further outlines the term pranayama and discusses the relationship between pain and breathing and the role that pranayama can play in pain care.

*Pratyahara*—the practices of pratyahara involve increasing internal awareness of body, breath, thoughts and emotions. Without thinking about it, we usually attend far more to external stimuli than internal sensations and processes. Recently, this internal attention is often discussed as interoception or awareness of physiological processes that normally proceed without our conscious awareness. Brain neuroscience suggests that the insula cortex in the brain is involved in interoception.[24] The insula not only receives physiological information, but also receives inputs from areas of the brain implicated in emotional processes. This aligns with pratyahara, since its practices include attending not only to the body, but also to thoughts and emotions.

The practices of pratyahara are similar to those of mindfulness meditation. Yet in yoga, pratyahara is practiced specifically as a technique in preparation for meditation, and is practiced during asana, and ultimately in life. Mindfulness meditation also differs in that it is based on Buddhist philosophy and beliefs rather than yogic beliefs. Pratyahara can be immensely valuable to assess and address in pain care. Throughout the book, we discuss the importance of cultivating awareness, in both the person in pain and the therapist. In Chapter 9, Rubenstein Fazzio takes us through an in-depth journey into pratyahara as it relates to pain and helping people in pain.

*Dharana*—this includes cultivating focus and concentration. The practices of dharana are specifically to prepare the yoga practitioner to meditate. Without skill in focus and concentration, meditation will not be successful. Dharana techniques can include focus on singular internal processes such as breath, on broader awareness of the ever-changing thoughts or sensations or on external stimuli such as when keeping one's focus on the flame of a candle. People in pain can have difficulty with focusing, concentrating, sustaining attention and even learning. As Pearson discusses in Chapter 5, there are changes that take place in the brain and nervous systems when pain persists that may lead to these reduced abilities. Practices that address dharana can have immense value in helping people in pain improve awareness, self-regulate and therefore influence the pain experience. Dharana plays a significant role in pain care, as we will further discuss in the following chapters.

*Dhyana*—this is meditation, moving from the outwardness of objects and mind into the inwardness of individuality, and moving into a feeling process that is not constricted by logical and concrete thought. In pratyahara we practice mindfulness of the mind and body, in dharana we practice attentiveness to a subtle object and in dhyana we practice effortless attention, gaining understanding and wisdom beyond body and mind.[25]

Meditation typically decreases the stress response, increases relaxation and can result in a sense of peace and joy. It can provide us with the capacity to adapt and sustain a sense of equanimity during times of challenge and adversity. In other words, meditation can help us be more resilient. We can appreciate the benefits this has for people in pain as well as for the health and longevity of the therapist. There may be immediate positive effects of meditation, yet it is the long-term positive effects of consistent practice of meditation that provide the desirable changes. Dhyana is more than a technique. It is a way of living.

*Samadhi*—the eighth and final limb is a state of wisdom, understanding and bliss in which one is connected to and is one with all that exists. This theme is referred to consistently throughout this book. In Chapters 14 and 15, Prosko and Sullivan respectively discuss the science surrounding the concepts and value of feeling a sense of unity, connection, worthiness and wholeness in pain care.

## Kriya yoga

Kriya yoga involves conscious volitional actions of our thoughts, words and deeds. It attends to the relationship between the activity of perception and the perceiver through a systematic approach in which one rotates prana or vital life force, mantra or sound and yantra or visualizations through areas of the spine and the energy centers or plexuses associated with these areas.

Kriya yoga moves the practitioner through levels of awareness to self-realization: beginning with awareness associated with disciplining one's body, mind and movement of energy, creating clarity of thought, fervency of action and peaceful self-discovery moving toward "self-mastery" in order to meet the higher goals of surrendering to one's own true nature as Spirit in form, living a human experience.

Kriya yoga has a long history of secrecy and was only passed on verbally from guru (teacher) to disciple (student). The phases of practice would expand and build upon one another and would only be given to the student when and if the teacher felt the student was ready to advance.

## Tantra yoga

Tantric teachings expound upon the philosophy and practices of both these paths of yoga and Samkhya. The word tantra refers both to a body of texts called "the tantras" as well as to the knowledge taught within these texts.[26] Wallis offers an understanding of the meaning of tantra as follows: "tantra spreads (tan) wisdom that saves (tra)."[27] Themes within tantric teachings include: focus on non-dualism, subtle body and experiential versus cognitive practices. The subtle body is emphasized through the teachings and practices. Through meditations, rituals, pranayama and physical postures, these energy centers, called cakras or granthis, can be activated and manipulated. Working with these energy centers frees the flow of prana, the life force, such that liberation from suffering may be realized. This focus on the individual is often spoken of as the person being the "microcosm" of the "macrocosm."

## Panca maya kosha model

In yoga, panca maya kosha describes a perspective with similarities to the biopsychosocial (and spiritual) view. In Sanskrit, panca means five, maya means body and kosha means sheath. Each individual is made of five aspects or bodies, each fitting together with the others, like a sword fits into a sheath. Table 4.2 provides details.

Table 4.2 Panca maya kosha model

| Kosha | Aspect | Function |
|---|---|---|
| Annamaya | Physical | Body systems |
| Pranamaya | Energetic | Life force |
| Manomaya | Lower mind | Autonomic processes, including thoughts and emotions |
| Vijnanamaya | Higher mind | Metacognition |
| Anandamaya | Peace, bliss | Connectedness and life purpose |

The annamaya kosha, the body of matter, is the first level of our experience. This kosha includes the physical components of the body, along with the needs of the body such as hunger and elimination.

The pranamaya kosha is the dimension of energy within us. Feeling sluggish, having tight muscles and being fatigued are all related to the pranamaya kosha.

The manomaya kosha is the mental body. It relates to our needs, desires, ambitions—to automatic actions related to these, rather than to contemplation of any of these or our actions related to them. Agitation and depression of the mind are related to this kosha, as is awareness of the automatic thoughts, habits and fulfilment of needs and desires, and awareness of aversions and grasping.

The vijnanamaya kosha is the higher mind, the part of the mind that is conscious and contemplative of other aspects of self.

The anandamaya kosha is the experience of bliss, which comes from fusion of the individual mind with the cosmic mind. This kosha can also include one's spiritual nature or feelings of a sense of purpose, meaning or connection to self, others or something greater, as discussed in Chapter 15.

Each of these sheaths/aspects are considered important in yoga therapy, both in assessment and application of practices and philosophy. Keep in mind that these sheaths are not separate and not looked at as layers that interact with one another; rather, they are integrated as one. Like all such perspectives, it is a model intended to help us better understand. Yoga therapy focuses on holism, understanding that the individual is an integrated whole. Therapy cannot impact one aspect without having potential effects on all other aspects. The therapeutic advantages of this view include knowing that we can impact any aspect of existence through any other aspect. This is an especially valuable model to use in pain care, since we know that pain is a complex biopsychosocial phenomenon and humans are complex organisms interacting with the environment. The panca maya kosha model in yoga therapy can serve as a biopsychosocial–spiritual framework from which to help people in pain in a more integrated way, as we will thoroughly illustrate in this book.

## Chapter 5

# Pain Biology and Sensitization

Neil Pearson

## Pain physiology

Understanding the physiological mechanisms related to pain is one of the foundations of success in the work we do assisting people in pain. This knowledge provides the rationale for realistic hope when pain persists, for greater compassion for the people we serve and for innovations in treatment processes and techniques. Without this knowledge we perpetuate beliefs that pain is immutable, that pain is either from the body or the mind and that the role of self-care is less important in pain management than the role of pharmaceutical or interventional medicine.

This chapter will describe key physiological processes involved in pain: from peripheral neurons, inflammation and neuropathic pain, to the dorsal horn, inhibitory neurons, microglia, neurotransmitters and ascending/descending modulation, to the brain. Sensory perception, saliency networks and the interactions of other key physiological systems on pain will also be considered.

Discussed in this chapter and book is an aspect of our human experience. Pain is complex and best understood from multiple perspectives.

## Introductory perspective of pain physiology

The pain we experience can be understood in many different ways and from many perspectives. You are provided here with a summary of the vast field of scientific inquiry, intended in part to demonstrate how real pain is, in part to provide some understanding of why and how pain persists and in part to stimulate understanding of how the practices of yoga assist the person living in pain. Consider as well that this information intends to provide you with hope, which you impart to your patients. Pain, like all human experiences, is impermanent. We are resilient.

As we dive deeper into body systems, and cells, and chemistry, we must remember that there remain many unanswered questions about pain, pain biology and pain management. Pain physiology is usually interpreted as an exploration within the "bio" aspects of pain. Expanding our view, and even altering our perspective to a panca maya kosha perspective, enhances our understanding that pain physiology is studying the person as much as our biology.

An additional lens through which to discuss pain is story. Story allows us to learn while accepting imprecisions and allowing for explanatory evolutions. Story can be incomplete, easily faulted, overly simple and open to argument. Yet, if the stories and metaphors you read in this chapter help you effectively serve people in pain more compassionately, then I will have told you a good one.

---

Consider these perspectives on pain while reading this chapter.

- Pain is a product of the brain. (Butler and Moseley)

- Pain is a complex and troublesome human experience, a whole lot like love. (Pearson)

- Pain is an unpleasant sensory and emotional experience associated with actual or potential tissue damage. (International Association for the Study of Pain)

---

Pain is a conscious experience associated with widespread altered physiology, including brain activity. When there is pain, we typically consider that this is arising in response to sufficient activation of peripheral nociceptive neurons, such that electrochemical messages are propagated through the spinal cord to the brain, activating brain networks and coming to our consciousness. Pain is complex. When we discuss pain as "associated with alterations of brain activity," we potentially oversimplify. Pain can occur without peripheral nociceptive inputs, it is influenced by many if not all aspects of the organism and we cannot state with confidence exactly when, where or how pain arises after neural stimuli excite networks of cells in the brain. In other words, our understanding is imprecise, and pain is complex. We can bring more clarity to our understanding of pain by combining pain physiology with the lived experience of pain. Let's start there.

If we think about pain, we recognize that when there is pain, we usually look for tissue damage. When there is injury without pain, we find this curious. When an individual's pain reports don't align with the extent of observed tissue injury, we question the person's reports or motivation. When an individual with extensive trauma and pain tells us how they used self-management techniques rather than pills to dramatically decrease the pain, we struggle to accept this as possible. Even with all this cognitive dissonance we rarely think about what you *think* about pain. When we do, our unquestioned beliefs can be contrary to what we know of pain biology, and even inconsistent with our own experiences of pain.

The physiological processes and anatomical structures involved in pain are equally complex. They include, but are not limited to peripheral neurons, inflammation and neuropathic pain, the dorsal horn, inhibitory neurons, microglia, macrophages, neurotransmitters and ascending and descending modulation, the brain, specific brain areas and networks, sensory perception, emotions, interoception, cognition, movement and stress processes. Pain interacts with multiple physiological systems of the organism, influencing societal, cultural, vocational, community and relationship factors. Across individuals, there are commonalities in pain experience and pain physiology, yet there are also vast differences in these processes between individuals, across time and contexts.

A chapter about pain physiology requires describing the associated anatomy—yet where do we start? By discussing the brain first, there is a risk of promoting a brain-centric view of pain and pain management—or "top-down" cognitive and emotional approaches and interventions that seek to change the brain as the only modulators of pain. If we start at the peripheral nociceptors and the tissue factors that can stimulate them, we risk sustaining views of a direct linear link between tissue health and pain—we might focus our treatments on fixing the tissues and solely on "bottom-up" approaches. If we start by discussing the autonomic nervous system (ANS), we risk focusing pain management only on stress management and engagement of parasympathetic processes. Even the discussion of pain as top-down and bottom-up, and as influenced by the ANS compared to the central nervous system (CNS) (as if any one of these can happen independently), can hold us back from evolving our understanding of pain, inhibiting effective innovations in pain management. As such, let's continue talking about pain a little more before we switch to details of pain anatomy and physiology.

## Acute pain and chronic pain

Many of the changes we experience when pain persists are also present in acute pain.

Have you ever noticed:

- how much it hurts to gently touch uninjured skin close to an injury, immediately after the injury? *Tactile allodynia.*

- changes in body image immediately after and over the first few days after an injury? Cartoonists vividly demonstrate the *distortions of body awareness and body schema* associated with acute pain when a rock lands on a head or foot.

- how much more hot water hurts when shower water hits your sunburned skin? *Thermal hyperalgesia or allodynia.*

- how much your ability to think clearly, or to focus, or to let go of excess muscle tension is impacted by the pain of an acute injury? *Diminished cognitive ability to influence autonomic processes.*

- how a toothache or headache changes how easily we become angry, how productive we are at work or how much we engage with others? *Emotional lability and social impacts.*

Human experiences have physiological correlates. As such, the resolution of these acute pain experiences is related to physiology. The physiological shifts during acute pain might then be considered elastic changes—they more easily return towards normal. On the other hand, when pain persists, the associated physiological and structural changes are referred to as plastic changes—requiring more energy and time to return towards normal.

This understanding is important when we consider that chronic pain management might most effectively commence prior to the three-month determination of the pain being chronic. When we observe early elastic changes persisting beyond expected timelines, or not resolving as usual, treatment addressing this physiology might be more effective.

We must recognize that the elastic and plastic changes are biopsychosocial, not only neurophysiological as they are often described. We might be angry or fearful or retreat from our friends during acute pain, yet these too resolve relatively quickly. Their persistence might be a clinical sign of an individual moving towards chronic pain.

Recent research suggests that physiological shifts in the immune system may be as important as those in the nervous system when pain persists. The polyvagal theory[1] provides a plausible explanation of a key role of the ANS in chronic pain. Brain scan research provides evidence of changes in activity and structure of the brain in people with diagnoses of chronic pain. Pain changes everything, whether it is acute or chronic. Maybe we should consider beginning "chronic pain treatments" earlier as much as we focus on treating people with chronic pain differently than those who have acute pain.

## Types of pain

Besides discussing pain based on time since injury, it can be helpful to discuss it in relation to the International Association for the Study of Pain (IASP) classifications[2] of the types of pain.

**Nociceptive pain**: "arises from actual or threatened damage to non-neural tissue and is due to the activation of nociceptors."

**Neuropathic pain**: "caused by a lesion or disease of the somatosensory nervous system."

**Nociplastic pain**: "arises from altered nociception despite no clear evidence of actual or threatened tissue damage causing the activation of peripheral nociceptors or evidence for disease or lesion of the somatosensory system causing the pain." Nociception is the neural encoding process of encoding noxious stimuli.

**Sensitization**: "increased responsiveness of nociceptive neurons to their normal input, and/or recruitment of a response to normally subthreshold inputs."

The first two pain types suggest the existence of a typical or normal physiological process associated with the pain when it is related to either injury of non-neural tissues (nociceptive) or to neural (neuropathic) tissues. This process is described below.

Sensitization and nociplastic suggest the existence of atypical processes associated with nociception and pain. When pain persists, physiology changes. The common changes are described below. From our expanding understanding of the complexity of pain, and before we discuss pain physiology further, we should consider what these definitions suggest for effective pain management.

- Nociceptive pain can be decreased by:

  - lessening tissue damage and restoring tissue physiological properties

  - lessening potentially damaging mechanical or chemical influences on non-neural tissues

  - decreasing the activation of nociceptors

  - blocking/altering the transmission of nociceptive signals to the spinal cord and brain.

- Neuropathic pain can be decreased by:

  - decreasing the lesion to the somatosensory nervous system

  - lessening the disease activity

  - decreasing the activation of nociceptors related to the lesion

  - decreasing the sensitivity of nociceptors related to the lesion

  - blocking/altering the transmission of nociceptive signals to the spinal cord and brain.

- Nociplastic pain can be decreased by:

  - restoring nociceptive processes towards normal homeostasis.

- Sensitization can be decreased by:

  - decreasing the responsiveness of nociceptive neurons to noxious inputs

  - normalizing the activity of nociceptive neurons so they no longer respond as if non-dangerous-to-the-tissues stimuli are dangerous.

In addition, the definitions/descriptions of two specific changes often related to sensitization should be considered.

**Allodynia**[3] is pain arising from stimuli that are normally innocuous. We often experience tactile allodynia when there is an acute contusion. Touch the skin close by to the injury shortly after it occurs, and there is often pain even from light touch. Listen to the stories of our patients who say that applying ice to the area of the injury actually causes more pain. Watch your patient with nociplastic shoulder pain grimace during a grip strength test or report pain from a movement that anatomically should not produce a dangerous increase in mechanical load to the tissue.

Persisting tactile and thermal allodynia are signs of nociplastic pain. So is mechanical allodynia. The neurophysiology of these is believed to extend far beyond peripheral nociceptive neurons and include changes at the dorsal horn, in descending modulation and therefore also in the brain. Thankfully, the neuromatrix model shows us that we can assist people with allodynia by changing inputs from the tissues, by changing descending modulation, by altering stress and by changing processes and activities of the brain.

**Hyperalgesia**[4] is pain of greater intensity than normal with the application of normally noxious inputs. This term has more importance experimentally than clinically. Most patients report pain from things that should not be painful, rather than more pain from things that previously were painful. And clinically, our goal is to decrease allodynia more than hyperalgesia.

Everything that is happening in the body, everything that is happening outside of it and all our cognitive and emotional processes influence not only the CNS but also the ANS. Understanding this relationship forms the physiological essence of the biopsychosocial view of pain. Pain and nociception can potentially be influenced by any aspect of our existence. As people in pain report, pain changes everything. As such, everything can change pain. Given this complexity, let's start with a summary of what we know about peripheral neurons.

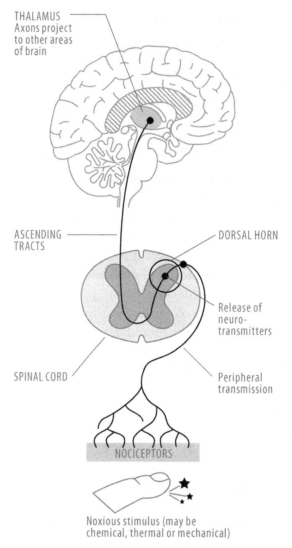

THALAMUS
Axons project
to other areas
of brain

ASCENDING
TRACTS

DORSAL HORN

Release of
neuro-
transmitters

SPINAL CORD

Peripheral
transmission

NOCICEPTORS

Noxious stimulus (may be
chemical, thermal or mechanical)

*Figure 5.1 Transduction, transmission and perception; a relay
system, demonstrating multiple targets for yoga therapy*

**Nociception** is the neural encoding of noxious stimuli.

**Nociceptive neurons** are peripheral or central neurons of the somatosensory nervous system that is capable of encoding noxious stimuli.

**Nociceptive stimuli** are typically stated as potentially dangerous heat/cold, mechanical stretch or compression forces and specific chemicals, for example those released from broken cells (e.g. adenosine triphosphate, ATP) and some of the chemistry of inflammation (e.g. bradykinins, histamines). Yet we have all experienced loud noises as painful, heartbreak as painful and sometimes bright light as painful. These experiences demonstrate how normally innocuous stimuli can be experienced as dangerous.[5]

**Peripheral nociceptive neurons** respond to nociceptive stimuli. They are believed to have a relatively high threshold for excitation. Uncontrolled pain,[6] unexplained pain,[7] inflammatory chemistry,[8] past experiences,[9] fear,[10] fight and flight processes[11] and even expectation[12] of pain all potentially decrease excitatory thresholds of peripheral nociceptors.

Peripheral nociceptors are always changing[13]—like all neurons. We might say they are under constant renovation, always updating component parts and altering their physiology in response to the neuron's internal and external environments, the organism's physiology and the person's external milieu.

Peripheral nociceptors are classified as: **A delta fibers**—lightly myelinated with conduction velocities of 5–20m/s; **A beta fibers**—myelinated with conduction velocities of 5–30m/s; **C fibers**—unmyelinated with conduction velocities of 1m/s.

Note that the difference in transmission velocity applies to the peripheral neurons, not to the spinal cord pathways or brain. As such, it is difficult to agree with the statement that the fast, sharp pain after acute injury and the second more dull and diffuse pain can be attributed to the signaling speed differences in peripheral neurons. Wouldn't the length of the peripheral neuron matter to this same attribution? And does it assume identical processing of C fiber and A delta fiber inputs in the brain?

- The more localized pain associated with A delta fiber stimulation suggests this information is processed in a cortical area with a detailed "map" of the body.

- Similar to all peripheral neurons, the threshold of excitation, and the signal latency period of nociceptors, are adaptable. When pain persists, the nociceptor threshold of excitation decreases, as does the latency period. This is related to hyperalgesia (but not a complete explanation of) and to reports of pain that does not quickly decrease after removal of noxious stimuli such as a single repetition of a painful movement.

- Some C fibers are categorized as silent nociceptors.[14] They normally do not respond to noxious mechanical stimuli and are recruited in the presence of injury, inflammation and intense pain. The existence of these silent nociceptors might be explained by long periods of inactivity, leading to "disuse" changes within the neurons. However, nociceptors seem ready and able to respond to nociceptive stimuli after periods without pain or apparent nociception.

- C fibers are involved in neurogenic inflammation.[15] In the presence of tissue injury, when a C fiber conducts a nociceptive signal to the dorsal horn, it also releases substance P and calcitonin gene-related peptide (CGRP) from its peripheral end into the injured (or previously injured) tissues—apparently beginning the process of inflammation regardless of pain. Yet neurogenic inflammation decreases when there is less pain. Some individuals have more swelling in rheumatoid arthritic joints on the side of their body not impacted by a cerebral vascular accident. If pain influenced neurogenic inflammation, then we should expect that in chronic pain there might always be an aspect of ongoing nociceptive input that could benefit from treatment.

## The spinal cord, dorsal horn and nociceptive pathways

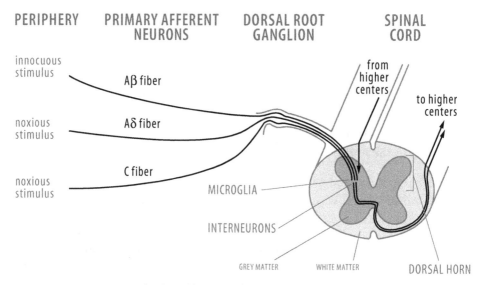

*Figure 5.2 At the dorsal horn, peripheral nociceptors, A beta neurons, interneurons, microglia and descending pathways all influence activity of each other and of the ascending nociceptive signaling*

Peripheral nociceptors from different tissues (skin, muscles, viscera) enter the spinal cord and terminate in an area called the dorsal horn. The dorsal horn is organized by tissue source of the afferent neuron and by sensory function, yet recent research provides evidence of much greater complexity.[16] This organization is part of the explanation for the greater difficulties in localizing the tissue source of the nociceptive input when it arises from viscera versus muscles versus skin.

- **Nociceptive A fibers**: Primarily terminate in laminae I, II and V.

- **C fibers**: Primarily terminate in laminae I and II, and from viscera in laminae IV and V.

## *Modulation of the excitatory signaling form peripheral neurons*

- A beta inputs from the skin are considered inhibitory to nociceptive signaling in the dorsal horn under normal situations (holding a painful area or rubbing it). However, when pain persists, normally innocuous A beta inputs can be experienced as noxious (allodynia) due in part to changes in the dorsal horn such as loss of inhibitory effects and phenotype shifts of A beta neurons such that they release substance P and CGRP on to post-synaptic terminals.[17]

- Descending neurons from higher brain centers provide input to the dorsal horn and the peripheral neurons. These inputs can be excitatory or inhibitory. The brain has multiple pathways and chemical processes through which it can facilitate and inhibit spinal cord transmission and thus modulate nociceptive transmission and pain.

- Interneurons—most neurons within laminae I–III are interneurons.[18] These modulate sensory info at the spinal cord level. Interneurons can be excitatory or inhibitory. Recent research has shown the majority of interneurons as excitatory to nociceptive inputs, at least in rat studies.[19] This unexpected and replicated finding suggests that descending inhibition of nociceptive inputs to the spinal cord might be a powerful normal process. Thus, pain management might need to focus on increasing descending inhibitory control of interneurons and nociceptors, as well as decreasing nociceptive inputs from the body and altering nociceptive process in the brain.

## Neurotransmitters

Neurotransmitters are endogenous molecules involved in neurotransmission—signaling between neurons at a synapse or between neurons and other cells such as muscle cells. Neurotransmitters communicating between neurons are released from presynaptic axons into the synaptic cleft, where they bind to specific receptors (ion channels) on the post-synaptic neuron. This may lead to excitation or inhibition of the post-synaptic neuron depending on the neurotransmitter and the post-synaptic receptor. Research shows that persisting nociceptive stimuli can lead to an increase in release of neurotransmitter into the synapse and increase density of excitatory ion channels on the post-synaptic neurons.[20] This resembles the changes of long-term potentiation, which are observed in all types of learning.

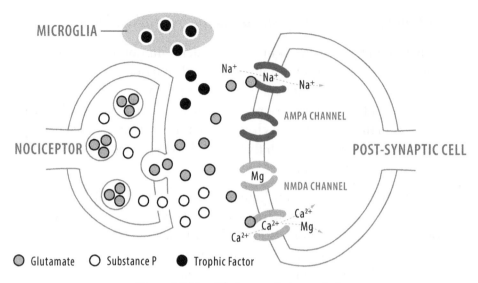

*Figure 5.3 Simplified synaptic transmission*

Pre- and post-synaptic cells constantly morph based on ascending, descending, systemic and local factors; this diagram highlights the most basic of ion channels, neurotransmitters and cells involved.

Glutamate and substance P are the primary excitatory neurotransmitters released by peripheral nociceptors, whereas glycine and gamma-aminobutyric acid (GABA) are the primary inhibitory neurotransmitters released from interneurons and descending neurons.[21]

Interneurons also release CGRP, cholecystokinin and substance P as excitatory neurotransmitters.[22] Each of these, and therefore interneuron activity and nociceptive signaling, are influenced by a broad range of factors at the level of the organism. For example, expectations of increased pain, nerve injury and anxiety have all been shown to increase cholecystokinin,[23] which is additionally antagonistic to exogenous opioids.

## *Neurotransmitters associated with descending inhibition of pain*

- **Serotonin**: Has both excitatory and inhibitory actions on nociception and is implicated in both pain control and in perpetuation of pain.[24]

- **Noradrenaline**: Inhibits presynaptic substance P release; also involved in sympathetic nervous system and preparing the body for movement.[25]

- **GABA**: Produces inhibitory effects on nociception through GABAnergic receptors; also the main inhibitory neurotransmitter in the CNS.[26]

- **Glycine**: An inhibitory neurotransmitter often decreased in chronic pain states.[27]

- **Endogenous opioids**: Endorphins, dynorphins, enkephalins, endo-morphins.[28]

## Spinal cord pathways

The spinal cord is not a passive group of wires through which signals travel between the periphery and the brain. Nociceptive signals are also processed within the spinal cord.[29]

Research shows both descending inhibitory and descending excitatory pathways from the brain to the spinal cord.[30] Descending signals constantly influence ascending nociceptive transmission, based on the relative amount of inhibitory versus excitatory signaling. More details of descending modulation are provided in the section "Brain and pain."

There are four ascending tracts that transmit nociceptive inputs to the brain. Each is influenced by the balance of descending excitatory and inhibitory signals being conducted by the neurons forming these tracts.

- **Spinothalamic tract**: This processes and transmits nociceptive, thermal and light touch stimuli, predominantly arising from laminae I and V, but also II, IV, VI, VII, VIII and X. The tract ascends to the contralateral thalamus and projects to specific cortical areas related to pain.

- **Spinomesencephalic tract**: Inputs arise from laminae I, IV, V and VI and terminate in various locations of midbrain including the periaqueductal grey (PAG) matter where they activate descending inhibitory (analgesic) pathways. Termination of some of this tract in the parabrachial nucleus that projects to the amygdala suggests a role in the emotional aspects of pain.

- **Spinoreticular tract**: Originates mostly in laminae VII and VIII. Some fibers terminate in the pons and medulla. The primary function of this tract is to influence autonomic centers, endogenous pain modulation and the motivational and affective aspects of pain.

- **Dorsal columns**: This pathway has a role in positional sense and two-point discrimination as well as transmission of visceral nociceptive information.

## Microglia

Glial cells make up 70 percent of CNS cells, including astrocytes, oligodendrocytes and microglia.[31] Oligodendrocytes are similar to Schwann cells, providing myelination to the neurons. Microglia and astrocytes are cells of the immune system that can be excitatory or inhibitory to nociceptive signals in the spinal cord and the brain.[32] Research shows that nerve injury creates an increase in the release of proinflammatory chemistry from macrophages, as do other factors such as stress and decreased physical activity.[33] Increased physical activity not only decreases the proinflammatory chemistry but leads to phenotype shifts of some macrophages to become anti-inflammatory.[34] Understanding the role of microglia and of the balance of pro- and anti-inflammatory chemistry in altering both nociception and pain provides a plausible theoretical premise from which to develop innovations to therapeutic and medical interventions.

## Brain and pain

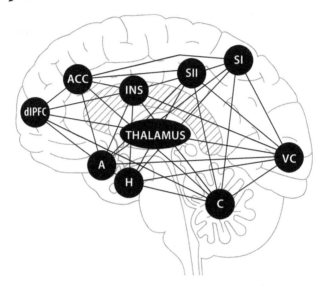

*Figure 5.4 Pain, chronic pain and salience "networks"*

Each are related to combined activity of many brain areas. These include dorsolateral prefrontal cortex (dlPFC), anterior cingulate cortex (ACC), insular cortex (INS), amygdala (A), hippocampus (H), thalamus, primary (SI) and secondary (SII) sensory-motor cortices, and at times the cerebellum (C) and the visual cortex (VC).

When nociceptive signals are transmitted to the brain, they travel to many areas of the brain. Science does not tell us where or how nociceptive signaling is experienced as pain. Yet when we consider pain biology and the lived experience of pain, the following *story* can explain parts of the relationship between nociception and pain.

Nociceptive signals from ascending pathways excite cells and networks in the brain.

The brain interprets the nociceptive signaling. This is typically below consciousness. Each brain area and its associated networks respond to the signals from its/their unique functional perspective. Certain brain areas and networks consider the nociceptive signaling from a perspective of sensory discriminative, cognitive-evaluative and emotional-motivational lenses. The nociceptive inputs and the subsequent activity within neural networks all seem to be considered in relation to saliency and in relation to all other current inputs and network activity, as well as past experience, current priorities and predictions of the future.

Under certain circumstances, pain (a conscious experience) is produced along with other autonomic biopsychosocial responses. The pain immediately becomes another input to be analyzed, and the cycle continues.

The individual in pain can consciously and purposefully analyze the pain—its saliency, sensory, evaluative and emotional aspects. The individual can also purposefully explore the relationship between the nociceptive stimuli and their pain.

In other words, autonomic processes and the conscious person are now responding to the pain.

Taking this story further we can consider that effective pain management might influence pain through the following.

- Altering the signals ascending to the brain, both nociceptive and non-nociceptive (e.g. flooding the brain with innocuous sensory signaling from the skin, joints and muscles, decreasing noxious mechanical and inflammatory signaling and gentle body movements).

- Altering brain processes involved in analyzing signals from a sensory discriminative, emotional, cognitive or saliency perspective (e.g. self-regulation, cognitive approaches and reframing pain).

- Altering perspectives on past history and future predictions (e.g. mindfulness and awareness practices).

- Reconceptualizing pain (e.g. knowledge of pain).

- Altering any other inputs to the brain from any system of the body (e.g. breathing techniques, body movement, calming sympathetic activity and digestive system).

- Conscious/purposeful/mindful/contemplative practices (e.g. focused awareness, open awareness and "taking the time to think about what we think about pain").

Current understanding is that experiences and brain processes are related to networks and that many networks overlap. In the case of pain, this supports that there is no pain center in the brain. Networks of the brain associated with the production of pain are not separate from other brain networks. There is overlap so that networks related to certain movements, certain memories, certain smells or sights or certain temperatures or weather can also be associated with pain. In apparent contradiction to this story of complexity and integrated functioning of networks, the following section will focus on evidence of key brain areas implicated within these networks related to pain, chronic pain and its management.

**Thalamus**—this has many nociceptive functions. It relays information to cortical areas involved in sensory, evaluative and motivational aspects of pain via projections to primary and secondary somatosensory cortices and via projections to limbic system. The thalamus also plays a role in descending modulation of pain.[35] Besides nociceptive inputs, thalamic activity is influenced by peripheral inflammation with decreased thresholds of excitation to nociceptive inputs.

**Primary sensory cortex (S1)**—this is chiefly involved in interpreting nociceptive signaling from a sensory discriminative perspective. Locating and accurately identifying the type of tissue injury is most precise in areas of the skin with the most detailed representation in the sensory cortex and far more accurate from the skin than from any subdermal tissues.

**Secondary somatosensory cortex (S2)**—this also receives nociceptive inputs (and non-nociceptive) from the thalamus; however, the neural areas for each body part are poorly represented. Projections from S2 to the limbic system have a role in recognition, learning and memory of painful events. Its precise role in nociception and pain is undetermined.

**Motor cortex**—this plays a role in pain modulation as well as sensory motor integration and control of both voluntary and imagined movements. Evidence supports increased nociceptive thresholds associated with motor cortex stimulation, along with analgesic effects on sensory discriminative and emotional aspects of pain.[36] Given the benefits reported by many people living in pain when they are able to sustain daily movement and exercise, it is not surprising that surgical motor cortex stimulation in humans has been shown to increase GABAnergic and opioid activity.[37]

**Anterior cingulate cortex**—this is a major part of the limbic system associated with emotional-motivational evaluation of nociception.[38] Its role in pain relates to involvement in attention, emotions, avoidance behaviors and placebo analgesia. Pain demands our attention.

**Insular cortex**—this has a role in interoception as well as nociception.[39] It is involved in body awareness and is influenced by contemplative practices such as mindfulness techniques. Based on the projections into the insula, it may also be involved in networks through which cognitions can modulate the sensory and emotional aspects of pain. Persistent pain is also associated with altered body awareness.[40] Some patients experience the area of body in which they experience pain as swollen, larger or smaller than usual or, "Like that part of body doesn't exist other than for the pain I feel." Even when skin sensation is intact or even allodynic, some report that it is difficult to "feel" the subtle non-pain sensations of the body. This experience may be an alteration of interoception via changes in activity of the insula or its associated networks. From a therapeutic perspective, of interest is that meditators have been shown to develop "thicker" insular cortices[41] and that some patients report that practicing mindfulness and improving their awareness of subtle non-pain sensations decreases pain. Further research is needed in this area, both to help identify the presence of altered body awareness in patients with chronic pain and to identify the role of the insula in meditative techniques that are associated with decreased pain and increased ability to experience the subtle non-pain sensations of the body.

**Amygdala**—this is involved in evaluating sensory signaling from an emotional perspective and is involved in emotional learning and memory. It is implicated in fear conditioning and in descending facilitation of nociceptive inputs via the PAG and rostral ventral medulla (RVM).[42]

**Hippocampus**—this has a role in learning, in modulating the amygdala and in both spatial and temporal awareness (differentiating past, present and future). There is believed to be a reciprocal influence between the amygdala and hippocampus that is important for people in pain. When the amygdala is more active, such as when a person is stressed or experiencing intense pain, the hippocampus is less active. This can have an impact on the individual's ability to learn new information or learn pain self-regulation techniques or exercises. As such, people living in pain often need more repetition to learn and more practice of new exercises or self-regulation techniques. The hippocampus also has a role in differentiating past from present and future. When we are stressed and in pain, getting stuck in ruminations of past and negative future predictions may be associated with the increased amygdala activity. On the other hand, if the person living in pain actively engages in awareness techniques (mindfulness is currently most common) these potentially increase temporal discernment (differentiating past, present and future). This focus on the present will not only decrease rumination and anxiety but also decrease amygdala activity. Given the decreased pain experienced by some patients in association with awareness practices, this is a plausible physiological explanation.

**Periaqueductal grey and RVM**—two of the more studied aspects of descending modulation. The PAG exerts powerful anti-nociceptive effects.[43] It receives inputs from cortical sites, the amygdala and the spinomesencephalic tract. The PAG activates the RVM, which is considered the common relay station for descending inhibition of nociception. It also receives input from the thalamus, parabrachial nucleus and pons (locus coeruleus). The PAG-RVM is believed to provide a key component of the mechanism whereby pain can be stopped due to homeostatic or experiential priorities (e.g. osteoarthritis hand and wrist pain disappearing as one lifts a crying grandchild). It has also been shown to preferentially inhibit C fiber inputs, decreasing the emotional-motivational impact of nociception while having less impact on the sensory discriminative perspective.[44]

**Cerebellum**—this is described as an area of the brain related to coordination and automatic movement control. It may become active when there is pain as part of the brain's processes to remove an individual physically from danger. Research also suggests it plays a role in the emotional aspects of pain, potentially demonstrating the brain's integration of body and mind.[45]

**Prefrontal cortex**—the dorsolateral prefrontal cortex (dlPFC) and anterolateral prefrontal cortex are involved in processes through which we exert control over pain and other physiological experiences. The dlPFC is also involved in placebo analgesia.[46] Experimentally, the experience of not being able to control pain is associated with decreased activity in these prefrontal cortical areas.[47] This may be an aspect of the neural correlate of learned helplessness and situation-created external locus of control. Research shows that in individuals who recover from chronic low back pain, these cortical areas once again become more active.[48] In practices such as yoga, this relationship between self-regulation, pain relief and recovering quality of life may be linked to shifts towards an internal locus of control and away from helplessness.

Most of the preceding changes are referred to as neuroplastic changes—the chemical, physiological and structural changes associated with learning within the nervous systems. The biological changes include neurotransmitter production, microglia functioning, ion channels, threshold of excitation, signal latency, axonal sprouting, axon die-back, receptive field changes, blood flow alterations within the brain and changes in connectivity and cortical thickness.

The lived experience changes in relation to persisting pain can be described as those changes associated with the development and maintenance and the recovery and resolution of chronic pain and all its biopsychosocial manifestations. When pain persists, it seems that the nervous systems (and the human) are practicing in a way that maintains pain through these "plastic" changes. The good news is that the nervous systems seem to get good at what they practice—we need to find ways to create new neuroplastic changes, ones that compete with and become more powerful than the ones associated with chronic pain. And as you will understand based on the neuromatrix model (see the "The neuromatrix model and pain" section), we can use any aspect of your existence to change pain.

## Other changes when pain persists

### Thinning cortex and persistent pain

Research indicates that when pain persists, some areas of the cortex become thinner and there is less functional connectivity.[49] When chronic pain resolves and individuals recover previous functioning, these cortical areas recover.[50]

## Persisting pain, depression and the brain

Research shows that when pain persists, changes observed on fMRI resemble those seen in individuals with clinical depression. This matches a clinical observation that people who are depressed report pain associated temporally with the depression and that people with chronic pain become depressed. However, we must take care when considering this idea (potential confirmation bias) that the fMRI findings confirm that chronic pain causes depression. There is considerable overlap in brain networks, and fMRIs have limitations. For example, Legrain et al.[51] showed considerable overlap in the brain regions responding when pain was experienced from physical noxious stimuli and from experimentally induced social rejection. They explain this by concluding that both experiences are salient, and both trigger multimodal processes involved in detecting, orienting attention towards and reacting to the salient event. The reason that the fMRI looks as if it is the same is because the fMRI is not able to differentiate the physiological differences between our experience of physical and social rejection pain. As such, the person can tell the difference between these, even though the fMRI cannot. In addition, these findings should not tell us to assess and treat people suffering from pain that we attribute to physical injury or psychospiritual suffering in exactly the same manner, but rather to consider that there are similarities and differences in how we should assess and treat across domains.

## Hormones and pain

Research to date is not conclusive regarding the interaction of hormones and pain.[52] Given the broad impacts of pain on the person, there is a potential for all glands and hormones to interact with the persistence of pain. Reproductive hormones and the thyroid have received the greatest attention to date. Some male patients with chronic pain have been found to have low serum testosterone and respond well with significantly less pain and decreased pain-related disability after testosterone replacement.

Some women with chronic pain report fluctuations of their pain temporally associated with other symptoms of menopause, and some report joint pain associated with menopause. Research suggests that estrogen fluctuations are involved in this;[53] however, given the varied research results, interactions for the individual patient will require individualized assessment and treatment planning.

Severe persisting pain can alter serum hormone levels, including cortisol, leading to more pain and other negative side effects such as osteoporosis and joint cartilage changes. Cortisol levels are positively influenced by emotional regulation, exercise and nutrition. Exercise influences pain through many other processes and systems, yet recent research shows a connection between the thoracic motor cortex and the adrenal glands,[54] which lead the authors to consider whether thoracic movements specifically improve health and resilience through a direct neural connection.

## Autonomic nervous systems

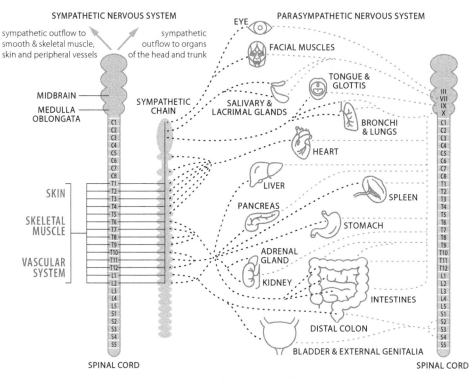

*Figure 5.5 The autonomic nervous system can be separated into sympathetic and parasympathetic aspects, as well as integumentary (skin) and enteric (gut)*

- The ANS includes parasympathetic and sympathetic systems and functions to monitor and control normally automatic physiology.

- The ANS includes the enteric nervous system. Digestion and elimination have strong bidirectional interactions in some individuals.

- The ANS is functionally integrated with the CNS. C fiber information is transmitted to both, and each has an influence on the other.

- The ANS receives inputs beyond what we usually see diagrammed in textbooks. As examples, skin is typically underrepresented, muscles are not included as important to the ANS, nociception is not shown and the primary influence of the brain on the ANS is represented by the vagus nerve.

- The diaphragm is not the only muscle normally under autonomic control that we can consciously influence. Nor are muscles the only aspects of the organism normally functioning automatically over which we can learn to exert control.

- The ANS does not work on a simple teeter-totter principle of reciprocal inhibition. Also, there is not a linear correlation in the increased or decreased activities of all of the organism's systems and organs when there are changes in the measured overall balance between sympathetic and parasympathetic activity.

The work of S. Porges[55] and of A. D. Craig[56] is expanding our understanding of the ANS. To date, through research we cannot make many direct links between their work and pain. However, Craig's work on interoception and Porges' work on the vagus nerve align with both the lived experiences of pain and with some of what we understand about pain physiology. For example, Porges, within his polyvagal theory, describes how the myelinated aspect of the vagus nerve can be viewed as important for protection and safety. From an overly simplified description, the theory suggests that the unmyelinated vagus nerve is involved in protection through immobilization, the sympathetic nervous system eliciting protection through fight and flight, and the myelinated vagus nerve is involved in protection through social engagement. If aspects of the polyvagal theory play a role in chronic pain, this theory provides suggestions for pain management similar to what a student might hear from a yoga teacher—let go of tension in your eyes, soften your tongue, relax your neck, create a sensation of compassion— all experiences related to social engagement and feeling safe.

Further research is needed to assess the efficacy of influencing the ANS as part of pain management and the relative importance and bidirectional impacts of changing autonomic functioning compared to conscious volitional actions. For example, what are the physiological differences in the ANS and CNS we can measure in the individual who can move with less pain after asking the question "Is this movement safe?" versus the individual who believes it is safe yet the movement hurts just the same. In other words, are CNS changes related to changes in pain beliefs sufficient to change ANS physiology in some people and situations but not others? Chapter 6 addresses the ANS in more detail.

## The neuromatrix model and pain

All of the above information on pain physiology can be summed by the following.

- Pain is produced by the brain. (Chapter 1, of course, reinforces that pain is experienced by the human.)

- Pain is influenced by everything, including but not limited to nociception neurons, the spinal cord, other sensory inputs, thoughts, emotions, past experiences, future predictions, ANS, CNS, hormones and immune cells.

- Pain itself becomes an input into the brain.

Melzack and Wall's "neuromatrix model"[57] provides a visual representation of this. Subsequent to the gate control theory,[58] Melzack and Wall envisioned a much more complex system of modulation of nociceptive signaling—one that explained much more of the lived experience of pain than a simple gating of signals at the dorsal horn.

This model predates considerable physiological evidence supporting that its biopsychosocial perspective of pain and of people living in pain was strikingly accurate. Simply stated, the model proposes that pain is produced not only by sensory inputs, but also by activity related to cognitions, emotions, voluntary and involuntary movement and stress. What is not obvious is that every output of the body–self neuromatrix immediately becomes an input. As discussed throughout this book, we can assist people in pain by influencing both inputs and outputs, and by how we respond to the outputs.

Equally important is that this model suggests that we can help people in pain by providing treatments to impact any of the three inputs or three outputs.

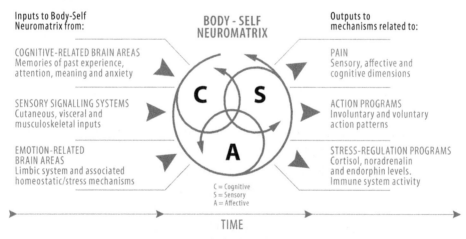

*Figure 5.6 The body–self neuromatrix*

The body–self neuromatrix model highlights the complexity and interactions of all aspects of our existence in the production, resolution and maintenance of pain.

*Source*: Adapted from Rey Allen, with permission

When we experience pain, it changes us—in complex ways and seemingly through every aspect of our existence. Each kosha, and each aspect of self, how we live in the world and all our relationships interact with pain.

Our physiology (according to science) and our pain are influenced apparently by everything, including:

- our conscious physical, cognitive and emotional reactions to pain
- whether we believe we can influence or control pain
- the responses of the autonomic process to pain
- whether these systems are tipped towards freeze, fight or flight
- the physiology of our immune and hormone systems
- slow breathing
- movement, and even specific types such as rhythmic movement
- mindfulness
- placebo
- touch
- expectations
- sounds, smells, light, taste
- sleep
- nutrition
- social connectedness
- emotions.

This list could go on, including more biopsychosocial factors, yet to summarize this chapter on pain biology, consider the following points.

Pain is real.

Pain is complex.

Pain is not immutable.

No matter how much we want a simple solution to this horrible experience of pain, pain biology provides guidance to a perspective that simple treatments are unlikely to provide effective solutions for the majority of patients. Enhanced understanding of physiological mechanisms is helpful, yet best success for people in pain arises from the ability to view pain, people living in pain and pain care from many perspectives beyond biology and physiology.

## Chapter 6

# Polyvagal Theory and the Gunas

## A Model for Autonomic Regulation in Pain

Marlysa Sullivan, Matt Erb

This chapter looks at the relationship of autonomic nervous system dysregulation and the experience of pain. Polyvagal theory will be explored to elucidate the connections between physiology, emotion and behavior stemming from underlying autonomic nervous system platforms. A translatory language between the neurophysiology of polyvagal theory and foundational yoga concepts will be considered to describe yoga practices for regulation and resilience of the autonomic nervous system for the cultivation of wellbeing and the mitigation of the experience of pain.

## Background: the autonomic nervous system provides a flexible response to the environment

The autonomic nervous system (ANS) is broadly divided into two branches—the sympathetic (SNS) and parasympathetic (PNS) nervous systems. The SNS is responsible for the mobilization of the systems of the body (e.g. cardiovascular, respiratory, endocrine) to meet any demand. This includes any response to real or perceived dangers or stressors in both the internal and external environment and is often referred to as the "fight or flight" response. The PNS is the counterpart to this mobilizing force, as it seeks to conserve resources, rebuild energy reserves and set the system for growth, healing and restoration. This system helps in processes of homeostasis and is often termed the "rest and digest" response. If, in the face of threat, the fight or flight is perceived to not be viable, an adaptive excess of PNS activity may occur and is often referred to as the "freeze" response.

While the accelerating (SNS) and decelerating (PNS) effects on target organs may seem to be contrary to one another, they are not antagonistic nor dichotomous. Rather, they interact to create a nuanced and complex response to inner and outer stimuli. Through their co-operation and co-mingling they offer a spectrum of strategies in response to stimuli ranging from optimal states of co-activation to either a withdrawal or increased activation of one of these branches for a continuum of control of the target organ.[1]

The heart demonstrates this variety of activation between the SNS and PNS, including: simultaneous activation of the SNS and PNS; reciprocal activation/ inhibition of each branch; co-inhibition of both.[2] This complexity allows for a fine tuning of response and ability to adjust to the various circumstances of the individual.[3]

A more general and systemic example of this interaction of the SNS and PNS can be illustrated through the image of driving your car and having another car turn in front of you in an intersection. You can feel your heart "jump" on and start to race. You put on the brakes, swerve and avoid a collision. Phew! Gradually, with some breathing, your heart slows as the SNS deactivates and the PNS reactivates. Had you actually had a collision, it is likely that in that moment, both high SNS and PNS were activated, called a "freeze" response, and if really severe, PNS may then exceed SNS and put you into complete "collapse" and loss of consciousness.

## The ANS as a systems-wide communicator for self-regulation and resilience

The ANS is key for systems-wide communication between the body and brain. It serves to both mobilize and restore the systems of the body with its vast connections to many bodily systems including: cardiovascular, respiratory, endocrine, digestive and immune. Consequently, the ANS is uniquely situated to assess, integrate and create a unified response for both mobilization and a return to restoration to help regulate the system in response to inner and outer stimuli.[4]

The idea of regulation, and more accurately self-regulation, indicates the conscious ability to maintain stability of the system by managing or altering responses to threat or adversity.[5] The ability to self-regulate is often described as *bidirectional* with both top-down (neurocognitive-focused) and bottom-up (somatic-focused) processes vital in moving from activation to restoration in response to inner and outer stimuli in a healthy manner.[6]

### ACTIVITY

Sitting or lying down, either close your eyes or create a soft focus. Notice the sensations in your body—places where there may be tension, tightness, stress, relaxation or openness. Notice your thoughts and emotions—the quality, speed, intensity.

> Top-down (neurocognitive-focused) example: Bring a visualization or word that brings a sense of ease, peace, comfort. Focus on that image or word and even begin to notice where you might feel the sensations in your body—what is the texture, form, color or effect of that intention? As you allow the energy of this intention to move into and through you, notice what happens to what you had felt in your body earlier—how does this interact with the places of tension, tightness, stress, relaxation or openness? How does this alter the quality of thoughts or emotions?
>
> Bottom-up (somatic-focused) example: Find a movement that brings into your body something that is needed or wanted—it could be something that soothes or relaxes the body or something that invigorates or grounds. It can be a single movement, a rhythmic flowing movement, a standing posture or a relaxing posture—that would fit your intention, needs or qualities that you want to cultivate. Practice that movement or posture for a few moments. Notice how this may alter the sensations of stress, tension or tightness in the body. Notice how this may alter the quality of thoughts and emotions.

The idea of self-regulation includes working with and managing the various components of the individual's response to psychophysiological challenges or adversity such as ANS activation, thoughts, emotions or behavior.[7] Working to improve self-regulatory strategies is thought to improve health and wellbeing in diverse conditions such as: irritable bowel syndrome, neuro-degenerative conditions, chronic pain, anxiety, depression and post-traumatic stress disorder (PTSD).[8]

This chapter will focus on the regulation of the ANS and its concomitant effects for physical, psychological and behavioral health. Regulation of the ANS involves balancing activation of the SNS and PNS such that the person can meet challenges and return to a state of homeostasis for healing, growth and restoration.[9] Resilience is significant to the discussion of regulation, as it signifies a timely response to challenges such that the individual's physical and psychological resources are conserved.[10] Resilience includes a unified response to stress that includes regulation of psychophysiological and biobehavioral components.[11] It is thought that ANS dysregulation plays a part in compromised resilience.[12] Additionally, compromised resilience has been linked to diminished management of chronic pain.[13]

## ANS dysregulation and pain

Before we move into a more detailed discussion of the ANS, it is helpful to look at the clinical picture of the relationship between chronic pain and ANS dysregulation. Here are some current understandings.

- Autonomic dysregulation can mean: excessive *or* insufficient sympathetic *or* parasympathetic dominance—meaning any state of relative imbalance, especially if prolonged.

- Imbalance between the SNS and PNS is considered to play a role in chronic pain conditions as it represents a dysregulated system with loss of adaptive function.[14]

  – There are possible associations between ANS dysregulation and nervous system sensitization.[15]

  – ANS dysregulation has been associated with pain intensity.[16]

- Chronic pain conditions such as fibromyalgia, rheumatoid arthritis, headache and irritable bowel syndrome include various expressions of autonomic dysregulation.

  – Fibromyalgia patients have demonstrated persistent ANS hyperactivity at rest and hyperactivity during stress.[17]

Autonomic dysregulation in chronic pain may be a part of the pathogenesis, a biomarker or a combination of the two.[18] It may be that chronic pain is the stressor leading to ANS dysregulation and diminished resilience or that ANS dysregulation itself contributes to the development of chronic pain through diminished resilience (see Figure 6.1).[19] Yet as shown in this diagram, the interactions are complex and bidirectional.

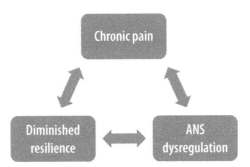

*Figure 6.1 Cyclical relationships between pain, autonomic nervous system, resilience*

## Connectivity and interdependency between nociceptive, visceral and autonomic input

There are many places within the nervous system structures where nociceptive, visceral and ANS input converge and may interact for the modulation, integration and response to inner and outer stimuli. In addition, it is suggested that a central network may assist in the unified autonomic, affective, motor and behavioral response to nociceptive, visceral and ANS input.[20] Places of convergence and possible interactions include:[21]

- spinal and trigeminal horns
- brainstem
- hypothalamus
- amygdala
- thalamus
- insular cortex.

## The vagus: an important link in pain?

The role of the vagus nerve as both a link between and way to affect change in the body, mind and behavior is not new. The writing of pioneers such as Darwin, Bernard, Cannon, James and Pert represent an evolution in thought and science that has viewed the vagus nerve as an important pathway in understanding the larger neurophysiological connectivity between physiology, psychology and behavior.

Some important considerations about the vagus and pain include the following.

- The vagus nerve carries sensory (afferent) and motor (efferent) fibers for both visceral and somatic tissues.

  - Approximately 80 percent of vagal fibers are sensory and are responsible for carrying information about the internal bodily state to the brain.[22] Information from the vagus nerve arrives at and is processed by the hypothalamus, the central structure responsible for regulating ANS activity—largely outside of conscious awareness. Due to bidirectional cortical communications with the thalamus (which is responsible for sensory integration, motor integration, arousal levels, pain modulation, emotion, memory and behavior) as well as with regions associated with self-referential processes (conscious awareness, pre-frontal cortices), portions of this afferent vagal information can be brought into the field of conscious attention—especially with training in body awareness.

  - Approximately 20 percent are motor and are responsible for transmitting the parasympathetic response of the heart, respiration, digestion and inflammation as well as somatic control of muscles related to hearing, voice control, swallowing and breath control.

» The motor component stems from two brainstem nuclei—the dorsal motor nucleus (DMN) and the nucleus ambiguus (NA)—with two different functions, as will be discussed below in the "Framework for connecting physiology, emotion and behavior: polyvagal theory" section.

- Vagal afferents play a part in the facilitation or inhibition of nociceptive input as they converge with nociceptive input along the path of the spinal cord and brain structures.[23]

- The vagus nerve may modulate and affect pain through projections sites to the insula, thalamus, amygdala and prefrontal cortex.[24]

- The vagus nerve may also modulate and affect pain through anti-inflammatory and immune effects.[25]

- The psychological impacts and interpretation of pain are a significant component of the pain experience. The vagus nerve has been shown to have influence on attention modulation and emotion regulation.[26]

- Vagal nerve stimulation has demonstrated an anti-nociceptive effect via its influence on the nucleus tractus solitarius, locus coeruleus and raphe nuclei and their ability to activate descending inhibitory neurons in the spinal cord, and influence on neuropeptides such as GABA, serotonin and endorphins and their receptors.[27]

- Greater vagal regulation of the heart—measured through heart rate variability as an index of parasympathetic control of the heart—has been shown to correlate with higher resilience to stress; differential activation in brain regions that regulate responses to threat appraisal; interoception (defined below); emotion and attention regulation; greater flexibility to respond to challenges.[28] Yoga practices for greater vagal regulation will be described later in the chapter. Other practices such as slow rhythmic/paced diaphragmatic breathing, humming, chanting and meditation have also been found to have an effect on enhancing vagal regulation or parasympathetic control of the heart.

- A close association has been found between lower vagal regulation and poor self-regulation; less behavioral flexibility; adverse health outcomes including increased mortality in diseases such as lupus, rheumatoid arthritis and trauma; chronic pain conditions such as fibromyalgia, musculoskeletal pain (including low back, neck, shoulder, pelvic), irritable bowel syndrome (IBS), headaches and rheumatoid arthritis.[29]

## The unique make-up of the vagus

The vagus nerve serves as a structural and functional bidirectional channel of communication between the viscera and the brain. This visceral awareness influences and is vital to the expression of emotions as well as for the concept of intuition. Along with the above-mentioned convergences with other neural processes, such as nociception, the vagus can be conceptualized as a vital link in the interdependence between body-wide physiology, emotions and behavior.[30]

The concept of interoception is significant to understanding the role of the vagus in regulation, resilience and the experience of pain. As mentioned above, the majority of the fibers comprising the vagus nerve are sensory. Therefore, the vagus is responsible for the transmission of much of the interoceptive input that is received by the brain from the body.

Interoception includes: the process of conveying information from the viscera; the receiving and integration by brain structures and connections; the pathways that enact a response by the human system; the emotional and cognitive perceptions of the individual.[31] This process of receiving, interpreting and responding to information—including bodily sensation, emotions and thoughts—can help us to clarify and refine our understanding of the relationship between sensation, emotion and autonomic state.[32] As a person becomes more accurate in sensing, interpreting and processing bodily and affective states, the greater their adaptability, capacity for self-regulation and resilience in restoring a state of homeostatic balance.[33]

With such an extensive and multifaceted capacity, the vagus is well situated to assist in the broad goal of regulation and resilience of the system, including in pain states.[34] Influencing the underlying autonomic neural state of the individual through vagally mediated pathways may contribute to altering the individual's experience of and response to physical and emotional stimuli including both nociception and the pain experience itself.

## Framework for connecting physiology, emotion and behavior: polyvagal theory

The vagus nerve, as a conduit for both interoception and the formation of an integrated motor response, is central to polyvagal theory (PVT).[35] PVT describes the connections between physiological state, processes of the mind and behavioral attributes emerging from the establishment of underlying ANS platforms.[36] As a result, the capacity to shift physiological state, including ANS "platforms" (which is a simplified construct for core ANS circuits and relative patterns of activation) enables the accessibility and emergence of different psychological and behavioral attributes.[37]

Neuroception, described as the subconscious detection of safety or danger in the environment, influences underlying ANS platforms with its concomitant and integrated effect on physiological, psychological and behavioral states.[38] Interoception can be seen as part of the process of neuroception as it takes into account information from the viscera. This detection of safety or danger in the internal and external environment is important in the pain experience, as it affects physiological response—including homeostatic processes influencing self-regulation and resilience—as well as healthy, adaptive psychological and behavioral responses to inner and outer stimuli.

PVT moves beyond a bimodal construct of the ANS with the PNS and SNS. PVT describes three distinct "neural platforms" and five global states arising from their co-mingling and co-activation with integrated physiological, emotional and behavioral characteristics.[39] These neural platforms are hierarchically activated in response to perceived threat or safety in the environment and are named for their characteristic behaviors.

The experience of pain is inherently based on the psychobiological construct of threat, fear or danger and the organism's drive for safety and survival. PVT presents a theoretical view of these behavioral drives that can aid understanding pain as an adaptive, protective defense mechanism. The addition of yogic theory assists in moving beyond the necessary reduction of the complexity of pain to any one neural structure, while still underscoring the importance of these biological substrates.

## Three neural platforms and five global states
### 1. Social communication/the ventral vagal complex (VVC)
This neural platform includes the vagus nerve, along with the motor components of the glossopharyngeal nerve, spinal accessory nerve, trigeminal nerve and facial nerve. This integrated network slows the heart to a resting state and controls the muscles of the head, face, middle ear, pharynx and bronchi.

This neural platform is named social communication, as it connects visceral state, facial expressivity, receptive and expressive domains of communication and mechanisms for monitoring external and internal conditions. It is theorized to be associated with optimum functioning in the presence of the detection of safety where prosocial behaviors and positive psychological states fostering human connection and engagement, such as compassion and love, are suggested to be more likely to emerge. In addition, this state of optimal functioning may provide a stronger physiological foundation for a flexible and adaptive response to stress, including regulation and resilience of the system.[40]

## 2. Defensive mobilization/sympathetic nervous system (SNS)

This neural platform is the aforementioned SNS, "fight or flight" response. When the VVC fails to detect safety in the environment and/or threat is perceived, mobilization of this protective system is initiated. This sets the stage for responding to real or perceived danger in the environment and toward the goals of safety and survival.

The emotional and behavioral attributes most likely to emerge from this neural platform are related to fear, anger or anxiety as the person orients to real or perceived threat in the environment—such as the experience of pain.

## 3. Defensive immobilization/dorsal vagal complex (DVC)

This neural platform represents the component of the vagus nerve responsible for a dramatic slowing and inhibition of the systems to the least amount necessary for survival. This pattern of activation is proposed to arise from the detection of immense danger or terror and, while adaptive like the SNS, may be considered the most primitive or passive response to stress.

The emotional and behavioral attributes associated with this neural platform include a spectrum of immobilization, shutdown or disembodied and dissociative states including death-feigning, collapse, "freeze" and loss of consciousness.

## 4. Safe mobilization/co-activation of VVC and SNS

This state is proposed to arise from the co-activation of the VVC and the SNS. It is termed safe mobilization, as it is present in circumstances such as play, dance, exercise and creative thinking. The VVC creates a foundation of safety, while the SNS mobilizes the body's resources for healthy and desirable demands.

The emotional and behavioral attributes associated with this co-activation include those of creativity and activity where the system is mobilized while maintaining positive emotional and prosocial states. This safe mobilization is important in fostering regulation and resilience. Yoga practices that utilize active postures while promoting calm states, experiences of connection and calm breath are an example of this state.

## 5. Safe immobilization

This state is proposed to arise from the co-activation of the DVC and VVC. It is termed safe immobilization, as it is present in circumstances such as childbirth, conception and nursing where the VVC promotes a foundation of safety while the DVC generates a safe immobilization of the system. It has been shown that the same circuits may be co-opted for different purposes in the presence of different neurotransmitters, for example oxytocin in this example, versus vasopressin in an adaptive freeze response to threat.[41]

In response to perceived threat or safety in the environment, one of these neural platforms is activated with its concomitant and connected physiological, emotional and behavioral attributes.[42]

When safety is perceived, a unified state of physiological restoration may be fostered. Positive emotions such as peace or calm and behaviors of connection and compassion are made more accessible or likely to emerge. When the defense strategy of the SNS is activated, an integrated physiological, emotional and behavioral strategy for the mobilization of resources to respond to demand emerges. When the defensive immobilization strategy of the DVC is implemented, the combined physiological, emotional and behavioral strategies for active responses are inhibited.[43]

Understanding how the underlying neural platforms relate to and are a part of concurrent physiological, emotional and behavioral characteristics—and the influence of vagal regulation on these processes—offers a novel approach to exploring both the contributors and possible interventions for pain conditions. Through learning to identify and shift autonomic states we may be able to affect an underlying component of pain as has been proposed in conditions such as IBS or fibromyalgia.[44]

## Yoga and regulation of the ANS

A growing body of research supports yoga practices for autonomic regulation, positive influence on ventral vagal nerve activity, interoceptivity and positive psychological and behavioral states. These findings include yoga's effect on the following.

- ANS regulation has been demonstrated as a result of yoga with various populations—including individuals experiencing pain. This has been measured through heart rate variability as an index of increased PNS activation on the heart.[45]

- Improvement in interoception—including the construct of body awareness.[46]

- Improved psychological resilience, and self-concept, and lessening of dysfunctional coping mechanisms.[47]

- Combined effects that benefit attention, affect and ANS regulation.[48]

- Emergence of attributes such as compassion and eudaimonic wellbeing.[49]

Theoretical mechanisms describe yoga as a comprehensive framework that includes both top-down (neurocognitive-focused) and bottom-up (somatic-focused) practices that cultivate self-regulation and resilience for physiological and psychological health and wellbeing.[50]

## Philosophical context of yoga for ANS regulation and resilience

*The Self is the source of abiding joy.*

*Taittiriya Upanishad*

To understand the application of yoga for ANS regulation and resilience, it is essential to look at the philosophical perspective and worldview that forms its context. Yoga teaches the realization of awareness from which the individual experiences attributes such as tranquility, unwavering connection and equanimity. The person in pain can discover an aspect of their experience whereby they encounter the rising and falling of bodily sensation, thoughts, emotions, beliefs and worldly stimuli without overly identifying with them.

The recognition of an underlying abiding equanimity amidst the fluctuating stimuli of the body, mind and world can create a broadening of the field of attention and a larger context for the experience of, and reaction to, sensation. Learning to shift attention and focus to the various sensations that are present in any moment and are concurrent with the experience of pain may help the individual in the alleviation of their suffering.

The systematic methodology of yoga practices orients the person toward this realization of awareness with its concomitant equanimity. Thus, it is important that yoga practices are undertaken within the whole of this cohesive and synergistic framework that they arose from.

Vital to this realization is the discrimination between those aspects of experience that are constantly changing from those that are unchanging and immutable. A methodology of inquiry is taught to differentiate these concepts of the changing from the unchanging. Prakriti is the term that encompasses all malleable and fluctuating components of the body, mind and environment. Purusha represents an aspect of the unchanging experience of awareness through which unwavering equanimity arises. Purusha may be conceptualized as the "Observer of the observed," the Self or source of being and consciousness itself. An essential step of the yogic process is this differentiation between prakriti—that which is constantly changing—and purusha—that which is constant and unchanging.

To understand prakriti, and separate it from purusha, three substrates known as gunas are defined that combine and work together to create the various manifestations of body, mind and world. These are termed sattva, rajas and tamas, and each is responsible for the emergence of physiological, psychological and behavioral attributes as follows.

- **Sattva**: Clarity, illumination, calmness.

- **Rajas**: Activity, mobilization, agitation.

- **Tamas**: Form, stability, inertia.

Everything that is prakriti is comprised of these gunas in varying proportions, including each individual's body and ego (personality, psychological content, "self"). As such, the person can step back and inquire into any stimuli of the body, mind or world to explore the gunas of which it is comprised. This determination of sattva, rajas and tamas assists in the understanding of the aspects of experience that are impermanent—prakriti—from those that are unchanging—purusha.

When the gunas are in balance, healthy body and mind states are supported. Sattva provides vitality, health, contentment and ease; rajas provides enthusiasm, motivation and mobilization of systemic processes such as digestion; tamas provides stillness, stability, focus and strength.

Rajas and tamas are taught as the most likely potential sources that obstruct one from the realization of awareness and the concomitant unwavering equanimity. Rajas when unbalanced by the other gunas underlies and promotes states of activation such as fear, anxiety and anger. Tamas when unbalanced underlies and promotes states of delusion, obscuration, numbness, depression and fatigue. Sattva can also manifest in unbalanced forms as unhealthy detachment and avoidance and "addicts one to joy" (*Bhagavad Gita* 14.9).[51]

## EXPERIMENT: JOURNAL AND MEDITATION

Sitting or lying down, take a few moments to settle in and bring your attention to the breath. Create an intention—visual image, word, affirmation—that brings a sense of safety or calm.

Then bring your attention to a bodily sensation, thought, emotion or life situation—something that you want to inquire into or are working with.

As you bring your attention to this—notice any bodily sensations, thoughts, emotions, beliefs, awareness of relationship with others or life in general that emerge. Notice if you can bring your attention here and still stay connected to the intention of safety or calm.

Begin to look at and tease apart the aspects of your experience in the body, mind, relationship to others or life that are made up of the qualities of:

- **sattva**: clarity, calm, illuminating

- **rajas**: activity, activation, agitation

- **tamas**: stability, obscuration, fatigue.

What aspects of bodily sensations, thoughts, emotions, beliefs or relationships are clear and calm; agitated or activated; stable, dull or fatigued?

Notice how these three qualities of experience of the gunas rise and fall—fluctuate—from moment to moment. Also notice the potential to experience an underlying or overarching abiding and steadfast equanimity that can simultaneously observe, allow and experience.

## The importance of sattva and of mastering the gunas

Sattva is emphasized at the beginning of a practitioner's practice as it offers a glimpse into the experience of what arises from realization of awareness. This is of particular importance to working with the person experiencing pain. Offering an experience of equanimity, tranquility, peace, ease or connection alongside the experience of pain has the potential to shift and broaden the individual's perspective and to create a different relationship to sensation. These sattvic experiences are key to helping people in pain find renewed capability and inspiration for wellbeing.

While sattva is a positive experience, it is still a guna and part of prakriti, which will inherently change—it is a fleeting occurrence. As such, yoga teaches that beyond sattva is a steadfast joy and unwavering equanimity that comes from being firmly established in awareness. This realization of awareness enables the person to experience the rise and fall of the gunas and the shifting phenomena of the body, mind and world and stay connected to a sense of peace within. It is this understanding that enables access to equanimity within the pain experience.

> *as the mountainous depths of the ocean are unmoved when waters rush into it, so the man unmoved when desires enter him attains a peace that eludes the man of many desires... (Bhagavad Gita 2.70)*[52]

In the *Bhagavad Gita*, Krishna explains that the person who "transcends" the gunas finds a capacity for unwavering equanimity without preference for any guna (14.21). Being situated in the recognition of awareness, the person is able to watch the movement of the gunas without becoming overwhelmed or misidentified with them. The person finds the capacity to be content amidst the variable and opposite realms of experience such as suffering/joy; blame/praise; honor/disgrace (14.22–27).

It is this equanimity beyond the gunas that creates a resilience to life. Being able to watch the gunas without becoming them enables the person to remain at peace and develop a healthy relationship to the ever-changing stimuli of the body, mind and world.

This is of particular importance in working with pain. As one aspect of pain self-management, the person in pain learns to find access to equanimity through sattva and then to remain firmly established in that peace or ease alongside their pain. From this vantage point, the person can inquire into how to change their relationship to pain and to the physical sensations, emotions, thoughts and circumstances that co-mingle and contribute to the experience of pain. The person becomes able to explore the gunas that underlie the experience of pain and to experience the myriad fluctuations of body, mind and world while connected to equanimity.

## Relationship of the gunas and neural platforms

Both PVT and yoga provide a framework from which to understand the connection of physiological, emotional and behavioral processes. Through affecting these underlying neural platforms (PVT) or gunas (yoga), there is potential for unified shifts within the interconnected domains of physiology, emotion and behavior. For the person experiencing pain, yoga serves as a guide for exploring the connectivity and relationships between physiological states, the physical and social environment, emotions, cognitions and behavior—while simultaneously teaching powerful tools for regulation and resilience.

The gunas and neural platforms can be conceptualized to share certain attributes. As such, it is suggested that the gunas and neural platforms can influence the accessibility, likelihood and/or activation of one another. When a guna predominates (such as sattva), certain neural platforms are likely to become activated (social communication–VVC). Likewise, when a neural platform is activated (social communication–VVC), certain gunas may become predominant (sattva). While this explanation is reduced as a way to break the concepts apart, in reality the relationship between the gunas and neural platforms as synchronous and parallel processes is likely more accurate.

This relationship is further described as follows:

### 1. Social communication/sattva guna

The behavioral and emotional attributes that are described as emergent from this neural platform and guna include: connection; steadfast peace, happiness or joy; compassion; equanimity; contentment.

## 2. Safe mobilization (SNS and VVC)/
## rajas in balance with sattva and tamas

Just as the SNS provides a mobilizing and activating force within the container of the VVC for play and creativity, raja guna promotes activity and excitement within a base of sattva for clarity and tamas for stability. These co-activated states (of neural platforms and/or gunas) allow the person to experience the mobilization needed for creativity and right action within a container of clarity and stability. In other words, rather than the SNS or rajas overwhelming and creating disturbance to the system, they are positive, motivating forces for change, action and creativity.

## 3. Defensive mobilization (SNS predominance)/raja predominance

The description of what emerges from this neural platform and guna includes fear, anxiety, or anger as the person orients toward safety and responds to real or perceived threat or danger. This neural platform, or guna, provides a continuum of mobilization from well-adapted responses to threat in the environment to maladaptive reactions—such as ANS dysregulatory states of SNS predominance with its adverse effects on the systems of the body.

## 4. Safe immobilization (VVC and DVC)/
## tamas in balance with rajas and sattva

Just as when the VVC and DVC co-activate, there is the emergence of bonding and intimacy—tamas guna promotes stability and stillness within a container of mobilization of body and mind resources (rajas) and insight (sattva). This integration of tamas with the other gunas enables the discipline needed to notice habitual patterns that contribute to the pain experience, as well as the focused work needed for change. In addition, the container of the VVC can ensure that tamas or DVC does not overwhelm the system into dissociative states or shutdown.

## 5. Defensive immobilization (DVC)/tamas predominance

The description of what emerges from this neural platform and guna includes delusion, inertia, obscuration and fatigue. While this can be a well-adapted response to extreme threat, it can also become maladaptive when it overwhelms the system or is maintained for prolonged times. In a recent theory paper, Kolacz and Porges looked at the plausibility of this neural platform held over time as a contributor to chronic disease states such as IBS and fibromyalgia.[53]

With these shared emergent attributes, it is plausible that by cultivating one (neural platform or guna), the other becomes more accessible or apparent. Sattva predominance would help enable VVC activation and VVC activation would enable sattva predominance.

As such, yoga practices can be oriented to influence the gunas and their neurophysiological correlates as conceptualized in relationship to the PVT platforms. Moreover, yoga teaches the capacity to experience the continuously shifting platforms and gunas while continuing to connect to unwavering equanimity through the realization of awareness. This construct has implications for influencing the mind-body relationship to the pain experience.

## Yoga model for regulation and resilience in pain management

A paper that we recently published presented this theoretical convergence of the gunas with PVT to demonstrate yoga as a model for regulation and resilience.[54] This theory can similarly be understood and applied to helping manage or mitigate the experience of pain with emphasis on the following.

- Importance of helping to downregulate the SNS by facilitating sattva guna and the VVC neural platform. This may help strengthen the capacity for the person to discover calm, restorative states of the body and mind.

- Facilitating capacity to move between neural platforms and guna states, as well as fostering the ability to return to sattva and the VVC. This can assist learning to shift from distressing states within the pain experience toward states of ease more readily. Through repeated practice of accessing sattva or VVC, the client is empowered in their ability to relax their body and find calm states of mind.

- Widening the range of safe mobilization and safe immobilization by increasing the accessibility to sattva guna and VVC neural platforms amidst the experience of pain. This can facilitate a capacity to experience both pain and equanimity simultaneously. By becoming situated in sattva and VVC, clarity and insight into habitual ways of responding to body, mind and worldly stimuli that perpetuate pain may be discovered. For example, the person may discover chronic tensions, ways of holding their postures, reactions to bodily sensations, thoughts or emotions that contribute to their pain. This insight may empower the client to create healthier and more adaptive responses to physical sensations, thoughts, beliefs and life situations such that pain is alleviated or lessened. Resilience of the system is built as the person is able to more adeptly respond to stimuli and return to states of physical and mental restoration.

- Working with the idea of "transcending" the gunas and the impermanent and continuously shifting neural platforms whereby a foundation of unwavering equanimity emerges. Ultimately, this can enable the client to reduce identification with the embodied experience of pain, see it as both a teacher and a catalyst for transformation and thus cultivate a greater sense of stability, purpose or meaning. The person learns to nonjudgmentally observe and experience the gunas and neural platforms while connected to this equanimity. What emerges is a different way to be in relationship with pain itself and the very phenomena of life which may perpetuate pain. Over time, it also becomes possible for the client to shift the interpretation of sensations such that the perception of pain changes and the person is able to maintain equanimity within a pain experience.

## Practices of yoga

The practice of yoga provides both a lens through which we can explore pain and its interconnections with neural platforms and gunas, and a process through which to influence neural platforms, gunas and pain.

This reciprocal relationship through which gunas and neural platforms affect one another offers a lens through which yoga therapy practices can help to regulate systemic and integrated physiological systems, facilitate resilience and change the experience of pain. When yoga is practiced as a comprehensive system—movement, breathing, meditation, ethical principles—it combines both top-down (neurocognitive-focused) and bottom-up (somatic-focused) processes through yama/niyama, pranayama, asana and meditation.[55] When practiced as this cohesive system, yoga can be oriented toward the influencing of gunas and neural platforms for concurrent effect on physiological, psychological and behavioral health and wellbeing.

It is important in this perspective that yoga practices are not broken apart where asana is performed for "musculoskeletal imbalance," pranayama for "ANS downregulation" or meditation for "attention or focus." Rather, the practices are combined to optimize the relationships within the gunas and neural platform, such as strengthening the VVC and sattva guna while also creating a stronger therapeutic container to work with the spectrum of rajas/tamas and SNS/DVC. The result is a potential for healthier navigation of mind-body states which may contribute to pain and thus the possible alleviation or mitigation of pain.

These core practices of yoga will be described separately to help illuminate their effect on neural platforms and gunas. Despite this descriptive separation, they are best viewed, implemented and experienced as part of a unified approach to lifestyle as opposed to being discrete from each other.

## Yama and niyama

Yama and niyama serve as ethical intention setting through which the practitioner can begin to investigate how to strengthen sattva and the VVC. Using attributes such as non-harming or contentment, the person can investigate how their emotions, actions and behaviors either build or diminish sattva and VVC states.

These ethical intentions can be used to facilitate mind-body awareness and build sattvic or VVC experiences to create a foundation of ease, peace, safety, connection or restoration. In addition, these qualities can be utilized to change the relationship to other neural platforms or gunas that are part of the pain experience. The person learns to bring the experience of contentment, patience or non-harming to that of fear, pain, anxiety or depression. The potential to both notice the stimuli that activate these other gunas and neural platforms with their physiological, psychological, behavioral attributes and change the relationship to such stimuli can be learned.

The yamas and niyamas are key to this exploration of the habits of body, mind and behavior that perpetuate pain. The person learns to refocus attention to engage with the natural dynamism of life through a different perspective. This practice of deep listening, thoughtful sharing and enacting compassion for self and other in relationship is seen as supportive of VVC-related prosocial processes including cultivation of resiliency.[56] Ultimately, the person becomes able to experience rajas/tamas and SNS/DVC while simultaneously working with the intentions to experience sattva/VVC and/or the equanimity of awareness.

## Asana and pranayama

Pranayama such as alternate nostril breath or elongated exhales have been found to activate the PNS, facilitating VVC control of the heart.[57] This downregulation of the ANS promotes VVC/sattvic foundations as well as helping to widen the range of safe mobilization to safe immobilization.

Asana, including restorative practices or gentle flowing sequences, may also help to downregulate the ANS. The person in pain can work with a yoga therapist to find the unique postures or movements that build VVC and sattva.

Asana and pranayama can help the person cultivate sattva/VVC states, as well as building facility with moving in and out of these neural platforms and guna states by changing postures or breath patterns. The yoga mat serves as a "laboratory." For example, certain postures may facilitate learning to activate SNS/rajas while simultaneous use of the breath and yama/niyama balances that activation through accessing VVC/sattva. Such experiential learning enables the client to "train" the system unique to their patterns and needs, including capacity to be present to a wider spectrum of rajas/tamas or SNS/DVC, while still maintaining sattva/VVC; ultimately, the experience of abiding equanimity within.

## *Meditation*

Meditation practices include additional ways to support regulation and resilience of the system and change the relationship to pain. Awareness-building practices, affirmations, mantras, chanting for vocal toning and the exercise of prosody, and visualizations may all be used to support states of calm, equanimity and eudaimonia amidst the pain experience. In addition, yoga helps with resiliency building for future pain, stress, demand or any imbalanced states that may arise through the simultaneous practices of experiencing challenging postures while maintaining breath control, intention and a meditative state.

## Acknowledgements

We would like to thank Stephen Porges, Steffany Moonaz, Laura Schmalzl and Jessica Taylor for the work we did together in creating and publishing the paper "Yoga therapy and polyvagal theory: The convergence of traditional wisdom and contemporary neuroscience for self-regulation and resilience." This paper formed the background for much of what we expanded upon in this chapter in the context of pain.

*Chapter 7*

# Integrating Pain Science Education, Movement and Yoga

NEIL PEARSON

## Editor's note

There are different names for pain education—Explain Pain, Therapeutic Neuroscience Education and Pain Science Education. The content regarding physiology and biology is typically similar, yet some might provide pain education purely with the intention to help patients reconceptualize pain, while others might additionally intend to explain the rationale and benefits of recommended treatment techniques and plan of care. Further, those teaching "pain educators" differ in their instructions for how to use "pain education" as a guide for recovering movement. For example, there is agreement that pain is not an accurate guide for how much to move or exercise, yet disagreement on whether the patient should view pain as inaccurate and as such ignore it during movement or learn to discern it as one of many inaccurate protective mechanisms. These disagreements can be heated between groups. Some also state that the current pain science education is no better than any other process of pain education. To date, there do not appear to be any studies evaluating one type of pain education against others. Maybe we will need to consider that, like all pain care, there is not one best path of pain education. Pitting one against another might divert us from the important understanding that people in pain need to know that we have an understanding of their problem and of how to help. Context is important in therapeutic interventions. The beliefs of health practitioners and of people in pain are context. When a patient believes that their chronic pain or disability is immutable, therapeutic outcomes might be highly different than when both the practitioner and the patient conceptualize pain and pain-related disability as changeable and as an aspect of life over which they have some influence.

≈

Jnana yoga is known as the yoga of wisdom and development of discriminative knowledge. Providing opportunities to consider beliefs about pain and attitudes regarding recovery is an important process when working with people with persisting pain. Both pain science education and yoga, through their techniques and practices, provide repeated experiences through which the individual can explore and develop a deeper understanding. Having opportunities to think about what we think about pain can enhance wisdom and discriminative knowledge. This chapter will specifically explore pain science education, contemplative yoga techniques and movement practices as diverse educational opportunities for people in pain—and as vital treatment components of non-pharmacological pain management.

## Education is pain treatment

Knowledge is enlightening. It can be the foundation for change. Without it, we might not believe that change is possible, that pain can be changed and that both pain and pain-related disability are impermanent. Believing we already know what needs to be known, we stand our ground. We don't question our approach to daily activity, exercise or recovering movement, even when our approach is not leading to our desired improvements. If we are lucky, we might receive the expertise of someone who asks us to consider a different path, or maybe one might call it a detour in which the first step is taking the time to think about what we think about pain. Through a new perspective or different lens, we can acquire new knowledge and see more possibilities and new paths, and we can experience optimism that change and even changes in pain are possible.

Knowledge itself can change behavior. It can change how we think, how we relate to ourselves and how we act in the world. This is true for the knowledge we gain from health practitioners. Yet not all knowledge is the same. Whereas knowledge of tissue pathology can perpetuate disability,[1] knowledge of pain physiology can increase perceived and measured function[2] and decrease pain.[3] Some knowledge is passed on through verbal or written education, other knowledge is acquired by introspection and contemplation and still other knowledge is experienced through movement or the courage of trying something new combined with the grace of a positive result.

Education is a powerful treatment for people in pain. Yet similar to the lived experience of pain, the experience of acquiring knowledge is complex and individual. The practices of yoga, the experiences of movement and pain education are discussed here as conceptual change education and as treatments to improve outcomes for people in pain.

While writing this chapter and considering educational strategies addressing "the body" and others addressing "cognitions," it has been difficult to avoid dualistic language. We experience life dualistically, yet we are unitary. Pain is pain, and a human is a human. We can pull pain, or an individual, apart to understand them better. We can reduce the individual, the nervous systems, the brain and the atom to their component parts to study them. Pain is often considered from its sensory, cognitive and emotional aspects. The person can be considered from body, mind and spirit, and bio-, psycho-, socially. Yet we must endeavor to remember the unitary nature of each. This concept is as important in pain management as in understanding pain and people in pain, and it should be considered whenever we discuss pain.

Pain management is an equally important term to consider. A large body of basic science supports that pain itself can be changed, while many scholars/clinicians argue that a focus on changing pain can maintain a powerful conceptual limitation—until the pain decreases, I will not be able to improve my function or quality of life. Pain management as written in this chapter includes therapies intending to change ease of movement *and* quality of life *and* pain, while concurrently providing therapies to assist individuals in adapting to and coping with ongoing pain, impairment and ability.

## Jnana yoga

"Jnan" is knowledge; a cognitive event and a conscious experience.

Jnana yoga is considered the yogic path of knowledge. It is a path to less suffering, through using the mind to uncover truth behind the mind.[4] Distinguishing between illusion and reality, self and non-self, and permanent and transitory, Jnana yoga is considered the most difficult path to liberation.[5] The reasons for Jnana being the most difficult are not clear. We could ask whether this path involves techniques that are difficult to teach. Maybe fewer individuals have the life experiences that prepare them for this path. The requirement of staying still while contemplating adds an element that might interrupt success. Certainly, for many people with persisting pain, staying still too long is equally aggravating as moving too much. Beyond why it is most difficult, the inference is that Jnana is not equally effective for everyone, as is true of most pain management techniques.

Jnana yoga, using curiosity to explore the mind, the body and the universe, and doubting the reality of thoughts and perceptions, is stated to be the most direct path to truth.[6] Could Jnana be an equally effective path for some individuals in pain? Maybe knowledge and acquisition of wisdom provide an explanation for the dramatic improvements observed in a patient with over a year of intense pain and disability from what was diagnosed as complex regional pain syndrome (CRPS)? His explanation for the suddenly rapid changes was, "I figured out that I didn't need this much pain." Was this individual, who had been practicing mindfulness for many months and participating in a cognitive-behaviorally based pain management program, able to come to a new understanding of himself and his pain, and subsequently experience a remarkable recovery? The skeptical mind suggests something else occurred, yet an intense desire to release suffering, as one might expect in the presence of CRPS, is also vital to the Jnana practitioner.

Jnana yoga has four pillars including this desire to release suffering. The other three pillars are discernment, detachment and six virtues: the ability to remain calm, control over reactions to external stimuli, abandonment of anything not related to one's dharma, perseverance through suffering, faith in one's path and complete concentration/focus.[7] Considering this list, it appears that much prerequisite work is required for the practitioner of this path. Yet for the person in pain, strengthening these pillars and virtues may be exactly what is required. They offer a glimpse into the complex issues individuals face as part of their pain management.

If Jnana yoga is considered a treatment approach, it might also have adverse effects. The Jnana practitioner receives a caution while following this path. Acquiring knowledge without putting it into practice leads to arrogance and a false sense of spiritual pride.[8] Without continued curiosity and discernment, an individual in pain could easily accept the nature of the pain as both an accurate indication of tissue health and a definitive reason for a permanent disability.

Jnana yoga includes three practices—listen, contemplate, meditate.[9] Unlike Raja yoga, there is no physical practice. The practitioner is not encouraged to take the opportunity to listen, contemplate and meditate while moving the body. Rather, when practiced in isolation Jnana yoga is cognitive experience, using the mind as the agent of change. In contrast, within Raja yoga (discussed later), the effects of contemplative practices and kinesthetic experiences combine as change agents. This is not to suggest separation of body and mind, or that one can change the body without changing the mind or vice versa. For many though, the experience that their physical actions have created a difference in their body, that they can move with more ease, might be more powerful than developing a belief that moving with more ease is possible.

Jnana yoga is often not practiced in isolation. Yoga therapy expertise allows the integration of different paths and techniques of yoga, provided to assist the unique situation of the individual. The qualities of Jnana yoga, of curiosity, inquisitiveness and continuing to use the mind to question the illusions and delusions of the mind, are often brought into Raja yoga and yoga therapy. This is immensely important in all pain management. The individual needs to not only learn that the location, qualities and intensity of pain are not accurate indicators of what is happening in the body, but also to stay curious, as these same experiences create protective responses during movement and functional recovery.

When pain persists, increased pain can arise from small mechanical loads. Even movements that the individual knows are not dangerous to the physical body can increase pain. With this in mind, Moseley and Butler offer the effective strategy of the individual asking themselves when pain increases, "Is this dangerous, really?"[10] For some individuals, the answer is "No," and the movement then becomes less painful. Subsequent to a new thought, pain and function have changed. Yet for some, the result is "I know it's not dangerous, but it still hurts the same." This individual needs something more—maybe more time to contemplate or deeper understanding about pain physiology. Or maybe this is a practical example of the warnings to the Jnana practitioner. A deeper understanding is needed. An understanding that somehow surpasses the thought and logic and moves into a lived experience. The addition of repeated experiences in which moving the body doesn't worsen the pain could be an option to make the cognition a reality.

Jnana yoga is a difficult path. Sometimes there seems a disconnect between what is happening cognitively and what is happening physiologically, as if stress can induce fluctuations of body–mind connectivity. A life example is the individual who knows that there is nothing whatsoever dangerous about a brown spot on a banana skin yet experiences all the intense sensations of disgust and panic along with a difficult-to-control desire to either get it or oneself out of the house. Knowing a banana with a brown spot on it is not dangerous might not alter the physiological processes. If not, then changing cognition by itself is not enough to decrease the autonomic protective responses. Something more seems required. The (six) virtues of Jnana yoga provide some guidance. Specifically, the ability to remain calm, to control reactions to external stimuli, to persevere through suffering and to completely concentrate/focus on what we want—all these would be useful strategies that one might practice in order to influence this "brown-spot-bananaphobic" reaction. People with persisting pain are more likely to have fear of increasing their pain or of re-injury or losing their identity, yet much of the guidance of Jnana yoga aligns with techniques taught with interdisciplinary pain management programs. To become skilled in self-regulation, to improve ability to concentrate and to practice these even in the face of suffering may be part of the solution to using the power of cognitions to change autonomic physiology.

Given the importance of the six virtues in finding one's way to less suffering, the path of using Jnana yoga by itself would seem extremely difficult for many people with persisting pain. When pain persists, we can experience low self-efficacy,[11] difficulties in self-regulation[12] of breath, body tension, thoughts and emotions, unusually large reactions to potentially dangerous but low-intensity stimuli[13] and disconnection from life purpose and relationships.[14] Although all these changes might seem barriers to the success of Jnana yoga, the practices of the six virtues may be exactly what the person in pain requires in their path to recovery. Research shows that persisting pain is associated with alterations in body awareness, which could be "treated" with the pillar of discernment.[15] Connections between persisting pain and attachment style might be addressed through the pillar of detachment. As such, Jnana yoga may be both more difficult due to the complex impacts of persisting pain on the individual and an appropriate treatment path for some individuals.

For the individual with persisting pain, being guided to practice only Jnana yoga (or the non-asana aspects of Raja yoga) might be interpreted as ignoring the body or invalidating the pain. Pain, especially what we refer to as musculoskeletal pain, is experienced in the body. Some individuals might conclude that a cognitive practice, discernment and knowledge are not the answer to body pain, or that their pain needs to be addressed through treatment of the body. Others might believe that focusing treatment on the mind proves that the health practitioner believes there is nothing really wrong with them or their body. As such, Raja yoga, and therapies that specifically address the body as a change agent, may be more acceptable for some individuals. Moving the body, and exploration of it during movement, provides additional opportunities and a different lens through which to question beliefs, experiences and attitudes towards pain, the body and recovery.

Before we address using the body as an educational tool, we must consider another body—the significant and growing body of scientific research supporting the benefits of pain education and specifically pain physiology education. This, like Jnana yoga, includes a cognitive approach to pain management, while research indicates it is most effective when combined with movement therapy.

## Pain education

Health professionals typically provide patients with knowledge of relevant information about disease, injury and pain. This knowledge serves a number of purposes: providing a rationale for the prescribed treatment, increasing patient motivation to change behavior to promote recovery, decreasing fear and providing a common language with which to communicate between clinician and patient. In addition, research tells us that when an individual seeks an appointment with a health professional, they typically are looking for answers to four questions.

1. What's wrong?

2. How long will this last?

3. What can the health professional do for the patient?

4. What can the patient do for themselves?

For people with persisting pain, the answers provided by health professionals to these questions have been extremely slow to catch up with our current understanding of pain and treatment of people living in pain. Researchers and health professionals including Butler, Moseley, Gifford, Engle, Melzack, Zuzman, Louw, Jacobs, Blickenstaff to name a few have been influential in much-needed changes in pain education. Even so, patients continue to report receiving outdated explanations about pain, including that pain correlates well with tissue damage, that chronic pain is due to tissues that won't heal and that it is the health professionals' job to fix or cover up the pain. For many patients, answers have been confined to explanations related to tissue damage, scar tissue, degeneration, structural and biomechanical abnormalities and disease processes. These messages have been shown to increase fear.[16] They also negatively impact the subsequent three questions and answers. The patient might not even ask them when she believes the answer to question 1 means "This will never go away as long as this tissue problem lasts," and "If it is degeneration it will do nothing but worsen over time," and "Besides not making it worse, there is nothing I can do but rely on my health professional to fix this or cover up the pain."

For health professionals, answering these questions well requires them to listen to the patient's history and perform an objective examination. Equally important is understanding what the individual might actually be asking and then staying within one's professional scope of practice when we answer.

Each question can be interpreted in multiple ways when we consider the person with persisting pain, as in the following examples.

- "What's wrong?" can be answered by the professional as if the patient asked, "Have you seen people with this problem before?" and "Do you know how to help me?"

- "How long will this last?" can be answered by the professional as if the patient asked, "Do you think this is changeable?" and "How fast do you believe this will change?"

- "What can you do for me?" can be answered by the professional as if the patient asked, "What options do we have?," "How effective are treatments for this?" and "What's the plan?"

- "What can I do to help myself?" is not a question we should expect from most people in pain. Unless the person understands pain, they will likely see no role for themselves. Many believe that pain is a medical problem requiring a medical treatment. As such, our response to this often-unanswered question should begin with a statement to the patient, provided with conviction and compassion: "There are techniques and skills you can learn that will change this as well." This may be doubted, and it is our role to provide evidence to the patient. We can use "Explain Pain education" and "movement as education" to provide proof.

Two other questions we should consider when working with people in pain, especially when considering both Jnana and Raja yoga as treatment, are "How much pain is OK when I move?" and "How am I supposed to move more when pain caused by movement is my problem?" The complexity of pain makes both of these questions difficult to answer quickly and concisely. Simple solutions, such as "Use the pain as your guide," are rarely effective clinically and are not based on our current understanding of pain. More complex answers, aligned with science and with the lived experience of pain, can be found in the following sections.

## Pain science education

Lorimer Moseley wrote in 2007 that there is a need to reconceptualize pain.[17] Equally important is the need to reconceptualize the lived experience of pain and pain management. We need to ask health professionals to "think about what they think" about three things: about pain, about people in pain and about pain management and recovery when pain persists. Pain science education addresses patients similarly, providing them with knowledge with which to understand and potentially reconceptualize their beliefs and attitudes. Yet pain science education is not simply providing patients with information they do not know. Patients "arrive" with beliefs about pain and recovery. Successful pain science education requires new information to be offered that is often contrary to current beliefs. The process must provide new information in a manner that allows individuals to question their established beliefs about pain and their attitudes to recovery.[18] Faced with new information that doesn't match with current beliefs, individuals typically hold tighter to their beliefs, even when the information is provided in a compassionate and skilled approach.

Moseley's early research focused on people with chronic low back pain. He was able to show that the addition of one-to-one pain science education to standard physical therapy (PT) treatment provided superior outcomes in pain and perceived disability and that these changes persisted at one-year follow-up (2002).[19] In a 2003 paper he also showed that patients retained knowledge of pain neurophysiology for months after it was provided.[20] One possible explanation for this is that the knowledge was useful, that learning about how pain "works" sticks with the patient because the information can be used in life to move with more ease and experience less pain. In this same study, Moseley reported that health professionals underestimated the ability of patients to learn pain physiology. This of course remains a significant barrier to the acceptance of pain education. Most health professionals have never witnessed benefits from patients receiving education from a physical therapist. As such, regardless of the extensive research supporting this education as part of an effective pain management plan, many patients do not receive a prescription for it, even over 15 years since his early positive research findings.

Subsequent research using the Explain Pain principles has shown positive effects when provided by educators besides Moseley's team and for people with other chronic pain conditions, including whiplash-associated disorder and fibromyalgia.[21]

Research gaps exist. We do not have clear research findings providing the following:

- cost-effective dose or dosage of this treatment

- comparison of a single education session to shorter multiple education sessions

- ability of individual to generalize knowledge to daily living, to work behaviors and to varying levels of pain

- impact of inconsistencies between pain education and home exercise instructions

- impact of the education on medication use

- impact of the education within interdisciplinary pain management programs

- impact of providing pain education to individuals completing a therapeutic yoga program for pain

- most effective educational strategy or combination of strategies

- impact of adding large group (10+) education sessions in addition to one-to-one education

- how much training in pain science education is required to be an effective educator.

This long list of gaps is not intended to discourage practitioners from learning and using pain science education. However, the last gap is important to consider. One of the most common experiences of practitioners near the beginning of involvement in providing pain science education is receiving feedback that the message heard is that pain is all in the head. As we attempt to "physiologize" pain, it can take considerable practice to provide the education in a manner that clearly states "pain is real" and "it is not made up or all in your head." People in pain have often heard these unhelpful messages before. We should anticipate that they may be vigilant for invalidating messages about pain. With practice, the health professional providing the education can become more focused on adapting their message to the patient's subjective history and behavioral responses to education than to just passing on the correct physiological information.

## "Explaining Pain" process

Pain education differs in some ways between educators and researchers. The following is a summary of key aspects of this education.

- Due to the complexity of pain physiology, effective education requires one-to-one education individualized to the individual's history and presentation.

- One-to-one education can require more than one hour.

- The information provided includes the purpose of pain, the physiology of neurons, synapses, neurotransmitters and signal transmission, spinal facilitation and inhibition and an understanding of how pain is not an accurate indicator of tissue damage, that when pain persists the nervous systems change (neuroplasticity and sensitization) and that it is possible change the nervous systems' and organism's determination of danger (positive neuroplastic changes).

- The education is provided without reference to anatomy or focus on emotional or behavioral aspects of pain.

- The key to helping people reconceptualize pain is to provide the education using metaphors with references to pain experiences we have all endured or know. The use of story allows individuals to learn through an experience. Story is theorized to allow less resistance to new ideas than when told directly that one's understanding of pain is wrong or doesn't match with physiology.

- Verbal education is supplemented with diagrams to help explain certain facts such as neurons, nociception and downregulation.

Recent meta-analysis describes studies showing decreased perception of disability, decreased PCS (pain catastrophizing) scores, changed views towards pacing, changed attitudes towards recovery and some change in views on passive coping with education session lengths between 30 minutes and four hours. Interestingly, neuroscience education plus exercise has shown significant improvements, better than neuroscience on its own.[22] Overall, Louw[23] concludes from evidence that for chronic musculoskeletal pain disorders, there is compelling evidence that an educational strategy addressing the neurophysiology and neurobiology of pain can have a positive effect on pain, disability, catastrophizing and physical performance.

The primary messages of pain science education have similarities with Jnana yoga. Understanding that pain is not an accurate indication of tissue damage[24] is similar to finding the truth behind the mind. We realize through both processes that what we perceive is not necessarily precise information and that the pain we experience is influenced by everything. We learn about pain or contemplate it to know that pain is changeable (impermanent). Then, for most individuals, we must bring our new knowledge into life and into behavioral practice to attain that deeper learning. We experience through living and moving that pain truly is not immutable and that we indeed have the ability to influence it.

The acquisition of new perspectives on pain through pain education is similar to meditation practices and Jnana yoga. The subsequent contemplations in either process also have parallels. The individual, learning that "it's not really that dangerous," is better able to remain calm, to control adverse reactions to innocuous stimuli and to discern noxious and innocuous stimuli. Jnana provides the addition of contemplating one's current situation, including the pain, in relation to one's dharma or purpose in life. It also directly addresses the ability to observe the pain and to remain a detached witness, knowing that pain is part of one's current experience. Both processes can be difficult. They require capacity of the teacher to provide the student with an experience. Each individual is unique. This complexity again reminds us that not all educational strategies or Jnana techniques are equally effective for all individuals.

## Educational and learning styles: doing, observing, listening and reading

Jnana yoga and Raja yoga might be considered as different, based on their educational style or learning style. One provides more cognitive experiences and the other a range of biopsychosocial experiences. To date there are no research reports that discuss whether we should modify either yoga therapy or pain science educational strategies based on the individual's style of learning. In addition, research suggests, at least in children, that we cannot reliably assess an individual's most effective learning style.[25] Yet, since the different paths of yoga suggests different individuals are most suited to a particular path, this concept will be briefly discussed.

Neuroscience highlights that practice and repetition impact learning. Healthcare professionals have considerable practice learning in a lecture format and from reading books and reports. Many of the patients we treat have considerably less practice learning this way and possibly no similar practice since completing school. Our experiences as health professional students may have convinced us that verbal education is most powerful for all. Or we may be convinced that changing cognitions is the most powerful manner through which to change behavior. Yet is information and education alone sufficient for behavioral change? While knowledge is potentially a first step, it is not necessarily enough. Behavioral change is complicated and multifactorial, impacted by internal factors, attitudes, beliefs, motivation, ability, perceived threat, self-efficacy, social norms and sociocultural contexts. This aligns with the view of Jnana yoga as a difficult path and the recommendation to combine pain science education with movement therapy.

Lacking a reliable learning style assessment tool, we can ask our individual patient if he has a preferred learning style. We might even ask if he has noticed a difference depending on what is being learned. For example:

"Do you learn best by…

- doing

- observing another doing

- verbal guidance

- reading instructions?"

"I would like to teach you a mindfulness technique. Do you want me to let you experience it first, tell you how it will help, explain the science behind it or let you read instructions about how to do it?"

"I want to teach you some new things about pain that should help you move with more ease, and that might help decrease your pain. Should I guide you through an experience of this, explain to you why I think this will work, tell you a story of how this has helped another person or let you read instructions about it first?"

When pain persists, there have often been repeated experiences of trying new techniques and regretting it later. An individual's sense of safety, confidence and past experience might impact choice of educational approaches. Written and verbal education might be the safer ways to learn. Yet the lived experience of moving with more ease or of having less pain after a contemplative practice may be required to start to complete or deepen learning. Changing physical experience can be more convincing than changing what we think and believe.

Health professionals have not been taught to consider manual therapies, electrophysical agents or skin-needling techniques as educational tools. The ability of these interventions to change pain and change pain-free movement provides powerful education opportunities. As an example, when application of gentle joint mobilizations to a patient's neck leads to decreased pain and increased rotation movement, this is a perfect time to highlight to the patient, "That's fantastic, your pain changes." And, "Let's see if we can find some exercises or movements you can do to give you the same improved neck movement." By drawing the patient's attention to details of the experience, we convert a positive therapeutic intervention into an educational moment, highlighting that pain can be changed, and the individual can influence pain.

## Education through physical experience

No research reports consider whether people in pain can be effectively educated about pain using movement experiences as the primary educational tool. Experience can be a powerful change agent. During pain science education, patient stories are used as educational tools. Moseley championed these in *Painful Yarns*.[26] When individuals listen to these yarns, they might not notice that they are drawn in, as if experiencing the story and somehow part of it rather than listening to it. The story becomes more real, and often individuals can consider ideas or beliefs through story that they would otherwise resist. Much of the content of pain science education involves providing information that is contrary to individuals' understanding of the body, or pain, and of pain management. Through story, we can provide an experience that is inconsistent with current beliefs about pain and recovery. This is considered a key component of the success of this education. The question then is whether we can effectively use movement as an educational tool. Is education through movement advantageous in some individuals, for example when language or culture are barriers to learning through "listening" or "reading"?

Could we, rather than providing individuals with knowledge of physiology that supports the key messages of pain science education, provide individuals with experiences, both movement and contemplative experiences, that provide evidence supporting these same messages?

- Pain is changeable.

- More movement is possible without aggravating the pain or flaring up the pain even in the presence of tissue changes.

- The location, intensity and quality of pain are not accurate indicators of tissue damage.

- Pain and movement can be modified by the way we breathe.

- Pain and movement can be modified by muscle tension.

- Pain and movement can be modified by our thoughts.

- Pain and movement can be modified by stress and joy.

- Pain and movement can be modified by mindful movement.

The practices of Raja yoga provide an opportunity to explore more deeply the idea of using movement and physical experience as an education agent and of bringing the principles of Jnana yoga and pain education into the body. First though, the benefits of movement for people in pain and as part of pain management will be highlighted.

Persisting pain is associated with changes in practically every aspect of one's existence—relationships, work, identity, self-efficacy, locus of control, ability to tolerate and endure pain, fear of movement, body awareness, body image, breath patterns, muscle tension, the central nervous system, the autonomic nervous system, cognitions, emotions, range of body motion, balance... People in pain often state that pain changes everything. Moving with more ease might have equally broad influences on the individual and can potentially be used to impact many of these changes.

- Movement/exercise has an analgesic or hypoalgesic effect.[27]

- Movement helps us sleep.[28]

- Aerobic exercise is associated with modest improvement in neurocognitive functioning.[29]

- Movement may increase adrenal resilience by stimulating the adrenal glands via the thoracic motor cortex.[30]

- Movement alters proinflammatory and anti-inflammatory macrophages.[31]

- Movement stimulates the chemistry of neuroplasticity.[32]

- The interoceptive and sensory motor activity associated with movement has the potential to decrease distortions in body awareness and body image.[33]

- Movement can decrease anxiety[34] and help lift depression.[35]

Clinically we observe that movement also assists with the following.

- Movement can be used to desensitize to movement and weight bearing.

- Movement can assist with re-establishing one's sense of competence and internal locus of control.

- Movement has a positive impact on work ability, which in turn impacts identity, competence and social connection.

- Movement can help restore quality of life.

The available research evidence does not show superiority of one form of exercise or movement over another. One of my physiotherapy mentors likes to state that the best movement is what the person "will do." Yet once again, given the individual multifaceted nature of pain, and even though there is strong evidence for the benefits of recovery movement, it is difficult to imagine that movement is equally important for everyone's pain management success.

Many people in pain report increased pain as a result of movement.[36] Movements that shouldn't hurt are intensely painful, and then once the movement stops, the pain does not resolve quickly. These are the symptoms of sensitization, and some researchers point out that exercise physiology is not the same in all people with persisting pain.

- Exercise-induced analgesia may be absent in chronic pain,[37] at least in those with central sensitization.

- Pain and inactivity alter immune cells, including macrophages,[38] which produce proinflammatory reactions to increased movement, at least in rodents during the first one to two weeks of beginning to recover increased activity levels after extended periods of inactivity.

- Movement that is stressful can have a negative effect on the gut microbiome,[39] and on adrenaline via dysfunctional hypothalamic pituitary adrenal (HPA) responses.

- Some people with chronic pain have altered stress responses, suggesting they may benefit from more treatment or need to know how to recover from the stress of exercise.[40] It is important to find the optimal amount of stress during movement and recovery processes.

When movement is considered as a treatment for people in pain, like all treatments, adverse reactions are possible. Finding the right dose, the right movement, and layering in other treatments seems necessary for the success of movement as either education or treatment.

## Raja yoga

There are eight aspects to Raja yoga—each described here as separate although they can be practiced in combination with other aspects.

- **Yamas**: How you act in the world.

- **Niyamas**: How you treat yourself.

- **Asana**: Physical postures.

- **Pranayama**: Energy/breath regulation.

- **Pratyahara**: Awareness of inner sensations and experiences.

- **Dharana**: Focus and concentration.

- **Dhyana**: Meditation.

- **Samadhi**: Connecting to the divine and finding peace.

Raja yoga provides opportunities to learn through experience. The techniques practiced can be categorized as awareness, self-regulation and contemplation. Each is practiced in stationary positions and in movement. The practitioner is guided in techniques to assist with awareness of their breath, the sensations they feel in their body, their thoughts and their emotions. Regulation techniques guide in regulation of body, breath, thoughts and emotions while at rest and during positions and movements of varying difficulty. Contemplation techniques and guidance stimulate contemplation of each of these aspects of self, in addition to one's relationship to self and others and behaviors related to these relationships. Although the stated goal of these practices is to diminish suffering and connect to the divine, through repetition of the practices, individuals can learn more about the pain, more about how it interacts with body, breath, thoughts, emotions and relationships and more about one's influence over pain, as well as body, breath, thoughts and emotions. Opportunities and guidance are provided through which to think about what one thinks about pain. One can explore through contemplative experiences whether current thoughts, beliefs and attitudes about pain and pain management match with current experience. Yet this is not all self-guided realization. Yoga therapists guide individuals in techniques they have not considered or attempted before. The individual then gains more tools with which to help them with their pain and how the pain has impacted each aspect of their existence. Now the individual has more options. Yoga has not only shown the individual that it is possible to be more flexible, but has also provided a process through which to continue to improve flexibility.

Movement practices provide another opportunity to educate people in pain that pain can be changed, that movement can be increased. They are a type of Jnana yoga when they help to question the beliefs one holds about the body. They are a form of pain education when practiced as a technique of inquiry, with curiosity about one's own beliefs about pain, movement and the body. The novelty of yoga asana, the generally peaceful setting in which it is provided, the ritual in which the practice is provided, the volume and intonation of the teacher's voice and the permission to stop or modify when desired have potential influence on this process. When we can guide an individual to move without the usual aggravation of pain and let the individual experience that over time ease of movement can be increased, this is an important education agent.

Researchers explain that when there is pain, areas of the brain and processes of the nervous systems and immune system are responding as if there is credible evidence of danger.[41] Given this, pain during movement should be influenced by altering the determination of danger. Using the polyvagal theory as a guide,[42] activities of social engagement such as calming vocalizations and facial expressions, compassionate listening, diminishing muscle tension and slow, calm, rhythmic breathing all engage the parasympathetic nervous system and decrease evidence of danger. Focused attention to increasing the evidence of safety during movement and during asana provides a powerful approach to change and, when successful, to using movement as education.

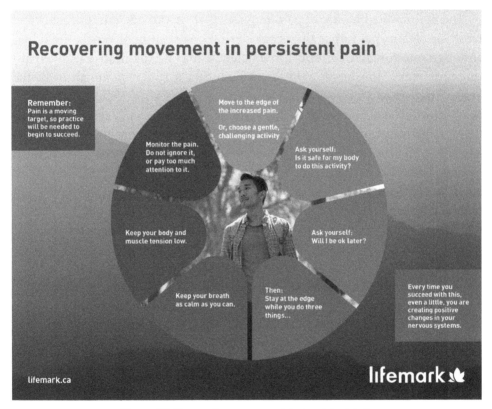

*Figure 7.1 Recovering movement in persistent pain*
Source: Reprinted with permission of Lifemark.

## Integrating pain science education and Raja yoga

There are many ways to integrate pain science education and yoga. One involves educating the practitioner in both pain science and the processes and goals of pain science education. The other is to provide pain science education to the patient prior to or concurrently with yoga. When a practitioner can explain to the person in pain that there is a physiological explanation for their change as a result of a movement or yoga technique, or for why changes have not occurred yet, this can increase motivation, confidence and persistence. Movement and yoga, as self-management techniques, require practice and become more effective with increasing skill. Through an understanding of science, and skill in pain science education, the practitioner can even use the experiences of yoga as a metaphor for teaching some of the key principles of pain science. Some individuals might be hesitant to fully engage in yoga techniques without understanding the physiological and/or psychological rationale first. Others will be less interested or not able to grasp the "how it works" until the experience of moving with more ease is "experienced."

The multifaceted nature of pain requires that we provide multifaceted care. Layering treatments rather than considering one treatment versus the other, although questionable in regard to efficiency, may be the most effective pain care approach. Movement, pain science education and yoga are all evidence based. They are all aspects of pain management, yet they receive less attention in health professional education than the medical, pharmaceutical and hands-on therapeutic interventions. These are the foundations of non-pharmacological pain care. They are also what must continue after the more expensive medical management is discontinued or inaccessible. By providing each of these in an integrated manner, we provide an integrated cognitive-behavioral and potentially biopsychosocial therapy for people in pain.

## Chapter 8

# Breathing and Pranayama in Pain Care

## Shelly Prosko

*Breath is the bridge which connects life to consciousness, which unites your body to your thoughts.*

Thích Nhất Hạnh

We often hear or use the term *just breathe*. When we are suddenly overwhelmed with emotion, we use idioms like "that took my breath away," or write words like "gasp" to describe intense emotions such as awe, fear or surprise. If a child is very upset and crying, or someone has just heard some shocking and tragic news about a loved one, we often notice the breath pattern has visibly changed—where the person may be gasping for air, holding their breath or breathing excessively with a shallow and rapid pattern. We naturally feel inclined to immediately attend to the breath by offering that advice to "just breathe" when we notice a person overwhelmed with emotion or experiencing sudden acute pain that results in a struggling breath pattern. As healthcare providers working with people in pain, we may notice breathing patterns are altered in people experiencing both acute and chronic pain. Conversely, when an individual's breath pattern changes, the person may experience changes in their pain, emotions, movement strategies and overall state of mind.

Intuitively and anecdotally, we likely agree that the breath can be a powerful agent of change and provide us with valuable information about our state of being. But what is science saying about the relationship between respiration and pain? Is there evidence to show that pain results in altered breathing patterns? If so, can changing the breath pattern change pain? What is the research saying about the benefits of yoga breathing practices and can we translate this to people in pain? Are these practices easily accessible and reproducible in the clinic setting? Are there any potential limitations or risk factors of breathing practices? This chapter will explore these questions and the potential role that yoga plays in pain care through breath awareness and regulation practices.

## Pranayama, breathing and breathing pattern disorders

Pranayama, the fourth limb of Raja yoga as discussed in Chapter 4, is commonly described as *breathing practices*. However, this definition falls short of the larger concept of pranayama. The more direct translation of pranayama is to control, regulate or extend the prana (life force or energy) within us. Breathing techniques can be a tool used to direct the prana or energy. In other words, the breath is the steward of the process of extending the life force energy within us.

One of my favorite definitions of pranayama is "the art of learning how to make the most effective use of every bit of air that we breathe in and the prana we absorb."[1] Optimal breathing is not always about breathing *more*; it is about breathing *more efficiently* to match the intent and demands of the current task. This may often mean actually breathing *less*. In fact, over-breathing or hyperventilation is one of the most common breathing pattern disorders (BPDs),[2] and there appears to be a link between hyperventilation (breathing in excess of metabolic demands) and pain, as we will discuss in this chapter.

For the purposes of this chapter, we will be using the terms *yoga breathing practices* and *pranayama* interchangeably. We will also differentiate between breath awareness and regulation practices.

### Breathing

Breathing is a complex system that has numerous functions. The most obvious role of breathing is to move air in and out of the lungs for gas exchange. However, there are many other roles, such as the following examples.

- Voice production requires air passing through the larynx on exhalation.

- Smell requires air passing through the nostrils on inspiration.

- Breathing influences vascular and lymph circulation and gut motility.[3]

- The respiratory diaphragm contributes to regulation of intra-abdominal pressure and is part of the core strategy system—the movement of the diaphragm during breathing influences spinal and rib mobility, movement efficiency, posture and balance strategies.[4]

It has been shown that breathing can also influence aspects of our existence on more than just a biomechanical and anatomical level. For example, the breath:

- is closely linked to interoceptive processing and can inform us of the physiological condition of our body[5]

- may influence and be influenced by our emotions,[6] mental state and cognition[7]

- may influence and be influenced by our autonomic nervous system (ANS)[8]

- can connect our "conscious awareness to the state of body"[9]

- can influence pain.[10]

Conversely, our posture, movement patterns, emotions, thoughts, ANS state and pain can influence breath. Consequently, any changes in breath further contribute to changes in the aforementioned systems, feeding into the complex interaction of breath and many aspects of our existence.

In other words, respiration is a "complex psychophysical system with multiple functions"[11] and can be a powerful agent of change.

Perhaps the breath has the power to influence all koshas and all koshas can influence the breath. What about the link of breath to anandamaya (spiritual kosha)? Many ancient wisdom traditions believe there is a meaningful connection between breath and spirit. Interestingly, the English word "spirit" is derived from the Latin word "spiritus," which means "breath," and the ancient Greek word "pneuma" is translated as "breath" and "soul" or "spirit." Or perhaps it is not so much a *link*; perhaps breath and spirit are one and the same.

The control of respiration is complex and can be voluntary and involuntary. It includes interdependent neural and chemical processes that take place in the periphery, brainstem and higher brain centers. An overview can be found in any respiratory physiology textbook and may be beneficial for the reader who is unfamiliar with these regulatory mechanisms to review.

## Breathing pattern disorders

An appropriate or healthy breath pattern may be defined as the most efficient pattern that uses the least amount of muscular effort and energy in order to meet the metabolic demands of the task for optimal tissue oxygenation. BPDs have been discussed in the literature for decades and are distinct from pathological pulmonary diseases. There is no one agreed-upon definition of BPDs, however a working definition used by Clifton-Smith and Rowley is "Inappropriate breathing which is persistent enough to cause symptoms, with no apparent organic cause."[12] These may include the following patterns: upper chest dominant with chronic overuse of accessory muscles of respiration; dynamic chest hyperinflation, which can result from persistent inadequate exhalations; chronic hyperventilation, which results from breathing in excess of metabolic demands. Over-breathing or chronic hyperventilation is one of the most common BPDs that can lead to hypocapnia or low carbon dioxide arterial pressure ($PaCO_2$) or low-end tidal carbon dioxide (PET $CO_2$), resulting in respiratory alkalosis. Respiratory alkalosis has been shown to induce a sympathetic dominant state in the body, leading to a cascade of responses such as increased muscle tension or spasm, paresthesia, vasoconstriction, ischemia and a reduction in the release of oxygen into the tissues (Bohr effect).[13] This sympathetic dominant state may further contribute to pain, fatigue and anxiety.[14] Instructing people to "take a deep breath" therefore may not always be a helpful cue if this coincides with a rate that leads to over-breathing or hyperventilation.

Capnography can be a practical way to measure PET $CO_2$ clinically; however, it is important to keep in mind that hypocapnia may not necessarily always lead to these symptoms[15] and these symptoms may be present without hypocapnia. There may be other mechanisms contributing to BPDs for people in pain.[16]

The Nijmegen Questionnaire was originally introduced in 1982 to detect patients with hyperventilation symptoms that might benefit from capnography feedback. However, the creators of the questionnaire recently clarified that the Nijmegen score is not indicative of hyperventilation syndrome (HVS) or hypocapnia, rather it can be used as a screening tool for dysfunctional breathing related to subjective complaints of breathing related to stress and anxiety.[17]

"The Nijmegen Questionnaire mainly reflects the subjective, psychic dimension of breathing and its response to stress" and is not used as a diagnostic tool for HVS.[18] The questionnaire can be used to help guide the clinician as to who may benefit from breathing regulation practices.

## Breath awareness versus regulation

It is worthwhile to differentiate between breath awareness and breath regulation practices as there is value in both as they relate to pain care.

### BREATH AWARENESS

Breath awareness is simply noticing the breath without trying to change anything. Awareness practices provide people with a way to practice controlling attention and sustaining focus. A breath awareness practice may consist of observing the following qualities of the breath: the rate, pace and depth; rigid or smooth sensations; the temperature as it enters and exits nostrils; length of inhale versus exhale; if there is a continuous flow or a pause between the inhale and exhale; how the breath moves in the body. The position in which the practice is performed may change the experience for the individual. Try it for yourself! Explore a breath awareness practice in prone versus supine versus sitting.

It is advisable to start in a position and state of rest or relative ease. It can be performed throughout the day (even for one to two minutes). Subsequently, the person will be more aware of how the breath pattern or qualities change when in a position or state of discomfort, such as when performing a movement that hurts. The person can self-evaluate the breath, which may provide information about their current state, like if there is tension in body, mind or emotions.

Breath awareness practices can also give the person an opportunity to start to notice the correlation between breath, tension and pain. This gives them a direct experience of the complexity of pain and can provide them with an experiential form of pain science education. In other words, the person can use breath awareness practices as pain education via direct experience.

## EXAMPLE

Peter* has lived with persistent low back pain for over 20 years. After only one session of a breath awareness practice for approximately three minutes, he discovered later that day that he held his breath every time he bent forward and transferred in and out of his car and from sit to stand. He later noticed that this also coincided with increased muscle tension and guarding around his entire trunk region. After consistently practicing this short breath awareness practice daily for four days, Peter also noticed he held his breath when just thinking about stressful situations and this seemed to correspond with his back pain worsening. He also described a moment when he was angry and frustrated and he noticed his breath was very shallow, rigid and "up in the chest" with muscle tension around his low back and belly. He said it felt like he couldn't get enough air and like he was suffocating. These breath awareness experiences were the first steps required for Peter to understand the value of breath and the link it has to his thoughts, emotions, movement and pain experience.

* Patient's name has been changed to protect confidentiality.

In the *Patanjali Yoga Sutras*, breath awareness is one of the five areas for focusing attention. See Chapter 9 on pratyahara and the science surrounding awareness and awareness practices, which can include breath awareness, for people in pain.

### Breath regulation

*Prachchhardana vidharanabhyam va pranayama.*

*The mind is also calmed by regulating the breath, particularly attending to exhalation and the natural stilling of breath that comes from such practice.*

Yoga Sutra 1.34[19]

Breath regulation is manipulating or controlling aspects of the breath. This may include changing the breath rate, pace or length of inhale and exhale, manipulating one's attention or focus by intentional breath visualization or manipulating breath pattern (abdominal/belly versus costal-lateral or posterior-lateral expansion versus upper chest).

There are many types of breath control practices in yoga. It is beyond the scope of this chapter to describe them all, but the following is a list of some commonly used in the pain research as well as common practices that myself and colleagues often find useful for people in pain: calming and balancing breath practices such as bhramari (bee's); dirga (three-part); nadi shodhana (alternate nostril breathing); abdominal or belly breathing; Longer-Smoother-Softer; prolonged exhalation; and paced slow breathing are commonly used, as well as energizing or "calming alertness" practices such as ujjayi (victorious). The description of many of these practices can be found across yoga literature. We will briefly outline a few below.

Slow-paced breathing (SPB) or deep slow breathing (DSB) are most commonly used in pain research.

- **SPB**: Half the individual's normal rate. If the person's normal breath rate was 14 breaths/min (bpm), then the slow pace would be 7 bpm. Initially, this might be very uncomfortable for the person, causing more anxiety and threat to the nervous systems, and may not be calming at all. Often, I will start with Longer-Smoother-Softer as described below, and work towards a slower pace that is most comfortable, enjoyable and even peaceful for the person.

- **DSB**: Five-second inhale and five-second exhale (6 bpm). Once again, following an external pace may not be comfortable or feel safe for the person initially and may not be successful at changing pain. With practice, perhaps the person's physiology would eventually respond favorably (calming). However, not enough research has been done with people living with persistent pain to confirm this, as we will later discuss.

- **Prolong exhale**: Work up to inhale:exhale of 1:2 ratio. We can start with simply extending the exhale by one second and only add another second when the individual feels comfortable. It may take around five cycles at each length until 1:2 ratio is reached. Example: if inhale is four counts, the exhale would eventually be eight counts.

- **Longer-Smoother-Softer:**[20] Pearson describes cueing the breath to be slightly longer, smoother and softer (not "deeper"). This can often help people be more calm and patient with the breath without rushing or forcing it. Allowing the exhale to "last and linger" and the inspiration to be slow, like one is "sipping" the breath, can be useful cues. I often find the cue "take a deep breath" or "breathe deeply" can lead to over-breathing or inspiring with too much effort and recruiting the accessory muscles of respiration when not required. Of course, as with any cue, whether or not you use the cue will depend on the intent and the subsequent effectiveness towards the desired outcome. This type of breath can be used in conjunction with other breath practices such as nadi shodhana, belly/abdominal breathing or ujjayi.

- **Breath visualization**: Visualize the breath filling and expanding various areas of the body: low back, belly, side ribs, back ribs, front chest or ribs under armpits, or any region of the body. The three-part breath, for example, can be practiced where the person visualizes the breath filling and expanding the belly, then the ribs, then the upper chest on inhale; then emptying upper chest, ribs and belly on exhalation. Often people with low back pain tend to keep the area surrounding the low back rigid. Gentle cues that guide and allow the breath to move the rigid, protective and guarded areas can be helpful. Different positions in which the breath practice is performed often provide a different experience.

- **Alternate nostril breathing (nadi shodhana)**: Using a finger to gently close a nostril to block one side of the nasal airway, the person inhales through one nostril, changes the block to opposite nostril and exhales through the other nostril. Repeat on the opposite side and continue to alternate. A modified version is practicing only through visualization, without actually using the fingers to close off the airways.

## EXAMPLE

Peter was taught the Longer-Smoother-Softer breath regulation practice in a position of rest and comfort. Then, he was instructed to try this practice during times he noticed he was holding his breath. He reported it helped him move more easily, with less tension, and it often reduced his pain. This also gave Peter an experience that showed he could influence the ease of movement and his pain through changing his breath, giving him a sense of agency and heightened self-efficacy. It was a method he could also practice independently throughout the day.

Peter started to also use the Longer-Smoother-Softer breath when he noticed his breath being held during times of overthinking or ruminating about his pain or stressful situations. He reported that the practice significantly brought him back to the present moment and eliminated the elaborative stories in his mind, including that the pain was uncontrollable. It often corresponded with a reduction in pain. He also used this breath practice when he noticed his breath was shallow and rapid during moments of anger or frustration (when he felt like he was suffocating). He reported that the longer exhale helped him feel more centered and calm with a feeling of "letting go" and even subdued his feelings of anxiety.

In these above examples, Peter was successfully using a breath regulation practice to self-regulate (body tension, movement, mind and emotions).

In summary, if we begin with breath awareness, it can provide both the clinician and the person in pain with insight into the person's needs and whether or not breath regulation is indicated. If the person in pain can regulate, this can improve their chances of changing the pain experience.

## What is the research saying?

The following section will review the literature surrounding the effects of yoga breathing regulation practices in general, the influence of pain on breath and the effects of breath regulation practices on pain, with proposed underlying mechanisms and research gaps and limitations.

## Research on effects of yoga breathing practices

In 2017, Saoji *et al.* published a narrative review of the research surrounding the effects of yoga breathing regulation practices.[21] The review included 68 studies that used a variety of yogic breathing practices such as nadi shodhana, surya anuloma viloma, chandra anuloma viloma, ujjayi, bhramari, kapalabhati and bhastrika. The review outlined that these yoga breathing practices influenced neurocognitive, psychophysiological, biochemical, cardiorespiratory and metabolic functions in healthy subjects. It also showed a variety of positive outcomes for people with anxiety, cardiovascular disease, respiratory disorders, stroke, diabetes and cancer. The review included one study that measured the effects of slow breathing (50% of the individual's normal rate) on pain.[22] A reduction in pain intensity and unpleasantness ratings was reported by the healthy subjects but not by the subjects with fibromyalgia living with persistent pain.

To date, there is no research on the effects of specific pranayama practices on people with persistent pain. However, breathing regulation practices such as SPB and DSB are often used in yoga therapy and are the most commonly used practices in the research surrounding pain and respiration. So although not always described as pranayama in the literature, SPB and DSB could be considered yoga breathing practices.

DSB has been found to increase respiratory sinus arrhythmia (RSA), heart rate variability (HRV) and baroreflex sensitivity[23] and to reduce chemoreflex sensitivity.[24]

Ujjayi breath is a pranayama practice consisting of a slow, deep and rhythmic pattern through the nostrils that employs partial closure of the glottis resulting in increased airway resistance, which has been hypothesized to stimulate vagal afferents,[25] therefore contributing to the regulation of the ANS.[26] Additionally, it is hypothesized that slow, rhythmic breathing at six breaths/min or fewer results in a shift of the ANS to a parasympathetic dominant state,[27] also by stimulation of vagal afferents.[28] These vagal afferent pathways, mediated in the thalamus, send information to regions of the brain involved in self-regulation processes such as emotional control and attention.[29] We can see the potential benefit this may have for people in pain, as described above with Peter.

We are highlighting slow rhythmic breathing, as the majority of the research found is based on this pattern; however it is also interesting to note that faster paced breathing may have benefits such as enhanced memory and sensorimotor performance.[30] Faster paced breathing such as kapalabhati[31] and bhastrika[32] appears to enhance sympathetic nervous system (SANS) activity; however, bhastrika appeared to enhance parasympathetic nervous system (PANS) activity in one study in the Saoji *et al.* 2017 review.[33]

Although the relationship is not clearly understood, fMRI studies show that changes in both depth and rate of breathing appear to be associated with signal changes in numerous brain regions, including the basal ganglia (BG).[34] Other research suggests that the BG are involved in the processing of our motor, emotional, cognitive and autonomic responses to pain.[35] This is conjecture, but perhaps manipulating the breath rate and depth could influence various responses to pain via the BG, therefore contributing to modulation of the pain experience.

Nadi shodhana has been shown to result in reduced blood pressure, increased HRV and PANS activity[36] and changes in cognitive parameters that influence sustained attention.[37] A randomized controlled pilot study by Schmalzl *et al.* found that a group of healthy young adults participating in a breath-focused yoga practice that included alternate nostril breathing had improved sustained attention compared to the movement-focused group.[38] For an overview of the research surrounding the effects of alternate nostril breathing, the reader is encouraged to review Schmalzl *et al.*'s chapter, "Research on the Psychophysiology of Yoga," in *The Principles and Practice of Yoga in Health Care*[39] and Saoji *et al.*'s narrative review.[40]

Sudarshan Kriya Yogic (SKY) breathing program has been studied and includes four components: ujjayi, bhastrika, chanting om and Sudarshan Kriya (unique form of cyclic breathing). Authors propose that the mechanisms involved in the "calm alertness" often associated with practicing SKY breathing may include stimulating the PANS, inhibiting stress response systems, balancing cortical areas via thalamic nuclei and promoting release of oxytocin and prolactin. For a detailed description of their neurophysiological model, see Brown and Gerbarg.[41]

## Limitations

Yoga breath practices such as breath awareness, SPB, DSB, alternate nostril breathing (or other nostril manipulation) and bhramari breath practices may be more easily reproducible with higher reliability in consistency of performance of technique by participants and delivery of method versus yoga breath practices such as ujjayi, bhastrika, kapalabhati or SKY breathing methods that include more specific and involved instructions where the healthcare provider would require special training in order to teach these practices safely and consistently. For example, the SKY breathing method used in the research by Brown and Gerbarg is taught in a 22-hour course. The researchers suggest that a trained instructor is required to teach the breathing techniques, "to convey the subtleties and to ensure they are done correctly" and that "follow-up sessions are strongly recommended to correct and refine each person's practice."[42]

The authors of the Saoji et al. review express some of the limitations of the review, including that "no attempt was made to establish the statistical validity of the data presented in the literature"[43] and that the studies lack methodological rigor. Given the overall numerous and promising benefits of yogic breathing, they state that further research that includes larger studies and better methodological designs surrounding yogic breathing research are warranted. Furthermore, we are unsure if the benefits in these studies can be translated to people in pain. I would add that research surrounding the effects of specific yoga breathing practices on various parameters in people with persistent pain is also warranted.

## Research on influence of pain on breathing

In a systematic review on pain and respiration, Jafari et al. found that healthy subjects exposed to sudden noxious stimulus resulting in acute pain demonstrated patterns of increased respiratory frequency, volume and inspiratory flow rate.[44]

With sustained pain, the findings were relatively consistent, showing hyperventilation with increased minute ventilation that appeared to be from deeper breathing or faster breathing or a combination of both.

However, changes in breathing patterns in people living with persistent pain are less clear and less researched. Glynn et al. was the only study in the Jafari systematic review that included people with persistent pain. Hyperventilation was observed as the breathing response during a painful procedure clinically.[45] Past research has shown that hyperventilation was also noted in anticipation of pain without an actual noxious stimulus applied.[46] Jafari et al. summarized that "these hyperventilation effects do not seem to depend on the stimulation of nociceptive receptors, but rather may reflect the influence of feelings of fear, panic, and uncontrollability in response to a potential or actual aversive event such as pain."[47] In other words, hyperventilation or breathing *too much* may actually be a stress response that occurs in situations where stress, fear and pain are uncontrollable.[48] The exact neurophysiological mechanisms underlying these respiratory responses to acute or chronic pain are not clearly understood.

Both hyperventilation and upper chest breathing appear to be common patterns associated with pain. Altered breathing patterns have been associated with neck pain,[49] orofacial pain,[50] pelvic pain[51] and back pain.[52] It is interesting to note in the Smith *et al.* study that breathing pattern dysfunctions were shown to be associated with back pain more than obesity or physical activity.[53] Keep in mind that these are associations, and no causal relationships have been found.

## Effects of opioids on respiration

The endogenous opioid system influences many physiological processes including respiratory control. Research shows long-term opioid use may result in a variety of abnormal breathing patterns such as ataxic breathing, Cheyne-Stokes, obstructive sleep apnea and central sleep apnea.[54] It has been shown that 70–85 percent of people using opioids suffer from sleep-disordered breathing and may experience under-breathing from a reduced respiratory drive, with subsequent hypercapnia.[55] This is opposite to the findings previously mentioned that suggest people in pain tend to over-breathe or hyperventilate, often resulting in hypocapnia. The mechanisms are not completely clear, and more research is needed to determine the risk factors for hypercapnia in those who use opioids for pain management. The key message here is that we do not have enough information available to assume that every person living with persistent pain (particularly those with opioid-induced breathing dysfunctions) would benefit from breathing practices that involve slowing down the breath rate. Any potential adverse effects have not yet been researched.

In summary, acute pain significantly changes respiration, but more detailed research is needed to outline the relationship between chronic pain and respiration.

Clinically, however, I have observed some common breath qualities and patterns in people with persistent pain. For example, I find that people with persistent back pain tend to brace the trunk by co-contracting surrounding trunk muscles. This may be from a perpetuating fear of moving the spine, perhaps because of the belief that they need to protect it from damage or they have been instructed to keep it "neutral" with the abdominals braced as part of "core stability." This protection pattern does not allow the breath to naturally move the abdomen nor expand the rib cage and results in a rigid, shallow, rapid and less efficient breath pattern both at rest and during general mobility. When the diaphragm is not appropriately participating as one of the key synergistic muscles in the dynamic core strategy system, movement strategies can also become less efficient. Remember, the respiratory diaphragm is meant to move throughout its excursion in order to fulfill its many roles, including its role in the core strategy system, movement efficiency, posture and balance strategies.[56]

People with persistent pain also appear to have a tendency to brace and hold their breath when moving in ways that are painful or when anticipating pain. These altered breath patterns can potentially further contribute to perpetuating the pain experience. As discussed by Pearson in Chapter 5 an altered breath pattern may be one of the many outputs of the human system that serves as a protective response. Each protective output (including the altered breath pattern) subsequently then becomes another input of threat into the system. If we can regulate the breath so that its input into the system is no longer a threat, perhaps we can change the pain experience.

## CONTEMPLATION EXERCISE

What is your own experience? How does your breath change when you experience pain? If you change your breath, does your pain change? Next time you experience pain, observe and explore your breath and see what happens.

## Research on effects of breathing regulation practices on pain

Slow and controlled breathing practices are often used to reduce pain.[57] The systematic review on pain and respiration by Jafari *et al.* summarizes that the majority of experimental and clinical research suggests that paced slow deep breathing (SDB) may indeed help to reduce pain. However, upon thorough review, there are still many gaps and limitations in the research with inconsistent findings and underlying mechanisms unknown.[58]

### *Clinical research*

Eight clinical studies measured the effects of breathing practices on acute pain. Three studies included people with painful conditions such as people with chronic low back pain (cLBP), children with cancer and burn patients. The cLBP group showed no change in pain after 30 minutes of daily SDB for 15 days; however, pain reduction was more prominent at three months in the cLBP group compared to the control group.[59] Elkreem showed that pain was significantly reduced after one session of a breathing practice in children with cancer pain; however details of the breathing method used were not outlined.[60] Three sessions of slow abdominal breathing with a ratio of 2:4 inhalation:exhalation was found to reduce pain during dressing changes in burn patients.[61]

## Experimental research

Nine experimental studies were included in the Jafari *et al.* review. Six studies included the effects of SDB (six bpm or less) on acute pain and three studies compared the effects of inhalation versus exhalation on acute pain. Four of the studies showed SDB significantly reduced pain. Interestingly, one study found that only the relaxing instructions of the SDB technique significantly increased pain thresholds compared to the attentive SDB instructions, which were not effective.[62] Most of the research involves healthy subjects except for Zautra *et al.*, which included people with fibromyalgia (FM). The healthy subjects reported a reduction in pain with SDB, but the people with FM did not. A reduction in negative affect was reported across all subjects.[63] It is suggested that pain is reduced during the exhalation phase of respiration; perhaps because of the link between reduced heart rate and enhanced parasympathetic dominance during exhalation. However, the three experimental studies that measured pain during inhale versus exhale during SDB showed varied results. One study showed pain reduced on inhale,[64] another study showed pain reduced on exhale[65] and another found no difference.[66] These inconsistent findings warrant further research and also highlight the complexity of the mechanisms underlying respiratory-induced hypoalgesia.

## Potential underlying mechanisms

There are many mechanisms hypothesized to be responsible for respiratory-induced hypoalgesia, but none are yet clearly understood.

The baroreceptor system appears to be a plausible contributor to modulating pain via the cardiovascular and respiratory systems. The baroreceptors detect blood pressure changes and information is sent to the nucleus of the solitary tract (NTS) in the brain. The NTS connects to brainstem nuclei, and output from these nuclei can regulate heart rate via sympathetic or parasympathetic (vagal) efferents.[67] The NTS also sends information to other brainstem and cerebral areas that can influence cognition, emotion and pain control such as the thalamus, hypothalamus, anterior cingulate cortex and periaqueductal gray, to name few.[68] Perhaps this provides insight into how Peter's thoughts, emotions and pain changed after engaging in a breath regulation practice. The baroreceptors also play a key role in respiratory sinus arrhythmia (RSA).[69] The baroreceptors detect the drop in blood pressure during inspiration, resulting in increased heart rate. Conversely, upon exhalation, the baroreceptors detect an increase in blood pressure, resulting in reduced heart rate via vagal efferents. SDB causes more pronounced fluctuations in blood pressure resulting in higher HRV and RSA.[70] It is hypothesized, therefore, that slower paced and deeper breath patterns may contribute to pain modulation in this way.[71] However, the role of the baroreceptor system in pain control is complex and the mechanisms remain unclear.

The baroreflex may have less influence on pain in certain conditions or situations such as stress, emotional states or certain pathologies.[72] I would add that the proposed mechanisms may not necessarily translate accurately to people with persistent pain, particularly if their physiological systems are not comparable to the healthy subjects used in the research.

Research from Martin *et al.* concluded that slow breathing reduced pain compared to normal or fast breathing. However, the study suggested that this was not due to changes in either parasympathetic activity or spinal nociception. The nociceptive flexion reflex (NFR) used to measure spinal nociception was not influenced by breathing and the HRV was not associated with changes in pain or the NFR. The authors suggest that respiration-induced hypoalgesia may not require parasympathetic involvement and they hypothesize that slow breathing might reduce pain by top-down modulation, that is, descending activity from the brain to the spinal cord that inhibits nociception.[73]

Additional research suggests other modulators may potentially be responsible for respiration-induced hypoalgesia such as relaxation,[74] distraction from pain,[75] expectation,[76] placebo, noradrenergic pathways and endogenous opioids.[77]

Although our clinical experience may demonstrate that certain breath practices may help reduce pain, we need to appreciate and acknowledge the complexity of the underlying mechanisms. It does not mean we abandon these practices, rather it should inspire us to ask deeper questions in order to expand our options and better guide how we help people in pain.

## Limitations and gaps in research

- Expectation bias: subjects and clinician believe that it will work.

- Methods not exclusive to breathing practices (relaxation instructions also included in methods).

- Heterogenous pain populations (examples in above research: cLBP, cancer pain, burn pain, all types of pain from people admitted to emergency, labor pain, bypass surgery, chest tube removal).

- No consistency in type of breath methods studied.

- Poorly described breathing method: sometimes the breath practice and the delivery of breathing instructions were not described.

- No objective measurements of breath practices were reported, other than breath rate, to know whether subjects were following the breath practice correctly. Breath depth and quality may also be important factors in pain modulation[78] and should also be measured.

- It is unknown if SDB is relaxing or comfortable for person. Often the SDB rate is a percentage of the individual's normal rate.

- It is unknown if breath practice played a role in distraction.

- The vast majority of studies do not include people living with persistent pain. In the experimental studies, the response to a noxious stimulus was measured in healthy subjects. In the clinical studies, acute pain experiences during "painful procedures" in a variety of populations were measured; therefore, the outcomes are not generalizable to the persistent pain population for the reduction or management of persistent pain.

Jafari *et al.* conclude: "In summary, several clinical studies suggest a beneficial effect of SDB on pain, but more well-documented studies on homogeneous patient groups that control for expectancy, demand characteristics and distraction effects are clearly needed."[79]

It would be interesting to study the effects of a regularly practiced breath method on pain in the persistent pain population over an extended period of time, as most of these studies consisted of one to three sessions or took place over a small number of weeks.

As mentioned, although the breath regulation practices included in the above pain research were not specifically identified as yoga breathing practices or pranayama in the studies, they are breath practices commonly used in yoga. Furthermore, it may be advantageous to include additional specific pranayama methods in this research, as it may help with the consistency and reproducibility of breath types and delivery of instructions of the breath practices.

Clinically, for over two decades, I have seen immense value and benefits of breathing regulation practices for people in pain. I believe that further research in this area would contribute to enhancing safe, accessible and effective delivery of non-pharmacological pain care.

## Clinical relevance of yoga breathing practices in pain care

Yoga breathing practices can play a valuable role in pain care and help people in pain reduce and manage their own pain. As we have seen, breathing and pain can influence one another in complex ways and the mechanisms are not clearly understood. I think it is important to understand the complexity of the relationship and the many interdependent factors and systems involved and not make assumptions that we think we know why a breath method helps someone in pain, when it does. Perhaps the effectiveness lies in the interplay of the breath with all koshas within the context of the relationship between the person, the clinician and the environment.

The breath may help reduce body tension and influence mechanical efficiency and overall movement patterns so people move with more ease. The breath can influence physiology, calm the nervous systems—reducing incoming threat messages—and influence the stress response and emotions such as reducing fear and anxiety, resulting in increased confidence to move. Breath awareness practice might heighten interoception and emotional awareness, which can then enhance one's ability to self-regulate. These may all contribute to changing the pain experience.

Is it possible that isolated breathing practices delivered outside the yoga framework would not be as effective or beneficial? In a yoga therapy setting, it is not just about prescribing a particular breath rate, quality and pattern, but attention is also given to all five koshas and eight limbs, adding both top-down and bottom-up influence to the pain experience.

Furthermore, no one breath practice seems to be superior for people living with persistent pain. The practices must be individualized to meet the unique needs of the person. The type of breath practice chosen for the person in pain and the outcomes of the breath practice are context dependent. The person's sense of safety (and therefore pain experience) may be influenced by the anatomical position in which they are performing the breath practice, their beliefs and expectations about the practice, their current physiological state, the external environment (light, sounds, temperature), the therapeutic relationship between therapist and individual, the therapist's tone of voice and language used, the therapist's current physiological state and even the therapist's beliefs and expectations about the practice.

In summary, breath practices in pain care are:

- accessible and practical. The breath can be accessed anytime, anywhere; it is always available to the individual

- low-cost treatment options. No equipment is needed, and they are easy for healthcare providers to deliver and free of charge for the person in pain to use independently once instructed

- non-invasive interventions

- relatively simple techniques that can be reproduced with potentially powerful impact to change pain and other aspects of our physiology that may influence pain

- time efficient: simple practices can be instructed and performed in a few minutes

- active forms of pain care, fostering patient self-empowerment and self-efficacy

- potentially safe options with low risk for adverse side effects when practicing introductory breath practices, not advanced pranayama

- a method of pain science education by allowing the person in pain to directly experience that by changing their breath, they can change their pain (refer to Chapter 7)

- awareness practices that can give the person in pain a tangible way to evaluate their current physiological state including emotions and tension in the body or mind. The breath is the link to access the ANS. It is the portal to the conscious awareness of the state of your body[80]

- a path to awareness and regulation of the breath, leading to potential change in other aspects of your existence, including the pain experience.

## Conclusion

I believe there is tremendous value in addressing the breath and integrating yoga breathing practices in pain care. Breath can serve as a powerful tool to provide insights into one's current physiological state and can be a profound agent of change. Breathing practices can be an accessible, easy, safe and effective treatment strategy to modulate pain that can give the person in pain a sense of self-efficacy and empowerment in their pain care.

## Chapter 9

# Body Awareness, Bhavana and Pratyahara

LORI RUBENSTEIN FAZZIO

As discussed in the prior chapter, through practices of pranayama we can influence the physiology of the body including neurocognitive, psychophysiological, biochemical, cardiorespiratory and metabolic functions and ultimately shift from survival-based reactivity to thoughtful responsiveness.

Observing the breath not only brings the mind to a one-pointed focus, but also draws attention away from the sensory experiences of the external world and inward towards the internal sensory experiences. This drawing of the senses inward is pratyahara, the fifth limb of ashtanga, as described in Chapter 4. This *withdrawal of the senses* is the transition from the outer limbs of yoga to the inner limbs.

*Svavisayasamprayoge cittasya svarupanukara ivendriyanam pratyaharah.*

*Pratyahara is conscious withdrawal from the sensory world by detaching the cognizing mind from objects of the senses.*

Yoga Sutra 2.54[1]

Pratyahara is the process of *becoming aware* of the sensations in order to recognize and regulate our reactions to them and then ultimately cease our responses to them. This practice of detached observation of sensations can reduce the emotional and cognitive alarm response that may exacerbate the pain experience. Such practices that nurture volitional control over the senses result in reduced suffering (duhkha). Without such practices, the habitual response to pain and discomfort is to "make it go away." This natural aversion (dvesha) to discomfort can be protective at times, as in the case of touching a hot stove. The reaction to the intense heat sensation is to quickly withdraw the hand to minimize the burn. However, in the case of persistent pain, it is thought that the learned hypervigilant alarm response contributes to the chronicity of the pain, thus the heightened aversion becomes a source of the dysfunction.[2] Dvesha, according to

Patanjali, is one of the five obstacles to awareness. These five obstacles are called kleshas and include:

- **avidya**: ignorance

- **asmita**: ego, I-am-ness

- **raga**: attachment

- **dvesha**: aversion

- **abhinivesha**: fear of death, fear of change.

While Patanjali presents the kleshas in the context of *obstacles to awareness*, in the case of persistent pain, dvesha could be considered as aversion to the experience of discomfort. In order to transcend the pain, we must *become aware of it* and welcome it in order to dismantle it. This chapter will discuss awareness from both the yogic and medical perspectives and how awareness is affected in chronic pain sufferers and will offer a novel practice for the management of persistent pain.

## Awareness

What is awareness? Did you notice the various uses of the words "aware" and "awareness" in the preceding paragraphs? One refers to a state of knowledge and the other refers to a state of sentience, or consciousness. "Become aware *of*" involves intentional placement of attention on an object. One can be aware of one's self (self-awareness), of space (sense of direction), of knowledge or intuition (knowing and feeling), of expectations (sense of responsibility) and of sensations such as warmth, cold, tension, hunger, thirst. These all involve awareness of an object. In such cases the terms "placing attention," "noticing" and "becoming aware *of*" could be used interchangeably. However, in the context of "becoming aware" without identification with a particular object, there is a striking difference. When we dis-identify with the objects we can shift towards "being awareness" itself. Imagine that you are a movie screen upon which various images are displayed. When your attention falls upon the images displayed upon the screen, that which is present in your awareness is the changing images. These images are akin to the plethora of thoughts that reside in our awareness in any given moment. If we dis-identify with the images and thoughts and rather sense *being* the movie screen upon which the images are being displayed, we can settle into awareness itself. It is here, in awareness itself, where we can sense the essence of yoga according to Patanjali.

Yoga Sutra 1.2: *yoga citta vritti nirodhah.* "Yoga is the restraint of the fluctuations of the mind."[3] Through the quieting of the mind we seek to experience our true nature or purusha. However, as Patanjali describes in Yoga Sutra 4.20, it is impossible to be consciously aware of purusha. Yoga Sutra 4.20: *Eka samaye cobhayaanavadharanam*. "Nor can both the mind and the illuminating process be cognized simultaneously."[4] While we can't consciously be aware of purusha, being aware of awareness itself is akin to sensing the essence of this true nature that resides within each of us.

There is no pain in awareness itself. Have you ever noticed that when you are in pain you are aware of the pain? What, exactly, is aware of the pain? When you are cold you can be aware that you are cold. You are neither the pain nor the cold because the very fact that you are aware of them means that you are not these things. Who are You? Oftentimes people in chronic pain identify with the pain. They may identify as a chronic pain patient and make statements such as "my pain." Instead, consider the perspective "I am experiencing pain." Or, to take this further as is often presented in mindfulness practice, "Pain is visiting me." You are not your pain. Pain is an experience.

If we welcome pain without trying to change it, without trying to make it go away, we can actually use it as a means of cultivating awareness itself and remembering our true essence of being—to invite in and be with all sensations from the perspective of the unbiased observer, from the perspective of being the movie screen itself.

## Body awareness and chronic pain

Body awareness is a multidimensional mind-body construct that involves proprioception, interoception and exteroception and is influenced by thought processes including beliefs, memories, attitudes, affect, past experience, evaluation and attention. While a cohesive definition of *body awareness* is lacking, historically in medicine it was widely characterized as attentional awareness of internal bodily sensations. This understanding viewed heightened body awareness as maladaptive and was correlated with increased physical and emotional pain. The working definition of body awareness for this chapter is "the subjective, phenomenological aspect of proprioception and interoception that enters conscious awareness, and is modifiable by noted mental activities."[5] In order to fully understand body awareness from this perspective, we must first understand proprioception, interoception and exteroception.

### *Proprioception*

Proprioception is our sense that monitors equilibrium, motion and position of our body and limbs. It is thought to be controlled by mechanosensory receptors in joints, muscles, tendons and skin and the Piezo2 protein found in the receptors' membranes.[6] It involves integration of the vestibular, physical and neurological systems. For example, when you stand on one leg, notice how the body, particularly the ankle, makes constant adjustments to help you maintain balance. This is due to activation of the proprioceptors. Balance exercises help to refine this process, which helps you to maintain or recover your balance more easily when challenged.

## Interoception

Interoception (awareness of internal bodily sensations including respiration and heartbeat) is a highly complex process that has drawn the attention of neuroscientists interested in meditation. Interoception involves activation of the insula, an area of the brain also involved in empathy and compassion.[7] Psychopaths who commit heinous crimes showed reduced cortical thickness of specific regions of the brain including the left insula,[8] whereas studies done on monks who practice meditation show increased right insular cortical density.[9] It is theorized that practices that evoke increased interoceptive awareness may inherently increase empathy and compassion.[10] You may have noticed this effect yourself. Prior to yoga practice, we may be irritable, angry and tense. We may cut someone off in traffic on our way to a yogasana class or rush to make sure we get our preferred spot in the room. And after class, or after our personal practice, we may have less pain, move more mindfully and peacefully or perhaps even hold the door open for strangers with a smile and interact with others with love and gentleness. It is theorized that sustained non-evaluative attention on interoceptive processes increases neural connections and may have positive neuroplastic effects.[11] While these neurological findings are exciting, it appears that the underlying mechanisms may be much more complex. For more on compassion please see Chapter 14 and for more information on interoception I recommend checking out the work of Camila Valenzuela-Moguillansky and Bud Craig.

## Exteroception

Exteroception refers to the sensitivity to stimuli outside of the body as opposed to interoception, which pertains to sensitivity of our internal state. Exteroception includes vision, smell, taste, touch and hearing. Exteroceptive body awareness, or "body schema" as described by Valenzuela-Moguillansky,[12] refers to the integration of exteroceptive faculties with proprioceptive awareness that enables awareness of our body in relationship to space and movement.

## Evaluating body awareness

We can evaluate the quality of an individual's body awareness with screening questionnaires such as the Body Awareness Scale (BAS), Body Awareness Questionnaire (BAQ) and the Multidimensional Assessment of Interoceptive Awareness (MAIA).

The MAIA questionnaire evaluates one's ability to notice bodily sensations and identify them as comfortable, uncomfortable or neutral and quantifies the responses within categories of not distracting, not worrying, attention regulation, emotional awareness, self-regulation, body listening and trusting the body. In one study, patients with fibromyalgia demonstrated higher scores in noticing internal bodily sensations (interoception), however they demonstrated lower scores in the beneficial coping skills of not distracting and trusting. While these patients were more aware of sensations, they were not able to use this heightened awareness to regulate their suffering. Instead, they perceived the sensations as objects external to themselves from which they must guard and protect.[13] It appears that hyper-awareness of bodily sensations is related to maladaptive coping mechanisms such as rumination, catastrophizing and somatization and is associated with increased experience of pain.[14] However, mindful non-judgmental and non-emotional focus on the sensory aspect of pain can be effective in reducing pain and suffering.[15] In yoga, this non-judgmental awareness can be cultivated through vairagya (non-attachment) and abhyasa (practice) as discussed later in this chapter.

Currently, validated measures for body awareness are not able to discern between (a) anxiety-related hypervigilance towards pain and other physical sensations with catastrophizing interpretation bias and (b) a non-judgmental, meditative, "mindful" awareness of these sensations. Thus, the existing instruments perpetuate the persisting confusion about the benefits of focused attention either away (distraction) or towards internal physical sensations.[16]

No studies to date have evaluated changes in the BAS and MAIA score in the chronic pain population following mindfulness interventions, however similar approaches have shown positive outcomes.[17] Whereas heightened attention to bodily sensations coupled with fear avoidance is associated with negative emotional states of being, altered interoceptive and exteroceptive awareness and decreased quality of life, movement-based contemplative practices such as yoga re-establish healthy sensorimotor processing, foster coherent exteroceptive body awareness and are associated with improved quality of life. Currently, clinical trials are being conducted in collaboration with the National Center for Complementary and Integrative Health to evaluate fMRI data in relationship to attention to the body and thoughts during meditation, and such studies may inform further clinical applications.[18] I recommend following the work of researcher Camilla Valenzuela-Moguillansky for more information on this topic.

## Pratyahara

Pratyahara: gaining mastery over external influences.

Prati: against or away.

Ahara: things we take into ourselves from the outside.

Many medical studies have demonstrated that yoga and mindfulness interventions can be effective in reducing pain and improving quality of life in chronic pain sufferers.[19] How exactly these practices work is not fully understood in modern medical terms. While medicine continues to seek explanations as to how they work, let's look at what yoga instructs us to do. If we follow the logic of Patanjali and pratyahara, we must first heighten our awareness, purify and then regulate. In other words, in order to regulate our reactions to our senses, we must first become conscious of the sensory experience in any given moment, recognize our perception of it, alter negative perceptions and attitudes to positive ones (purify through pratipaksha bhavana) and learn to experience sensation without reactivity. While there are many practices outlined with respect to asana, pranayama and meditation, this critical step of pratyahara is not yet widely examined in modern yoga therapy. This chapter will discuss pratyahara as described by Patanjali and from a modern medical pain science perspective and offer a novel practice for individuals suffering from chronic pain.

In the cacophony of the world today we are bombarded with excessive sensory input throughout the day. As we practice focusing our attention, without reacting to sounds, sights, physical sensations and ultimately even thoughts, we cultivate pratyahara. We gain control over the senses. In yoga, this is the transition from external practices to inward practices on the path towards dis-identification with the activities of the mind (citta vrittis) and reconnecting with our true nature.

Pratyahara is often misunderstood as suppression of the senses. However, it is not an active suppression practice, rather it is the result of cultivation of inward focus. The act of closing the eyes, ears and mouth itself is not pratyahara, rather this act enables the practitioner to bring the attention inwards and prepare for pratyahara. Dr. Ananda Bhavanani points out that pratyahara is often misconstrued as killing or numbing of the senses.[20] Subduing the senses involves an external approach, whereas pratyahara is an internal approach. Merely closing off the external sensory organs (closing the eyes, ears, mouth), as in shanmukhi mudra, does not inherently cease the internal mental activity of the senses. Swami Gitananda further elucidates, "Pratyahara must also include an attempt to control and understand the *mind's reaction* to sensory stimulus."[21] Similarly, attempting to suppress pain does not cease the complex internal processes that perpetuate the chronic pain experience. Rather, it appears that the practice of observing the sensations with non-judgmental focus results in decreased reactivity to the senses and ultimately reduced pain and suffering.[22]

Many medical treatments for persistent pain focus on subduing the senses. Pain medications, surgeries, anesthetics and even distraction methods all focus on quelling the senses. Evidence over the past 20 years has shown that pain medications are ineffective in the treatment of persistent pain and in fact can result in increased pain, addiction and severe side effects.[23] Surgeries are often ineffective,[24] and anesthetics only offer temporary relief. In the late 1980s I worked as a physical therapist in an interdisciplinary inpatient and outpatient chronic pain clinic and our primary focus was distraction. We focused on reducing "pain behaviors" and increasing activity, and while it may have served some clients, overall it was frustrating for both the patients and the practitioners.

More recently, pain science has provided us with further insight that suggests an opposite approach may be more useful. Recent research seems to indicate that *focusing* on the sensory experience with discrimination or non-evaluative body awareness is more effective in reducing pain than suppression or distraction techniques and acknowledges that the entire process is much more complex than previously understood. Practices that involve this non-evaluative, non-regulatory body awareness such as body scans of Yoga Nidra and Vipassana ultimately can lead one to becoming aware of awareness itself.

### THE SENSES AND PRATYAHARA

There are four categories of pratyahara.

- **Indriya-pratyahara**: Mastery of the senses.

- **Prana-pratyahara**: Mastery of prana (energy).

- **Karma-pratyahara**: Mastery of action (Karma yoga of *Bhagavad Gita*).

- **Mano-pratyahara**: Mastery of mind from the senses.

In this chapter, we will focus on indriya-pratyahara and mano-pratyahara with respect to persistent pain. Sight (eyes), smell (nose), sound (ears), touch (skin) and taste (tongue) are the five physical senses (organs) as described in Western science and are the five cognitive senses (jnanendriyas) of yoga. The five jnanendriyas are the input from our external environment and they stimulate mental and emotional activity, much of which we are not typically consciously aware. When you see a rose in full bloom, the experience is not limited to seeing. In order to identify the rose as a rose, complex neural networks are involved through a process called visual recognition. Once recognized, the mind may perceive it to be pleasant. Or, noticing that the flower is about to die, you may feel sad. You may enjoy the sweet scent, which may remind you of a person, which, in turn, may activate memories. In fact, all of this can happen by just imagining a rose without actually seeing one with your eyes. As you can see, every sensory experience has the potential to activate a plethora of thoughts. By training the mind to observe sensations without judging, classifying, evaluating them, we can quiet these mental processes.

*Yoga citta vritti nirodhah.*

*Yoga is the restraint of the fluctuations of the mind.*

Yoga Sutra 1.2[25]

In addition to the five jnanendriyas, yoga describes five action senses called karmendriyas, which involve our output into the world. They include movement (feet), dexterity and grasping (hands), elimination (rectum), reproduction (genitals) and speaking (mouth). Metaphorically, we can recognize these in common pain-related phrases such as "run away from pain," "grasp for a cure" or "cry out in pain."

According to yoga, the ten indriyas do not define us, nor are they reliable:

While the external world keeps changing, the very senses with which we observe that world are able to have experience only within their own limited range. The eyes see only a limited range; the ears hear only a limited range; and so also with smell, taste, and touch. They all provide useful, though limited, inadequate information when seeking Truth or Reality. The way to find it cannot, then, be through the senses.[26]

To paraphrase, "the senses are not reliable."

As described by renowned neuroscientist V. S. Ramachandran, "Pain is an opinion on the organism's state of health rather than a mere reflective response to injury."[27] Mirror visual feedback (MVF), also known as mirror box therapy, motor imagery and virtual reality, have all been shown to be top-down mechanisms to modulate chronic pain, however further research is needed in order to fully support their effectiveness.[28] Motor imagery involves imagined movement, which has been shown to elicit the same fMRI activity as actual physical movement does.[29] MVF involves the use of a mirror such that the patient sees the reflection of their unaffected limb in the mirror and thus perceives its pain-free movement to be that of the affected limb. For more on this concept, refer to the work of Ramachandran, including his book *Phantoms in the Brain*.[30]

These examples all support the aforementioned statement "the senses are not reliable." Now, let's explore this further with respect to persistent pain.

Lorimer Moseley, a pain researcher in Australia, shares his pain story in many of his lectures, and you can access his entertaining TED Talk about this on YouTube.[31] He shares the story of bushwalking and feeling something touch his lower leg. He didn't pay much attention to this sensation as his evaluative process concluded that it was likely just a scratch from a twig. However, his evaluative process had been incorrect, it was actually a poisonous eastern brown snake bite that almost killed him.

Six months later he went bushwalking and felt something similar touch his leg. This time he experienced severe agonizing pain. And, this time it was only a scratch from a shrub. Why was the pain so severe the second time even though the injury was minor? Because the severity of the pain response was based upon complex evaluative thought processes that involve memory of his past experience. This further demonstrates how the senses are not reliable. Lorimer Moseley states, "Pain is an illusion 100 percent of the time. Pain is an output of the brain designed to protect you."[32]

While it is a logical protective mechanism for him to have heightened attention on sensations in the lower leg while bushwalking, if this hyper-focus were to persist, it would be considered maladaptive pain hypervigilance, also known as heightened body awareness, which is associated with catastrophizing, rumination and somatization, as well as increased pain sensitivity and disability irrespective of actual harmful stimuli.[33]

Non-judgmental mindfulness practices appear to counter this maladaptive hypervigilance, resulting in improved coping mechanisms, decreased pain intensity, improved function and improved mental state of being.[34]

There are a plethora of mindful body awareness practices, including yoga, Tai Chi, Feldenkrais, Alexander technique and body awareness therapy to name a few. Such practices have been shown to improve health and wellbeing and are typically cost effective.[35]

Many modern forms of practices that foster these qualities of non-judgmental bodily awareness exist within the field of psychology. These include Focusing,[36] Mindful Focusing,[37] Mindsight,[38] Somatic Experiencing[39] and somatic tracking. Most of these practices are basically modern medical adaptations of the Buddhist meditation technique of Vipassana.

Unprovided with such practices, people with severe persistent pain often resort to numbing their pain, be it with medications or through the process of bodily dissociation. Bodily dissociation has been understood to be a protective mechanism. However, the attempt to suppress sensation is not an effective road from duhkha (pain/suffering) to sukha (wellbeing). In yoga, the path from duhkha to sukha resides in dis-identifying with these ever-changing qualities (prakriti) and, in order to do so, one must first recognize them. In doing so, one may begin to recognize samskaras (habit patterns) that may be reinforcing the pain cycle. As one shifts towards witnessing the indriyas, non-attachment (vairagya) is cultivated. In yoga therapy for people suffering from persistent pain, the path from duhkha to sukha involves learning to witness the pain experience, letting go of unhealthy samskaras and cultivating awareness through vairagya (non-attachment).

In order to do this successfully, one must first recognize their habitual pain response. Typically, a person in chronic pain will have habitual responses, samskaras, that often feed into the pain cycle, creating more suffering (duhkha).

Samskaras are the deep thought patterns that guide our habits and way of interacting with the world. Just as a river eventually creates grooves in the rocks it flows over, making it easier for the water to flow without resistance, over time our repeated thoughts and reactions create patterns that become habitual and unconscious. For example, when experiencing hip pain, you may tense the area, shift more weight to the other leg and some muscles may become inhibited. While these compensations are intended to be protective, they often result in decreased sensorimotor control and function due to immobility, protective muscle spasm and disuse atrophy. As Chimenti *et al.* describe, "Pain can produce increased muscle contraction, tone, or trigger points, it can result in muscle inhibition or fear-avoidance behaviors resulting in disuse and disability or both facilitation and inhibition in opposing muscle groups."[40] Yoga practices can help us to become aware of these compensations. Becoming aware of increased muscle tension can enable us to consciously relax the area, becoming aware of habitual avoidance of weightbearing on one side can enable us to find more balanced postures and becoming aware of inhibited muscles can enable us to improve volitional motor control.

In essence, this process is self-study, or svadhyaya. While svadhyaha traditionally refers to study of yogic texts, in the therapeutic context it refers to self-study, self-reflection. What am I experiencing in this moment? What sensations are present? This extends beyond the physical. What emotions are present? Thoughts? How am I interpreting these experiences? Becoming *aware*.

As rehabilitation professionals and yoga therapists, we have the opportunity to provide a safe environment for patients to reacquaint with their bodies, learn to listen to the sensations with a neutral mind and respond rather than react. As mentioned, this process requires both abhyasa and vairagya, practice and non-attachment.

*Abhyasa vairagyabhyam tannirodhah.*

*Thought patterns (vrittis) are mastered through practice (abhyasa) and non-attachment (vairagya).*

Yoga Sutra 1.12[41]

In this context, vairagya refers to the non-judgmental witnessing of sensations and the non-attachment to the desire to label it, change it or make it go away. In short, non-attachment to making the pain go away. And this requires abhyasa, practice. From a neuroscience perspective, it involves creating new neural pathways for the neural output of the pain response. From the 1990s until now, research in neuroplasticity has expanded with fMRI studies focused on identifying the regions of the brain involved in pain. Similar studies have also been conducted to identify the changes in the brain from contemplative practices such as yoga and meditation. As a student of both pain science and the science of yoga, I have spent many years correlating these two sciences and lecturing on neuroplasticity. In the 30-plus years that I have been studying these sciences, I have witnessed a continuous evolution of the understanding of the neurophysiological basis behind them. After years of lecturing on neuroplasticity, pain and yoga, I now recognize that this reductionist approach is inherently flawed. These are complex processes and to dissect them does not serve. For more on the current understanding of neuroscience and pain, please refer to Chapter 5. For more on the evolution of this science, please refer to Chapter 3.

## Yoga therapy and altered body schema in people with persistent pain

As the nature of all prakriti, body schema is ever-changing and dependent upon many factors. Through mindful yogasana practice, we refine this body schema sensory awareness, resulting in improved mind-body function. To demonstrate this concept, consider the example of driving a car. When you drive the same car on a regular basis, you become aware of the size and maneuverability of that particular car. If you drive a different-size car, it is often awkward at first until you experience and learn the nuances of that particular car. When in India, I was awestruck by the ability of the bus driver to maneuver a huge bus down tiny busy streets with barely a couple of inches between the bus and the many obstacles in the road. The bus driver had developed body schema awareness of not only himself, but also the bus in relationship to space.

In contrast, people with persistent pain often have maladaptive altered body schema.[42] Associated with this is decreased sensorimotor control and increased pain.

Perhaps the most profound demonstration of alteration of body schema is the "rubber hand illusion" first presented in 1998 and replicated many times with multiple variations since then.[43] This widely used experiment involves a person watching a rubber hand being touched while their own hand is touched, yet out of their view. After a few minutes, the person takes ownership of the rubber hand in that they report feeling the sensation of touch when the rubber hand is touched, even if their real hand is no longer being touched. Their proprioceptive awareness of where their own hand is in space drifts from their real hand towards the rubber hand. This study has been replicated with a noxious stimulus applied to the rubber hand and the subjects report feeling pain even though the noxious stimulus is applied to the rubber hand, not their real hand. Thus, the illusion of a noxious stimulus created a pain response even in the absence of an actual noxious stimulus to the real hand.

In these studies, subjects reported that they could feel sensation when they believed that the hand was being touched even though it wasn't actually being touched. Similarly, in virtual reality studies, subjects who "see" that they have an avatar tail take on the movement of that tail as if it were theirs.[44] Again, the senses are not a reliable indicator of what is occurring in the physical body. Instrumental to this concept is that perception can have profound effects on both the sensory and motor experience. So, the question arises, can we alter the sensory and motor experience by altering perception? This question led me to create practices I refer to as Sensory Memory Visualization and the Virtual MRI.

## Sensory Memory Visualization

Memory (smriti) is one of the five fluctuations of the mind (vrittis) referred to in Yoga Sutra 1.2: *Yoga citta vritti nirodhah*. "Yoga is cessation of the functions of the mind."[45] Following the theory that persistent pain is "remembered pain,"[46] Sensory Memory Visualization attempts to replace this "remembered pain" with a happy, healthy memory prior to the onset of persistent pain. This novel technique was inspired by both shamanic medicine and a guided imagery protocol described by Dr. Murray Grossan.[47]

In 2013 I conducted a pilot study (n=37) comparing focused relaxed breathing to Sensory Memory Visualization in patients over age 50 who had suffered from pain for more than six months. We found that the majority of subjects in both groups experienced significant reduction in pain after only one 20-minute session and the subjects in the sensory memory group also demonstrated significant improvement in function.[48] Additionally, both groups did the Virtual MRI as an experimental evaluative tool to help us understand the subject's perception of their pain. A correlate was found between a change in what the subjects visualized during the Virtual MRI and reduction in pain with improvement in function.

## Virtual MRI

As mentioned, individuals living with persistent pain experience altered body schema.[49] They may perceive the painful area to be larger or smaller than it actually is.[50] The rubber hand studies demonstrate that perception of a noxious stimulus can create a real pain response. Could the contrary be feasible? Could changing perception alter the pain experience in such a way as to reduce pain? In essence, applying the concept of pratipaksha bhavana, cultivating the opposite vision/attitude (Yoga Sutra 2.33).[51]

Vijnanamaya (intuitive wisdom) is an element of the pancamaya yoga therapy assessment that helps us to understand how a patient understands their disease.

We may ask, "What do you think is the cause of your pain? What do you think you need in order to feel better?" I also ask patients to describe what they see or imagine in their body. Our small pilot study supported years of empirical evidence with patients in pain commonly reporting visuals in the painful regions as negative whereas non-painful regions were visualized as positive. For example, in painful regions patients often report seeing red and inflamed or grey and lifeless images. In non-painful regions they typically report seeing healthy images. I have found that guiding patients in this visualization inquiry can be helpful to better understand how the mind is interpreting the painful region and perhaps inform us of their body schema status. From there we can apply the practice of pratipaksha bhavana and cultivate a more positive image. I call this technique the Virtual MRI. An example of this practice is presented in Box 9.1.

---

### Box 9.1: The Virtual MRI

Choose an area where you currently have pain, have had pain or had an injury in the past. Visualize this body part as if you could see the internal landscape of that body part. There is no right or wrong. The image you see may be anatomical or abstract or you may see nothing at all. Notice the colors, textures, size or shape of what you see. How clear is the image? Does anything surround the image? Is this image free floating or is it attached to anything? As you visualize this image, notice if there is an emotion or thought that accompanies the image. Stay with this for a couple of minutes and observe what arises. Then, without moving, *imagine* moving the body part and notice what you experience. Is there a knowingness of pain associated with the movement, even though you are not actually moving? In your mind's eye, is there limitation or is there free movement? Does the image change as you imagine it moving?

Now, shift your focus to the same process on the opposite limb or, if you were imaging an aspect of your torso choose an aspect that does not have pain or perhaps has less pain. Repeat the two-step process on this side and notice any differences.

- Step 1: Visualize the internal landscape of the body part.

- Step 2: Visualize movement of the body part, without moving it.

    If you noted that the visual on the painful side was less clear or was associated with a negative perception, proceed to Step 3.

- Step 3: Manipulating the image's "psychic surgery." Alter the image in your mind to a more healthy, positive image.

For more information on this approach, see Fazzio and Langer.[52]

Clinically, I have found that many patients are able to reduce pain and improve function by merely manipulating the images they see in the Virtual MRI from images that carry negative emotions or thoughts to images that have positive meaning to the patient. The story of Dolly is one example of many patients I have worked with over the years.

## THE STORY OF DOLLY

Dolly was referred to me for physical therapy two years post C3-4-5 fusion (surgical fusion of cervical vertebrae three to five) due to cervical spinal stenosis. Prior to surgery, she experienced bilateral upper extremity radicular pain with neurological weakness. She presented with complaints of cervical pain and weakness in her hands and reported that she was often dropping things. The neurosurgeon had told her that the surgery was a success and that there was no medical reason to explain the persistent symptoms. Does this sound like a familiar scenario? A patient still experiencing pain or other symptoms after the problem was "fixed." The issue is that the problem that was fixed was not the only problem. Dolly received physical and occupational therapy for two years post-surgery, yet her symptoms persisted. The well-meaning therapists completed their assessments and implemented standard therapeutic protocols, including modalities to reduce pain, manual therapy to address the soft tissues in the region, exercises to stretch and strengthen and functional activities to improve posture and restore fine motor control. All of these treatments were focused on the physical body. How long do you think she should have expected to continue therapy before she saw results? Certainly, under two years. Dolly is a performer and the longer she was unable to work due to her disability, the more her career was in jeopardy. Despite all of this treatment, her symptoms persisted and, as time progressed, she became anxious and depressed, which further aggravated her symptoms.

The Virtual MRI revealed what appeared to be an underlying cause of her chronic symptoms. Physically she presented with active cervical range of motion limited to approximately 25 percent in all directions, C1-2 joint hypomobility, hyperactivity of the scalene muscles due to excessive use related to chronic obstructive pulmonary disease (COPD) and weak grip strength. During the Virtual MRI she perceived her neck to be a cement block. Through a specific awareness practice utilizing perceptual visualization, pain-free active cervical range of motion was restored to 75 percent. When she returned the following week, she reported that she was no longer dropping things. Her hand strength improved despite the fact that we hadn't included hand strengthening into her program yet.

The Virtual MRI attempts to guide patients to explore how their mind is perceiving the inner makings of their body. Ultimately, becoming more aware is a key aspect of yoga therapy. Oftentimes, people suffering from persistent pain will observe that merely imagining or visualizing movement creates anticipatory pain. Implementation of the aforementioned practices can be beneficial in enabling people in pain to become more aware in order to restore pain-free movement or movement with more ease and less pain. Once a person is able to visualize or imagine pain-free and easeful movement, they are often able to actually move more comfortably.

If there were a pill that offered such results, doctors would regularly prescribe it for their patients with persistent pain. While there are no known negative side effects, these awareness and visualization (bhavana) practices are not a panacea. Practitioners need to be prepared to safely support a patient should traumatic association arise during the visualization process. Disturbing images may trigger heightened uneasy emotional states or unhappy memories. In addition, patients who have difficulty visualizing may find these practices frustrating. While these practices are promising alternatives for people living with and suffering from persistent pain, more research is needed in order to determine parameters for successful implementation of these practices. Ultimately, awareness practices are the foundation of yoga therapy and the essence of mind-body therapies.

## Chapter 10

# Ingredients for Pain Care

## Nutrition and Yoga

MATT ERB

## Overview

As is apparent from our exploration thus far, pain, like the whole of life, is complex. Nutrition is no exception. Living systems are self-organizing and interact intimately with their environment, maintained by a continuous flow of physical matter, energy, and information. Food is one avenue of this flow. As physical matter, food may be seen through the lens of its composition of fiber, proteins, fats, carbohydrates, and specific nutrients. As energy, it is seen as the chemical energy derived from the process of reorganizing the molecules of food via chemical reactions. It may also be seen through the lens of energy medicine where everything is vibrating and interacting at various frequencies on the quantum level. Finally, the field of "nutrigenomics" sees food as information. Food contains and communicates thousands of codes and properties that can "turn on or turn off" the expression of DNA and genes. It also carries vast amounts of information from other living systems such as bacteria.

In yogic teachings, nature, the world, and all beings are a single interconnected, ongoing cyclical pattern of emergent, arising and dissolving movement; everything is related and in relationship. Examining and understanding the complexity of our relationships with others, with ourselves, and with other levels and layers within our life experience is fundamental to yoga. As such, exploring our relationship to food, nutrition, and eating, and how that relationship interacts with the pain experience, is the focus of this chapter. As you read, you are invited to contemplate and intuit your unique relationship to food, eating, and the many ways in which food can enhance or detract from your wellbeing.

## What we know
### Pain, stress, inflammation, and the immune system
Pain is normal and generally not a matter of *if*, but *when*. In yoga, the word "pain" may be seen as not just physical pain, but also in the context of mental

pain or anguish, emotional pain or suffering, and spiritual pain or despair. In the framework of the koshas, pain may have representations across multiple layers within the whole of human experience. Considering such complexity, pain can be seen as any aversive experience associated with actual or potential threat or harm across physical, sensory, emotional, cognitive, social, and spiritual levels.

So, what does pain have to do with food and nutrition? A good starting place is to look at a context that supports understanding a comprehensive and integrative view of stress and, ultimately, of pain. While stress is often understood as psychological (mental and emotional), stress can also be introduced into the organism from across many other levels: environmental, physical, chemical, social/relational, spiritual, nutritional, and more. Our physiology has an innate capacity to adjust to and respond to stress, and it also has limits. The greater the combined stress load across interacting levels, the more susceptible we are to developing a myriad of health issues, including the development of chronic pain.

Next, the physiology of pain is linked to both inflammation and the immune system. Inflammation is a necessary part of your body's response to foreign invaders such as viruses and bacteria, to irritants such as harmful chemicals, and to damaged tissue as is the case with physical injury. In such cases, the process of inflammation signals to the body that tissue repair and other healing processes are needed and is considered beneficial. However, if this process does not shut itself off, it can lead to other problems, including loss of normal function.

In addition to these commonly knowns sources of inflammation, other factors include food allergies or sensitivities; environmental toxicities from air, water, or food; dysbiosis (bacterial imbalance or overgrowth in the gut); as well as high, excessive, or prolonged psychological stress linked to changes in the levels and processing of the well-known "stress hormone," cortisol.[1]

One of the features of inflammation is that the chemicals, peptides, and other cellular substances involved can increase nerve sensitivity such that normally non-painful stimuli contribute signals that get interpreted as pain in the spinal cord and brain. The pain process involves several components such as "nociception" (sensory signals or "danger detectors" from the body) that could reflect real or potential tissue damage and regions in the spinal cord and brain that involve processes of interpretation and appropriate behavior/response. A variety of conditions and agents contribute to this sensitization including the release of inflammatory mediators. These include substances known as "cytokines" and "prostaglandins." These have a sensitizing effect on nociceptors and other pain-related processes in the body and brain.[2] In essence, inflammation in the tissues of the body and the nervous system are increasingly being shown to play an important role in the development and persistence of many pathological pain states.[3]

So, how is the immune system involved in this? Immune cells interact with different types of nerve cells to alter pain sensitivity and are now believed to mediate the transition from healthy, adaptive pain, to the unhelpful, maladaptive chronic pain state. When injury, strain, or stress occurs in the tissues of the body, local immune cells get activated and traveling immune cells may also be sent to the area of injury. These immune cells increase the activity of nociceptors. Through the release of the inflammatory mediators, and additional interactions with neurotransmitters, the immune cells and neural cells form a unified network to facilitate the body's defensive response. In chronic pain states, this sensitivity can get "stuck on."[4] In such cases, a normally adaptive and healthy set of protective responses that is intended to promote tissue repair and defend against invaders goes awry. The complete picture of the complexity of the mechanisms through which chronic pain states emerge remains unclear, but these advances in understanding can lend insight into a more comprehensive approach to treatment, including strategies to reduce inflammation and improve immune system function. This is where the growing concept of "food as medicine" as rooted in principles of nutrition, gut health, and mindful awareness applied to eating, stress, and one's mind-body relationship with food comes in. Given additional links between food consumption, inactivity, obesity, and pain,[5] working with these relationships from the whole-person yogic perspective to improve wellbeing provides a more cohesive approach than our often-fragmented medical system usually offers.

## Connecting the dots to nutrition

Good nutrition can be seen as one important facet to address for people dealing with chronic pain. There is no such thing as a "chronic pain diet" and caution is urged if such a message is conveyed. Research into the role of nutrition in the treatment of pain is in its infancy and, even if it were well established, would still be best explored though individuality as opposed to a cookbook recipe. Having acknowledged this, there are numerous studies examining how substances in certain foods can assist the body in managing inflammation, boosting the immune system, and supporting positive mood states, as well as reducing sensations of pain by influencing the underlying chemistry associated with these processes. A few examples are given below.

- Omega-3 fatty acids, for example, as found in fish oil, flaxseed, and certain types of squash, may reduce inflammation and pain associated with various conditions including arthritic conditions.[6] Omega-3 fatty acids are either plant-based (known as alpha-linolenic acid, ALA) or derived from fish oils (known as eicosapentaenoic acid, or EPA, and docosahexaenoic acid, DHA). Omega-3s were even shown in one study to be as effective as over-the-counter nonsteroidal anti-inflammatory drug (NSAID) medications like ibuprofen at reducing chronic non-specific neck and back pain, with no side effects reported.[7]

- Ginger has been found to have pain-relieving properties. Clinical research shows that taking ginger can modestly improve pain in some patients, for example pain from inflammatory osteoarthritis, and may be comparable to ibuprofen in a dose of 500mg twice daily.[8]

- Quercetin is a bioflavonoid found in red wine, tea, onions, kale, tomatoes, broccoli, green beans, asparagus, apples, and berries and has anti-inflammatory effects and may influence immune system function.[9]

- Tryptophan, an amino acid that is found in many foods including dairy products, turkey and other poultry, chocolate, and some seeds, may be helpful in a number of conditions including influence on pain chemistry. Given that there is also a link between poor sleep and chronic pain, and tryptophan has evidence for beneficial impact on sleep, overlap for supporting both is a consideration.[10]

It is important in viewing a sample list like this to not think that the solution to pain will be found if you consume any one or combination of these or other supplements that may influence pain, inflammation, and the immune system. It is also important to remember that in many cases, part of any positive influence derived may arise from the placebo effect and be attributable to mind-body psychophysiologic mechanisms rooted in conditioning, belief, and the empowerment and self-efficacy that comes from taking an active role in one's health.

The concept of nutritional medicine has been documented as far back to the time of Hippocrates in the 400s BCE, although the precise origin of the quote "let food be thy medicine and medicine be thy food" that is attributed to him remains unclear. Unfortunately, what is a sound concept has been hijacked in a way that leads some to suggest that food and diet can cure everything, when yogic complexity reminds us that our human experience is not so simple. Supporting the wellbeing of your body's physiology through good nutrition might be seen as one part of the soil in which the seeds for an improved relationship to the pain experience may flourish.

### Exploring a whole-foods diet—avoid SAD

While there is some limited information suggesting pain-relieving effects of certain foods and substances for various conditions, given the uniqueness of each individual and their body's biochemistry, it is far more useful to explore general principles of contemporary medical nutrition. A good starting premise is to eat as much of a "whole-foods diet" as is possible. A diet of minimally processed foods that remain as close to their natural origin as is possible at the time of ingestion, and that is predominantly plant based, is associated with health promotion and disease prevention and is a uniform component of seemingly distinct dietary approaches.[11] This also points to a general recommendation to eat more fiber and less refined sugar and flour, the latter two of which contribute to inflammation, insulin resistance, and obesity.

Post-industrial changes in food production such as the refinement of whole grains, processing of sugars and oils, and changes in the quality of meat from animal husbandry have led to "new foods." These are often highly processed and make up a high percentage of all food consumed in the US, often called the SAD (Standard American Diet). "Shopping the perimeter" is a common guideline, as the center aisles of grocery stores are largely comprised of highly processed foods. If a label has more than four or five ingredients, pause to consider other options. To underscore the reality of SAD, author Michael Pollan in his book *Food Rules: An Eater's Manual*,[12] created a number of other catchy concepts such as: if it cannot rot, do not eat it; do not eat anything your great-grandmother wouldn't recognize as food; do not eat breakfast cereals that change the color of the milk; do not get your own fuel from the same place your car does!

A general recommendation for a healthy plate of food, as opposed to the specificity that often comes with the endless fad "diets" being advertised, can be found in the resources of The Center for Mind-Body Medicine's "Food As Medicine" professional training courses. These basic recommendations are consistent with the "anti-inflammatory" and "Mediterranean" diets. In essence, these represent whole-food plans that counter SAD and that have published research on health benefits ranging from longevity, improved cognition, lower cancer risk, cardiovascular benefits including for metabolic syndrome, reduced inflammation including in arthritic conditions, improved mood, decreased depression, and more.[13] Finally, to support the immune system, include foods containing the essential nutrients of vitamins C, E, B6, A, and D, folate/folic acid, iron, selenium, and zinc.

As previously noted, there are no specific studies examining the influence of these diets specific to a population of persons experiencing chronic pain states. While such research is needed, extrapolation of existing science as has been laid out supports the logic that it is an important part of health and wellbeing. This reflects additional "entry points" for positively impacting the underlying and inter-related inflammatory, immune, and biobehavioral aspects of pain. Combining healthy food choices with stress management, mind-body integration, and the other efforts laid out in this book will optimize potential for healing to emerge "from the inside out." This reflects addressing root causes, as opposed to merely seeking temporary relief.

## Healthy eating and digestion

Good nutrition is dependent upon good digestion and subsequent absorption of nutrients from the gastrointestinal (GI) tract. There are many processes, factors, and steps influencing the transport of nutrients into our bloodstream. This includes saliva production, adequate chewing for breakdown of food particles, gastric acid and bile production, a healthy mucosa (inner wall of the digestive tract), the balance of bacteria in the gut, digestive enzymes, and more. Stress, medications, food sensitivities or allergies, parasites or foreign bacteria, and poor diet choices all influence these processes. Perhaps one of the most talked-about aspects of this in recent years is the potential for disruption to the "microbiome," the unique populations of various bacteria that support the biological processes of the human body. More on this in a bit, but first, back to digestion.

Digestion is a complex process, and actually begins in the head! The "cephalic phase" of eating reflects the anticipatory phase, linked to needs (true hunger) as well as wants (pleasure). Planning your meals involves many factors from availability, convenience, resources, the energy expended in obtaining and preparing the foods, prior experiences and preferences, mental and emotional state, and more.

The act of eating activates and involves imagery. Whether we are aware of it or not, digestion involves and starts with the state of the mind, not just the body. Supporting all stages of digestion is an important and necessary part of good nutrition to support the body's needs.

### EXPERIENTIAL ACTIVITY

Take a moment, close your eyes, and imagine your favorite food. What do you notice happening in your body as your mind anticipates this food? Or, imagine cutting a juicy lemon into quarters and taking one up to your mouth and biting into it—do you notice puckering, salivation, or other physiological responses in your body?

## Emerging topics

As we move into additional detail about yoga, nutrition, and pain, the following topics are worth a peek:

- stress and comfort eating

- sugar, inflammation, and addiction

- the microbiome

- toxic food

- botanical medicine.

Let's dive in…

## Stress, "comfort eating," and cortisol

Most people can relate to the fact that stressed is desserts spelled backwards! How often do we reach for the cookie when stressed out? Comfort eating can be seen as a behavioral response to stress. Cortisol, a major hormone associated with mobilizing the body's resources for demand, increases appetite, biases food selection to high caloric foods, increases blood sugar and insulin, supports weight gain, and increases our risk for diabetes and metabolic syndrome.[14] Cortisol is released from the adrenal glands and controlled by a brain–body neuroendocrine axis known as the HPA (hypothalamic pituitary adrenal) axis. In the short term, cortisol can assist in the control of inflammation, but in chronic stress states it may compromise inflammatory processes, compromise digestion, and increase food intake and weight gain, and it may also link to the development of food sensitivities and allergies due to connections to stress eating, food choice, and gut inflammation.[15]

Normally, in an acute stress situation, food intake and digestive processes are decreased in favor of fight/flight responses. In chronic stress states, intake of nutrient-dense foods if available increases and is linked to weight gain and evolutionary adapted responses to famine. In other words, humans frequently respond to stress with a "primitive famine response." Research has demonstrated that sad moods lead to increased food consumption, especially of "hedonic" or "comfort" foods.[16] Given additional links between stress, cortisol, inflammation, and insulin processing, eating high amounts of processed sugar and flour during times of high stress, a frequent combination, has stacking negative effects. When faced with a stressor, the HPA axis is activated, and cortisol, adrenaline, and norepinephrine are released into the system to mobilize the body's resources for an adaptive response. Cortisol inhibits insulin production, preventing glucose from being stored such that it is immediately available. These also contribute to other parts of our fight/flight stress response. Once the stressor passes, these systems and hormone levels return to normal. Unfortunately, chronic psychologic stress can leave this process stuck on and dysregulated, contributing to maladaptive patterns, which often include eating high-sugar foods, increased inflammation, and weight gain, and in some cases leading to the development of an increasingly recognized condition known as metabolic syndrome that is associated with weight gain and heart disease.[17]

Yoga is often utilized to assist in regulating the burden of stress in our lives and has been found to positively impact the biological underpinnings of stress.[18] Inquiry into how stress and eating interact is a useful tool in your yoga lifestyle renewal kit.

## EXPERIENTIAL ACTIVITY

Bring to mind recent times you were stressed. Contemplate how the stress state affected your relationship to food. Now consider which yogic practices may help you to modify that response. Ask yourself, "What am I really 'hungry' for?"

## Our collective sweet tooth

The average American consumes 82 grams of sugar daily. That is 19.5 teaspoons per day, or 66 pounds per year.[19] In contrast, both the American Heart Association and World Health Organization recommend limiting sugar intake to 25 grams (6 teaspoons) per day for adults and, depending on age, as little as 12 grams (3 teaspoons) for children, due to links to inflammation, heart disease, and metabolic syndrome, not to mention growing links to mental and behavioral health issues.[20] This is 5 percent or less of daily caloric needs from added sugar. It is easy to exceed such limits considering that one can of soda has up to 50 grams of added sugar. Given that processed flours in the form of simple carbohydrates have similar influence on our physiology, we may be exceeding recommended limits even sooner than we realize.

Sugar is processed in the body with direct parallels to alcohol processing in its craving patterns, withdrawal symptoms, and addictive biology.[21, 22] Sugar consumption has been shown to have addictive properties, linked to dopamine and reward centers in the limbic regions of the brain. Sugar is known to elevate serotonin levels in the short-run, which is seen as a short-term fix for stress and anxiety.

How is all of this relevant to pain? High sugar intake increases inflammation potential throughout the body and inflammation is intimately linked to pain biology. Stress itself may increase inflammation, contributing to potential for pain, and coping patterns in relation to the stress and/or pain experience may intertwine. While not seen as causal, reducing sugar, flour, and processed food intake, in conjunction with other facets of the comprehensive approach laid out in this book, may improve the overall internal environment, increasing potential for the emergence of improvement in the underlying brain–body patterns of chronic pain.

> ## EXPERIENTIAL ACTIVITY
>
> In yoga, mind-body metaphor can be a useful tool for exploration. Contemplate: Where do I find "sweetness" in my life? What hidden need underlies my sweet tooth? Are there yogic practices that represent healthier ways to create the feeling that is produced when I consume sweets and other comfort foods?

## Eat your bacteria?

Did you know that 1–3 percent of your body weight is comprised of bacteria? For a 200-pound adult, that is between 2 and 6 pounds of body weight![23] The collective environment of bacteria in and on the human body is known as the microbiome.

The microbiome reflects a fascinating area of expanding research that may hold additional relevance to pain biology, as well as numerous other health issues. Gut microbiota are composed of dozens of different species of bacteria, some of which are considered healthy and some harmful. These bacteria play an important role in many vital health functions including: processing nutrients from food; assisting absorption of electrolytes and minerals; breaking down indigestible food substances; producing healthy fatty acids; developing and maintaining a healthy gut lining (intestinal epithelium), a primary barrier to foreign invaders; managing inflammatory processes in the body; breaking down toxins and carcinogens; providing direct support to the immune system—noting that up to 80 percent of our immune system is located in the gut.[24]

What we eat (discussed above) and how we eat (discussed below) both have a major impact on the microbiome.[25] Evidence exists that high sugar and processed carbohydrates in the diet leads to inflammation, dysbiosis (imbalanced microbiome states), and aberrant immune activity and is linked to a number of chronic diseases.[26]

While lifesaving and critical to medicine, antibiotics also contribute to dysbiosis that can persist for years if unaddressed.[27] The impact of other medications on the gut and microbiome is also being described. This includes opioids and other pain management medications.[28]

Specific species of bacteria impact specific health conditions.[29] Research into the role of the microbiome in pain conditions is relatively new. Associations between fibromyalgia, a well-known chronic pain condition, irritable bowel syndrome, and dysbiosis have been reported.[30] Increased intestinal permeability where the lining of the gut breaks down allowing foreign substances to enter systemic circulation (often referred to as "leaky gut syndrome") has been shown in both fibromyalgia and complex regional pain syndrome (CRPS), including in the absence of obvious GI symptoms.[31] Animal studies have demonstrated that oral administration of probiotics may diminish pain of visceral origin. Further research is needed in human subjects, especially those with pain from conditions such as irritable bowel syndrome.[32] For example, administration of Lactobacillus reuteri targets an ion channel in enteric sensory neurons, which may mediate its effects on pain perception.[33] This may be linked to autonomic nervous system processes, which is another important connection to pain mechanisms. An additional example of links between dysbiosis and specific pain conditions was found in a study on chronic pelvic pain in both women and men.[34]

The microbiome has been shown to impact neurotransmitter production, including serotonin, which may have an impact on peripheral pain perception.[35] Pain, mood disorders, and functional GI disorders such as irritable bowel syndrome often co-exist, and links between stress, the brain–gut axis, and the microbiome are being examined within these correlations.[36] This is consistent with the teachings of bidirectional interactions in both ancient yoga and contemporary mind-body medicine teachings.

A good overview of evidence, mechanisms, and links between the microbiome and disorders of the central nervous system including pain has been delineated.[37] Evidence for anti-nociceptive processes linked to specific bacterial strains has been found, including evidence that bacteria activate sensory neurons throughout the body that modulate pain and inflammation.[38] Of strong interest to this topic is a study that found that the intake of a common bacterial strain known as Lactobacillus acidophilus had a similar analgesic efficacy in treating abdominal pain as did a standard dose of morphine via the expression of mu-opioid and cannabinoid receptors in epithelial cells.[39]

Probiotics are food sources and dietary supplements that deliver healthy strains of bacteria to our digestive tract. Prebiotics are food substances that these bacteria thrive on. Interest in the use of probiotics and prebiotics as a means to restore and maintain health is growing.[40] Individualized assessment and replacement may be ideal, however not feasible for most, and thus many choose to take a general approach to gut health including the use of over-the-counter probiotic supplements, which are now widely available.

There is a potentially beneficial role that probiotics may play in various pain conditions, including musculoskeletal diseases such as various types of arthritis.[41] Taking probiotics with prebiotic foods, that support and "feed" the beneficial role that the bacteria play, such as the production of short-chain fatty acids, is recommended. Such efforts are best considered in context of the larger lifestyle renewal that comes with a yogic approach to wellbeing including the implementation of stress-management skills.

**EXPERIENTIAL ACTIVITY**

Connecting with body awareness, intuition, and your inner capacity to come to see yourself honestly and clearly is an important part of the yoga adventure. Sit quietly with the eyes closed, breathe with a soft and relaxed belly, become aware of the sensations of your digestive tract, and contemplate "What is my gut telling me today? Is there anything that I am not digesting well?" You might even have a conversation with your microbiome to discuss co-creating improved health, effectively recruiting new allies in your journey through pain.

## Toxic food?

There is no obvious data linking chemical exposure from food to pain. However, the topic of organic is often raised in any discussion on food and nutrition. There is evidence that organic foods carry higher nutrient density and nutritional value. One meta-analysis demonstrated that organic dairy and meat has been shown to have around 50 percent more omega-3 fatty acids, and significantly higher vitamin E and iron content.[42] As noted earlier, omega-3 fatty acids have been shown to be useful for chronic neck and back pain and linked to anti-inflammatory effects. Another meta-analysis of over 300 studies demonstrated that organic crops ranging from broccoli and carrots to apples and blueberries have higher concentrations of antioxidants and other potentially beneficial compounds, lower cadmium metal levels, and four times lower pesticide levels than non-organic crops.[43]

If it is within your budget, and accessible, exploring organic foods to reduce exposure to chemicals from pesticides and herbicides may be beneficial for general health, as these chemicals have been shown to disrupt endocrine function and increase cancer cell load,[44] and a large recent prospective study of 68,946 participants revealed that a higher frequency of organic food consumption was associated with reduced risk of cancer.[45]

If you are interested in exploring this topic further, the US Environmental Working Group publishes lists based on the top most contaminated fruits and vegetables to help you decide where to put your resources. For seafood, which is a major source of exposure to mercury and heavy metals, the Environmental Defense Fund's Seafood Selector is an excellent source for guidelines. Chemical use in farming varies by country and geographic region so be sure to look for similar lists in your region, such as the European Food Safety Authority who periodically publishes updated data for the European Union. Finally, you are encouraged to not add extra stress, worry, or anxiety around the questions of organic food, as that theoretically may be more harmful to your overall wellbeing!

## Spice up your life?

If you like spices and herbs, there is some support that they impact our health via chemical and cellular influences. While an overview of some of the more commonly used ones will be presented, it is beyond the scope of this chapter to give personalized recommendations on the use of these. Again, you are encouraged to do your own research and to work with a qualified professional for personalized assessment. You are also advised to check for food/herb/drug interactions. There are numerous websites today that assist you in this goal. Side-effect profiles are usually mild and related to GI upset. A comprehensive source on the topic is found in the *Botanical Safety Handbook* (2nd edition).[46]

Cayenne and other pepper plants contain capsaicin. Capsaicin is often extracted and available in topical applications that absorb through the skin, binding to specific receptors that can deplete substance P,[47] a neuropeptide that assists in conveying sensory information from the body to the brain. Substance P is well known to be involved in pain physiology by facilitating transmission of nociceptive information to the brain as well as promoting release of inflammatory cytokines.[48] Inhibition or depletion of substance P may reduce the brain's access to noxious sensory stimuli. This may be useful for joint and arthritic pain conditions, neuropathic pain, and pain associated with the shingles virus (post-herpetic neuralgia).[49] Another common product for pain is arnica, which is available in creams, gels, oils, and homeopathic remedies. One study using arnica gel for knee osteoarthritis showed improvements over six weeks with twice a day application.[50]

Ginger, mentioned earlier, contains substances that inhibit inflammation, including prostaglandins and leukotrienes. A systematic review of six studies (two for osteoarthritis, one for dysmenorrhea, and three for experimentally induced acute muscle pain) found that ginger reduced subjective pain reports.[51] The authors found the quality of the studies to be mixed and concluded that the efficacy of ginger to treat pain remains insufficient. They added, however, that the available data provide tentative support for the anti-inflammatory role of ginger, which may reduce the subjective experience of pain in some conditions.

Turmeric, in the same plant family as ginger, has growing popularity and research support as a medicinal food supplement. Turmeric contains curcuminoids, one of which is curcumin, which have been shown to inhibit inflammatory compounds such as prostaglandins, leukotrienes, and nitric oxide.[52] Studies have shown benefit for pain and symptoms from osteo- and rheumatoid arthritis.[53]

Mixed evidence exists to support pain management with the use of other herbal substances and supplements. Most are for arthritic and inflammatory pain in extremity joints, with a few for spinal pain and fibromyalgia. These include boswellia,[54] SAM-e,[55] willow,[56] Chinese skullcap,[57] devil's claw,[58] cat's claw,[59] and 5-HTP.[60] For headaches and migraines, evidence exists for butterbur,[61] feverfew,[62] and magnesium.[63]

Questions often arise around the use of cannabis and hemp-derived products (such as THC, CBD and other cannabinoid substances), kratom, and wild lettuce for pain treatment. Legality issues complicate the matter with the first two, and research is lacking on all of them, placing them outside the scope of this chapter.

More research is needed on these substances, including placebo control groups and determination of dose/frequency recommendations.

## The yoga lifestyle and nutrition

While gathering basic information on principles of nutritional medicine is valuable, perhaps more importance in your exploration of the role of nutrition in your wellbeing will come from exploring and better understanding your own individual *relationship* to food and eating and how this interacts with other levels of your experience—thoughts, beliefs, emotions, and the general mind-body connection. Yoga, while ancient, is increasingly supported by scientific rigor. The fields that inform psychoneuroimmunology provide us with the understanding that subjective constructs such as expectations, beliefs, thoughts, values, and emotions have identifiable physiological bases. As such, processes in the mind inform and shape our experience of physical health. Various yogic practices such as pranayama, asana, imagery, and meditation "enter" your biofield on different levels, having ripple effects across the whole of your being, including potentially positive impact on inflammation, immune function, pain processes, gut health, the microbiome ecosystem, and more.

## The yamas and niyamas

Yoga as a lifestyle involves looking at all limbs of yoga including moral precepts that guide your relationships to both self and others. These principles extend to other forms of relationship including to food and ultimately to the pain experience itself.

In review, the niyamas are intrapersonal actions or qualities to cultivate within oneself and include purity, contentment, austerity, self-study, and spirituality. The yamas are interpersonal actions to observe in support of healthy relationships with others, self, and the world in general, and include non-harming, honesty, non-stealing, conservation of energy, and greedlessness, which includes the concept of "non-hoarding." As we contemplate these in relationship to nutrition, food, and eating, the following questions represent a sample of applications.

- Is there any aspect of my relationship to food that brings harm to myself or others?

- Am I honest with myself and others about my relationship to food?

- Am I willing to look closely at underlying patterns of emotion, thoughts, and beliefs that influence my relationship to food?

- How are energetic relationships within my body–mind–spirit biofield affected by what I eat, how I eat, and when I eat?

- Do I eat more than is needed for my body's needs?

- Do I eat with awareness and mindfulness?

- Where and how do I invest the energy that I receive from what I eat?

- Do I eat in a way that supports clean, healthy energy for my body and how does this relate to my activity level?

- How does food and eating impact my relationships with others?

- What is my posture like when I eat?

- How do my breathing patterns interact with my relationship to food and eating?

- Do I exercise principles of compassion, acceptance, and loving-kindness with my own and others' relationships to food?

- How do my spiritual beliefs and practices interact with my relationship to food and eating? Do I exercise gratitude for the nourishment I receive?

- Am I willing to take a close look at my food choices and eating habits and their impact on my health and wellbeing?

- How do my food choices connect to and support the environment? Am I aware of the people and resources that went into the production of the food I eat? How do my food choices impact the karma and the interconnectedness of all life?

## EXPERIENTIAL ACTIVITY

Sitting comfortably, allow your eyes to slowly close. Become aware of your breathing and allow it to become gradually longer and softer… Allow your body to soften… Now, bring to mind the last meal you ate… Where were you? What do you see? What do you hear, smell, and feel? … Is there anyone with you? … Look closely at the food. What do you become aware of now? … What do you notice in your body? … Did you prepare this food yourself? If someone else did, where and how was it prepared? … Do you know where this food originated? Can you imagine the land or the people and other resources that contributed to its existence? … What journey did the food take to reach you? … And finally, what happened in the hours after you ate? How were you feeling? How did the meal affect your body and mind state? … When you're ready, slowly open your eyes and consider how this retrospective look at your last meal might inform your next meal…

## Mindfulness and food

These principles, as well as the other limbs of yoga, can be extended into the many other facets that we'll collectively call *mindful eating*. Applying the general principles of mindful awareness to every facet of nutrition and eating will assist in revealing not just hidden patterns in your relationship with food, but also possible connections to your pain experience and your body's unique needs in general. A few examples are given below.

- Eliminate distractions:
    - Are you multitasking or truly focused on the food choice and the act of eating? Can you set your phone aside?

- Relate:
    - Whenever possible, eat with people you love, and around a table!

- Sit down:
    - Sit down to eat, be mindful of your posture while eating. Ask yourself, am I upright, with my ears balanced over my shoulders, and my shoulders over hips?

- Listen to your body:
    - The more attuned one is to the subtle sensations, cues, and messages of the body, the more able one is to detect the influence of foods and dietary patterns and habits on the sense of wellbeing or dis-ease, including any influence on pain patterns.

It is also helpful to remember to slow down, check in with your mood, chew your food, eat until you are 80 percent full, and experiment regularly to explore and connect with your unique mind-body-spirit relationship so that you know what *you* need in each moment of your walk through this world. For some, simple ceremonies and rituals such as breathing, or saying a prayer of intention or gratitude will complement your mindful eating approach. These ideas assist in the ongoing creation of wellbeing that exists independent of temporary states of discomfort, equally of pleasure, and that takes into account awareness of our interdependence with others and the ecosystems that we interact with.

*Awareness experiments* may assist in learning more about your unique biochemical individuality in relation to food, including if you have developed food sensitivities linked to neuro-inflammatory and immune responses. Temporary selective elimination of certain foods, followed by reintroduction of that food, may allow you to see more clearly how your body responds. In an elimination program, foods are typically removed for a minimum of three weeks and then reintroduced to notice how you feel. During this time, noticing your overall pain experience including any emotional patterns connected to the food is useful. It is helpful to keep a daily diary of this process.

You may wish to devise your own awareness experiments and discover what your body is telling you. Remember the topic of complexity that we started with: such experiments do not occur in isolation, reflect only one small component of your overall experience, and may represent an entry point into one level of the complex living system that is *you*! Also remember that nocebo, the opposite of placebo, can sometimes be at work when we form negative beliefs and associations, and thus the point here is to explore and contemplate and not create negative associations that do not exist.

## Summary

Food, nutrition, and eating represent a complex topic that is ripe for exploration. While a growing amount of core research exists on the general topic of nutritional medicine for various illnesses and chronic disease processes, research specific to the experience of chronic pain is limited. This may be due to the fact that chronic pain can appear in endless manifestations with a strong contribution from each person's unique psychosocial and spiritual content and experience. Such complexity makes it even harder than usual to explore correlations as causal in research. Thus, no two recipes are the same. Much of what is presented here is intended to provide a solid foundation for nutrition and mindful eating irrespective of, but applicable to, chronic pain. Some information provided may be useful to address underlying biochemical facets of pain biology, especially as relates to inflammatory processes in the body. Pain is a highly individualized experience with a myriad of knowable and unknowable factors contributing to the manifestation in any given moment. As such, the true goal is to assist you in an ongoing experiment, rooted in the foundations of yoga lifestyle and the overarching goal of coming to know yourself—including your relationship to nutrition, food, and eating—better. In this, you will come to know what is true and right for your whole-being. May your exploration be fruitful!

## Chapter 11

# Transforming Psycho-Emotional Pain

Michael Lee

*Yogash citta vrtti nirodha*

*Yoga is the cessation of the modifications, or fluctuations, of the mind.*

Yoga Sutra 1.2[1]

In this chapter, we will explore the process of transformation in working with psycho-emotional pain.

Regardless of the setting or modality engaged, be it traditional, complementary, yoga based, or not, there are many creative and viable ways of working with psycho-emotional pain that are being practiced today. To engage the conversation here around transformational work, I will reference these approaches as two broad categories based on their underlying paradigm—a category in which the primary focus is on the treatment of symptoms and related conditions, and the other where the primary focus is upon whole-being transformation.

## Symptom management

Symptom-management methods often include practices, protocols, tools, and courses of treatment that can be employed to alleviate or lessen the impact of the symptoms and the associated pain. The goal of the practitioner is to minimize suffering in either the short or long term. If the approach is effective, the suffering experienced from the pain will be less intrusive in the individual's life, and so life may become more manageable or tolerable on a day-to-day basis. The symptom-management approach may be highly interventional, or it may be more integrative but still aimed at creating a specific outcome for the patient, for example giving a client a simple mindfulness technique to help them overcome bouts of anxiety. It is the most widely used approach in healthcare.[2] Success is measured in terms of positive change in the initial prevailing symptom or "condition" being treated. Such outcomes are generally easy to evaluate, and this could explain why these kinds of approaches are more likely to be chosen for research.

## Transformational approach

Whole-being transformation engages a process from which new insight or wisdom emerges. This produces a change in beliefs or values and new behavior results, and a different experience of life is engaged. The old way of seeing and experiencing life no longer makes sense and new beliefs and ways of engaging life are born. The moment the life-changing insight is integrated, a shift is activated. The full manifestation and life impact of this shift may or may not be immediate, but either way there is a new way of engaging life in place and a strong desire to move in this new direction is set in motion.[3] The new level of awareness accompanying this change acts as a compass for future choices and, although the process may take time to become fully established, a new way of being in life is in play. Things that previously mattered no longer matter, and other things previously ignored take on new importance. This new direction often changes some or most of the conditions that gave rise to the pain and suffering in the first place. In some cases, symptoms may completely disappear. The result of what is produced as a result of the shift is what is valued in transformational work. This outcome is often accompanied by less tangible and not so easily measurable outcomes that are relative to the individual. These may include such things as a sense of greater meaningfulness in life, increasing joy and happiness, or greater fulfillment in life.

## The two approaches side by side

It may be helpful to look at the two models side by side in terms of some of the key elements in each, as many of these elements will be referenced in the discussion that follows.[4]

Table 11.1 Paradigms of healing

| Symptom management | Transformational approach |
|---|---|
| Diagnosis and treatment | Co-created exploration of conditions arising and desired outcome |
| Focus on cause and effect | A unique, one-of-a-kind exploration |
| Desired outcome predictable | Accepting many outcomes possible |
| Power with clinician | Power shared in co-created process |

## Yoga and transformation

### Is transformation the purpose of yoga?

Sarbacker and Kimple write: "The various traditions of India have all recognized the great potential for self-transformation through yoga…to transform one's relationship with the world in profound ways…that one's capacities for action and perception are enhanced."[5]

In 1984 I experienced a profound and transformational life-changing experience through yoga.[6] My new insight was so significant and impactful that I decided to make my life's work helping others to change using yoga therapy as the vehicle to engage a transformational process. Since then I have engaged many personal experiences of transformation, supported many others, trained yoga therapists to deliver facilitated yoga-inspired experiences as a transformational process, dived deeply into the psychology and philosophy of yoga and Buddhism, and explored those elements of modern psychology and neuroscience that relate to the potential and power of yoga for transformation. So, in this chapter, the lens through which I will explore psycho-emotional pain is shaped by that experience, my subsequent learning, and ongoing study and work. Through this lens it is easier to see yoga as originally defined as a brilliant transformational process highly relevant to the world today. This is particularly so if experiences are structured to match current world phenomena and make use of much of what has been learned since Patanjali, and that fits with that transformational intention.

## Transformation as the essence of Patanjali's yoga

Let's examine transformation in the relation to the essence of yoga as expounded by Patanjali. In the second Yoga Sutra, quoted at the beginning of this chapter, it states, "Yoga is the cessation of the fluctuations of the mind."[7] The word "cessation" means an "end" or a "finish." In other words, no more fluctuations or modifications happening. "Fluctuations" and "modifications" imply a lot of movement and perhaps "false perception." In other words, when there are modifications happening in our mind, there is often a difficulty seeing things as they really are, so the mind strives to make sense of reality by constructing things differently. The fluctuations are the result of a restlessness and difficulty in focusing on any one state at any given time. Following a transformational experience however, there is greater stability, acceptance, and equanimity and an openness to "seeing things as they really are." And while it may not be possible in our modern world to live full time in such a state of being, once the journey has begun, there is usually no turning back. We must engage in day-to-day life with a rational mind to navigate modern life. But, at the same time, there is a deeper foundation to our awareness following a transformational shift. Our new insight and wisdom guide us when we encounter old habits and beliefs tugging at us.

Patanjali's eight limbs of yoga, in essence, outline a process of transformation—although many see them as "steps" on a path. My understanding is that his model is not linear and each of the limbs is not separate from the others. It is an integrated model. It describes yoga as a "process" and not a "prescription." It is a movement from an external world to an internal world that reshapes the body and mind.[8]

The external part of the process is outlined in the four limbs of yama, niyama, asana, pranayama. These might be seen as "preparation for transformation" or laying the ground. Putting in place one's intention in terms of what one wishes to create in one's life is helpful if one wishes to change. For example, if we desire peace, it makes no sense to harm others (ahimsa—non-harming, one of the yamas). When attention is paid to breath (pranayama) and we engage mindful asana at an edge, we begin to notice things in body and mind. Some of what we experience we may like, and some we may not. Here the practice of accepting things as they are (the niyama of santosha) is important for the process of transformation to continue. Pratyahara can be seen as the bridge linking the external and internal parts of the process together. External distractions and mental activity are disengaged and the focus shifts into present-centered direct experience. Concentration (dharana) is engaged and a deeper state of awareness evolves (dhyana), and new insight from seeing things as they really are is embraced (samadhi).

These limbs of yoga can be practiced in various ways in an individual practice and, traditionally, over a considerable length of time to attain wisdom. As we shall see in a model discussed later, a modernized approach to yoga therapy may in fact shortcut this process to the extent that it becomes possible in a very short time and hence takes on significantly greater therapeutic value in today's world. This is possible when the eight limbs are used as the cornerstone of a one-on-one facilitated yoga therapy process using an integrated transformational model based on yoga but drawing from other fields as well. And once the process of transformation is engaged, regardless of the method, it continues as Patanjali implicitly envisioned. It is "profound, fundamental, and irreversible. It is a metamorphosis, a radical change from one form to another."[9]

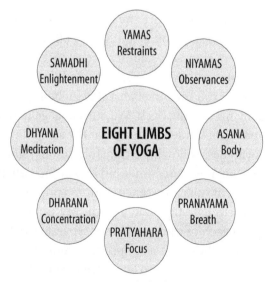

*Figure 11.1 Eight limbs of yoga*

## Metamorphosis and the Phoenix

The concept of metamorphosis is particularly helpful when we think of a butterfly emerging from the chrysalis. The ancient Greek myth of the Phoenix also describes transformation—the long-lived mythical bird in all its beauty flies into the "fire of transformation" to self-destruct but then rises again from the embers even more glorious and magnificent—a rebirth.[10] The transformational path is not guaranteed to be painless. It often necessitates accepting and embracing discomfort. This notion is counter-intuitive to the way we live in our modern world in which we seem to have an obsession with stopping pain at almost any price and doing so immediately however we might be able. Such mindset, while fueling some great science, can also lead to addiction and further suffering.

## The reality of psycho-emotional pain in daily life

Yet, suffering from psycho-emotional pain is, to some degree, a reality of life. As the Buddha articulated in the first of the Four Noble Truths—life involves suffering. It occurs in both subtle and not so subtle forms. Even when we feel "good" there is still often in place an undercurrent of tension or anxiety. We live in an imperfect world. From the time of our birth we are subject to the impact of those imperfections, some of us more than others. But regardless of the extent, it's a common problem. Very few humans, if any, go unaffected. As I work with clients in my yoga therapy practice, I see the pain in various degrees in just about every client.

Along with an intolerance of discomfort, we live in a society that is finding it increasingly difficult to either cope with or remedy our psycho-emotional suffering. Is it a byproduct of the complexity of living today and getting worse perhaps? I'm sure most of us notice this notion pop up in our casual conversations. People everywhere seem to not have "enough time." They are not engaging their passion except perhaps in short mini-vacations. Their lives lack purpose and meaning, and many will complain of the loss of values they see and feel around them. In the long term, living a life this way gives rise to a state of suffering. This may manifest or be diagnosed as stress, anxiety, or depression. Left unchanged, prolonged suffering may manifest in the extremes we see in the news for those unable to cope—school shootings, deaths from misuse of drugs and alcohol, domestic abuse and violence, homicide and suicide, and the list goes on… Is there any hope for the future, one might ask?

## Hope for change

I am more passionate now than ever before that change is possible. To transform our lives from an almost constant state of mental suffering to a life in which there is less suffering, more joy and greater meaning and fulfillment is possible.

All conditioned things are impermanent—when one sees this with wisdom, one turns away from suffering. (The Buddha)[11]

While such a quote offers hope, my hope is even further fueled by my direct personal experiences over the past 35 years both in my own life and in my work with my yoga therapy clients and students. Real and lasting change is possible.

### Conditions arising to support change

Change depends on the conditions that are in place supporting it. The conditions that "give rise" to the potential to experience transformation include presence, awareness, seeing and experiencing things as they really are, and a willingness to be open to engaging and learning from them. An awareness that there is no panacea or quick fix and that the solution that works for each of us is likely to be unique is also helpful in the process—particularly on the part of the facilitator.

And to reiterate, such change can be facilitated through present-centered, body-based process based on ancient yogic principles while also drawing from compatible elements of modern psychology, neuroscience, and educational processes.

Transformational change demands a present-centered focus rather than looking prematurely to the future or the past for answers to immediate issues. It engages direct experience rather than a cognitive process. Direct experience is awareness based in present time and it involves as much of a letting go as it does "doing" anything. It requires some tolerance to stay in the unknown to allow insight and wisdom to emerge rather than engaging the often almost overwhelming desire to "fix it now"—sometimes for both client and therapist.

The conditions for transformation to occur are something that either yoga therapist or individual can support in their own or another's life if such counter-intuitive mindset can be entertained and engaged.

## AN EXAMPLE OF SIMPLE TRANSFORMATIONAL PROCESS

Recently, in conversation with my brother-in-law, Joe, he asked me how the "transformational approach to yoga therapy" that I had developed was different to the allopathic diagnosis/treatment model in traditional healthcare. I'm often at a loss to explain this process in everyday language outside of my professional settings and it is clearly better understood experientially rather than cognitively. But I wanted to answer his question. So, with his agreement, I chose to give Joe a "mini-experience" of my work as a way of answering.

I asked him to close his eyes and bring his two index fingers together in front of his body and press them together. I then began to help him engage the experience more fully and coached him towards a more direct experience with a focus on body sensation and present-centered awareness. After a short while I asked what he noticed. He said he felt more present to the moment. He noticed his mind was not racing in many directions and thinking about many things. He was simply experiencing the touch of his two fingers. We continued for a few minutes more. I asked him to let his fingers come down and to remain with his eyes closed as I led him in a simple cognitive integration process. After he reflected on his experience, I asked him how it might inform his life. He said he noticed how "busy" his life had become recently. How he no longer had time for the kinds of things that made him more present to himself. And here, in a few minutes, he saw that more clearly. We discussed this a little and then I asked what he might want to do with this awareness. His answer was a little vague at first but with a little refinement of concepts and language and a few further questions he decided he would find his own 15 minutes of "quiet time" each day to be present to the moment and get clear as he had done in the exercise. He thanked me for helping him in a very short time to see the reality of what was happening in his life.

We spoke again the next day and he was excited to show me what he had done. He had been out in his garden and had pruned a large number of the overgrown bushes and trees and it looked beautiful. He was excited as he said he'd been avoiding working in his garden this year because his life had become too busy with much travel and family matters to deal with. But this morning he decided to engage in a little gardening following his 15-minute meditation time. I asked how it went. He said it was amazing. He had not been aware until now what gardening really meant in his life. It was more than just a love of gardens. It was a very important time in his life. A time when he could stop thinking and just be present to what was right there in the moment. It was another tool in helping him get clear. His mind slowed down and he felt rejuvenated and clearer about his purpose in life and what mattered and what didn't. "I can't wait to meditate and get out there again tomorrow," he declared.

The above story may be simple but it engages the essence of a transformational process. In yogic terms, the body was engaged as it is in asana or mudra, albeit a very simple one. There was a focus on awareness of breath (pranayama). An instructional dialog was aimed at inviting greater presence and observation of moment-by-moment experience and in so doing other distractions were reduced (pratyahara). As the experience progressed, a different state of being was reported, not unlike that engaged in the upper limbs of yoga (dharana, dhyana, and samadhi).

In essence, the process is also a form of "mindfulness." Once engaged, Joe became "concentrated" in his awareness. As a result, he gained insight that might otherwise have eluded him in his busy day-to-day life.

## Neuroscience and present-centered awareness in the transformational process

One of the key prerequisites for engaging a transformational process is present-centered awareness.

In our modern world we spend very little time in what Norman Farb and his team of researchers at Toronto University in a study in 2007 termed "present centered referencing" (being aware of what's happening now) as opposed to "narrative referencing" (thinking about the past or future in story form).[12] They were able to demonstrate, using fMRI, which states of awareness their subjects were engaging at any given time. The reality is that most of us don't spend much time in the present and the bulk of our time is spent thinking about either "immediate past," or "immediate future" happenings as the illustration from Farb's study indicated.

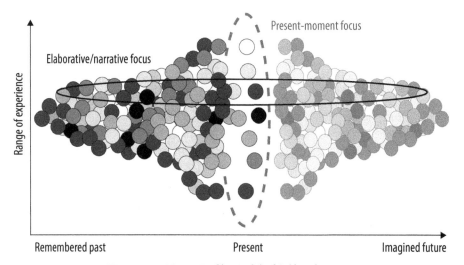

*Figure 11.2 Norm Farb's Model of Self-Referencing*

Source: Farb, N. A., Anderson, A. K. and Segal, Z. V. (2012) "The mindful brain and emotion regulation in mood disorders." *Canadian Journal of Psychiatry 57*, 2, 70–77. Reprinted with permission.

In relation to mindfulness, Farb and his team discovered that it was possible, through training, to induce more frequent and longer periods of time in the present. Furthermore, it was discovered that those able to drop in to present awareness possess a greater capacity to be able to shift easily back and forth at will between the two different forms of referencing. In my example with Joe, the way in which instructional dialog was delivered supported a focus on immediate present-centered awareness as opposed to engaging a "narrative." Besides training, however, another way of helping the yoga therapy client become present is skilled facilitation, which in my experience can be done for many clients in as little as ten minutes.

Another key element of the mini-experience with Joe was the relationship between us. He felt safe with me. A feeling of safety, along with authenticity, are key elements in the client/therapist relationship in transformational work. The experience was also open ended and client centered. I was careful not to imply that he was "expected" to engage in the experience in any stipulated way. This did not need to be spoken. It was made implicit by the tone and delivery of the process and supported by the relationship. From a psychological perspective, the approach was consistent with the theory of "unconditional positive regard" as defined in the work of Carl Rogers.[13] I did not make any formal "diagnosis" and simply took things as they came without judgment (unconditional positive regard). I heard and took seriously anything Joe spoke of and he felt safe to say whatever came to him without feeling judged or evaluated (empathetic listening).

I also utilized learning principles based on andragogy (how adults learn) in the educational process as opposed to pedagogy (how children learn) based on the adult learning theories of Malcolm S. Knowles.[14] One of Knowles' key principles in this theory is for the teacher/therapist to involve the learner/client in the learning process, in both the engagement of the learning activity and the construction of "learning plans" going forward.

Back in Patanjali's day, the way in which knowledge was transmitted was basically on a pedagogical top-down model. The teacher expounded theory and practice. The student listened and practiced, and understanding grew over time. The power was with the teacher and the student was generally a passive recipient in the process. This prevailing theory of education then was clearly demonstrated in the guru/disciple model with the power laying clearly in the hands of the guru. Modern learning theory, particularly if empowerment of the individual is at stake, utilizes models where greater power sharing and co-creation are evident. Practitioners of ancient traditions like yoga are often slow to adopt modern methods for fear of losing the essence of the tradition, when in fact these methods may enhance the underlying intention of the tradition, particularly in the modern world.

This mini-session with Joe was not set up as a professional yoga therapy session, in which I would have included longer, more complex, and engaging work, but it was delivered along the same principles that are inherent in the Phoenix Rising Method in yoga therapy.[15] In summary, this was an example of a transformational experience that included the principles underlying the essence of Patanjali's yoga while, at the same time, drawing from the advancements in psychology and learning theory. This, I believe, enhanced the progression towards the ultimate goal that Patanjali had in mind without detracting from it or devaluing it. For Joe, there was more "union" in his life—coming together of heart and mind.

## Our modern world needs transformation and yoga can accommodate

As our world continues to become more seemingly connected through social media and communication, we are becoming, on the one hand, more complex in the way our lives are managed and, on the other hand, more separated from ourselves. It would seem we may be losing our deeper and more meaningful "connection to self." Without it, we don't know or trust ourselves as we are, and so the seeds of discontent from which stress, anxiety, and depression emerge are sown. It could well be that our increase in suffering and pain in our modern world stems from this incapacity to "know ourselves." And connection to self seems to be more difficult to attain through a cognitive application of knowledge than it does through a more direct experience of self. Much of our modern work, even in yoga therapy, has become more cognitive and reductionist, and less experiential. Perhaps it's time to re-emphasize the importance of experiential learning in the yoga therapy process and delivery. So, then the focus becomes not so much on how much we "know" about the ancient traditions but how skillfully we might be able to experience in learning it, so as to apply the inherent wisdom and knowledge to change our way of "being."

## Where is the focus today—transformation or symptom management?

Not so long ago, and according to Freud, it was believed that the best we could do in therapy was support the client in a return to "normalcy."[16] It is clear that today people want more than "normal." If in pain, we may certainly wish to be free of it as a first step. But is this "normal" state enough in today's world? We yearn to be rid of emotional turmoil, we want to be free of our wounds from the past, we want to create a life without everyday anxiety and stress. We also strive now for happiness, for freedom from struggle and suffering, and for the capacity to live a meaningful and fulfilling life. The upsurge in yoga, meditation, and similar pursuits is clearly a result of this quest. But does the goal in these pursuits extend to transformation or stop short? Are we perhaps looking for another quick fix? And as we know from the discussion, if pain and suffering are to be "ended" as stated as the goal in both yoga and Buddhism, will a quick fix to alleviate the immediate symptoms help in reaching that goal? And is all yoga transformational or might it also offer a quick fix in some applications?

Much of the evidence-based research in yoga and yoga therapy to date has seemed to focus on the application of traditional practices and their effectiveness in alleviating the symptoms of psycho-emotional pain. Their relative success in this area has given yoga therapy a "leg up" in the mainstream world of healthcare and paved the way for the wider acceptance of yoga-based practices and processes. The titles of the studies clearly indicate the intent and will usually include "Yoga for…" or something similar like "complementary therapies for anxiety and depression."[17] Like all things, the rush to research in recent years has led to some great benefits but also some concerns. Has that success and focus on "yoga for…" and an almost exclusive focus on the treatment of specific conditions also resulted in stopping short of engaging yoga as a complex integrated process that is useful in facilitating an approach to change that is truly holistic, transformational, and long-lasting? And if the yoga in these studies is largely unconnected from Patanjali's paradigm of yoga, then what is it? As Lorenzo Cohen, chief of the integrative medicine section at MD Anderson Cancer Center, observes, "Many papers [on yoga] don't have enough of an in-depth description of what they mean by 'yoga.'"[18]

If yoga is thought of as "intervention" based on certain described techniques or practices rather than its "essence" as a transformational process, then this will result in a much different focus and process for the study and the outcome.

Medical practitioner and yoga therapist Dr. Ananda Balayogi Bhavanani, in a keynote address at the 2018 Symposium on Yoga Therapy and Research, termed this trend *yogopathy* and distinguished it from a more traditional transformational approach to *yoga therapy* based upon the ancient yoga psychology of Patanjali.[19]

## Limitations of yoga therapy for symptom management as a primary focus

Conditions "giving rise" to symptoms that can extend into disease are often many, varied, and different for each individual regardless of the same diagnosis being made within our traditional healthcare frame of reference. The idea of "conditions arising" or "dependent origination" as it is generally known is found in both Vedanta and Buddhist philosophy and has been a traditional focus in both of these ancient traditions.[20] In the application of yoga therapy therefore, the task is to understand the unique conditions arising and that underlie what is happening. This is best done through an acceptance of the prevailing symptom and an experiential exploration of the unique conditions giving rise to it. Transformation is possible for the individual when, and only when, they are able to accept and view reality as it really is and not as it might be experienced through or conditioned by past or future events created by the "fluctuations of the mind."

The Illness-Wellness Continuum, first created by John Travis, MD, in 1972 and still used today, shows how the human condition can be viewed on a scale ranging from illness to optimal wellness.[21]

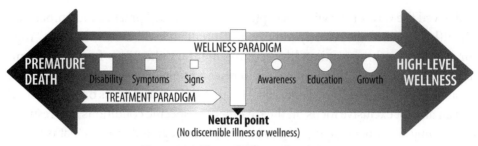

*Figure 11.3 Illness-Wellness Continuum*

Prior to the neutral point, symptoms are managed to return the person to a state of "no discernable illness" (Freud's "state of normalcy").[22] Transformation can occur anywhere on the model but seems to be most commonly experienced beyond the treatment area on the left side and through to the right-hand end of the scale.

Transformation generally occurs after some life-changing experience, which may be either pleasant or unpleasant or a combination. This "experience" of self may be in a therapeutic setting, facilitated by a skilled yoga therapist or other practitioner trained in transformational process work, but sometimes can be simply incidental to one's life journey and occur anytime and anywhere. For example, also known as "the Overview Effect," it is often experienced by astronauts on their journey in space.[23] It is the kind of experience that alters one's "insight" or perception as to what is held to be "true" now for the individual. As a result, the person's values and beliefs change and there is generally a new equilibrium established and no desire to return to the "old way" of seeing or experiencing one's life. There are two methods in different modalities that I will share below to illustrate ways to support transformational change relative to psycho-emotional pain.

## Memory Reconsolidation in psychotherapy as a transformational process

Bruce Ecker recently developed the theory of Memory Reconsolidation to explain an approach to psychotherapy in which the client may be transformed and a new way of being will result. Symptoms will no longer hold the same power.

Ecker makes the distinction between approaches that manage symptoms and those that are "pro-symptom" and "transformational."[24] "Pro-symptom" is explained as an approach that does not seek to address the symptoms as the focus but rather accepts the symptoms as the client's best currently available option given the circumstances. Acceptance of the manifesting symptom is seen as a starting point for the therapeutic process. They are embraced as a valid response to suffering, albeit ineffective.

This is discernably different than the stance that the symptom is something to be fixed or managed. Instead of attempting to mitigate the symptoms by offering antidotes, the symptom in Ecker's meta-theory is taken as a given. The aim is to support the patient in creating a "mis-match" experientially between a long-standing belief that fuels the symptom, for example the belief that "The only way to get love is to be needy or depressed," to a new belief resulting from experience facilitated by the therapist, for example "Right now I feel love and I notice I do not feel depressed. Right now this feeling of love comes differently without the usual associated feelings."

Once this mismatch between past belief and present experience is uncovered, it is postulated that there is an automatic neural disconnect and this affects the brain neuroplasticity to form a new way of seeing things from this point on. There is a transformation created by the mismatch and new belief for the client that not only makes better sense, but, given the new insight, becomes the only rational option.

The transformation may be instantaneous and the symptoms no longer exist, or it can go through a period of reconsolidation over time before becoming fully part of a new way of being. The therapist will often engage the client in an experience that may shed new light on the circumstances and result in a "reconsolidation" of beliefs, which in turn can bring about a complete "transformation." After such a transformational experience, the old symptoms no longer hold power and therefore do not impact the life of the person as they did before. Sometimes this shift is accompanied by what might be described as an increase in wisdom resulting from an experience. It is most likely to emerge at a time when the person is open, often vulnerable, but at the same time is feeling at peace from within and is simply seeing their life with new awareness and with greater clarity. Supporting these "conditions" for the possible engagement of a transformational experience is one of the key roles for the therapist engaging this approach. This new-found "wisdom" often grows into other areas of the person's life as well, and transformation in the future becomes easier for this individual.

## Transformation in Phoenix Rising Yoga Therapy

I developed the Phoenix Rising approach to yoga therapy in 1986 from my direct and transformational experiences of yoga.[25]

Like Coherence Therapy, Phoenix Rising Yoga Therapy is a pro-symptom and transformational approach to change. The method offers the client a yoga-based process that engages and is responsive to their moment-to-moment experience. It is a client-centered and therapist-facilitated process to engage direct experience (experience gained from immediate sense perception). This facilitated process, although clearly based on the essence of Patanjali's yoga, is not unlike certain potentially "transformational" processes as found in the present-centered focus in

Gestalt founder Fritz Perls' work or the client-centered approach of Carl Rogers.[26] From this experience clients will often gain new insight and awareness in a similar way to that discussed in relation to the Memory Reconsolidation process. The essential elements of the Phoenix Rising Method are also similar to those discussed earlier in this chapter in the example offered by my story about Joe.

In a recent study of the Phoenix Rising Method, the following reported themes emerged for clients each receiving a series of five Phoenix Rising sessions: mindfulness, self-awareness, *mind-body* connection, in vivo experience of new behaviors, client-directed, empowerment, and life changes.[27] *Participants noted greater insight into mind-body connection. They noticed the effect of cognition and emotion on the body, observed how the body can be used to improve coping through movement and breathing, and experienced different thoughts and emotions associated with different areas of their bodies.* In 2015, Phoenix Rising Yoga Therapy training courses were accepted as eligible for Continuing Education Units (CEUs) for therapists and counsellors in California. This was largely as a response to the growing interest in traditional therapies in "bringing the body to therapy" for the client and to facilitate greater client awareness and empowerment.

The Phoenix-Rising-trained yoga therapist supports the client in variations of assisted asana at an appropriate edge. An awareness of breath and a body focus help the client to transition to a facilitated engagement of pratyahara (elimination of distractions from sensory experiences outside the present focus). From here, the client has the potential to drop into a deeper state of awareness in the realm of dhyana (meditation) or samadhi (deep insight from a pure sense of reality and the wisdom that accompanies it) from which insight and wisdom emerge. Following this embodied experience, we end with a verbal and cognitive integration and a "reconsolidation" of learning.

Note that the yoga therapy process described above differs from a symptom-management approach to yoga therapy in which the focus is upon client assessment for the purpose of teaching or prescribing yoga practices rather than the use of a direct experience facilitated by the yoga therapist as the primary educational process. The engagement of direct experience is a transformational approach that engages the client in an "experience of self" through the application of a *yogic process* as distinct from engaging a *yoga practice*. Through the client's unique experience, both when engaging this process and with the integration of that experience into life, new direction is *discovered* rather than *delivered*.

The transformational change process may not be an appropriate option for everyone. Suffering may be such that temporary relief might be the only viable option in the short run. Others may, for whatever reason, prefer to disengage from any process that requires their involvement. It is important for yoga therapists using this approach to understand that they must use it within their scope of practice and must have the capacity to discern its appropriateness for a particular client.

## Changes going forward

Going forward, it seems that both the transformational approach and the symptom-management approach will exist side by side in yoga therapy. Much can be learned from both. It is also apparent that many psychotherapists are now aware of and eager to learn more about the facilitation of embodied approaches based on yoga. In traditional healthcare there is now more emphasis placed on the relationship between the practitioner and the client and the need for greater empowerment of the client to help overcome low adherence rates through more empowered relationships. This is happening in both traditional and complementary approaches. It is hoped that further research on the significance and impact of empowerment and adherence will provide clearer understanding of this important element of the change process and may well lead towards wider application of transformational models that are inherently empowering.

## Application of the transformational approach to daily life

Whether you are yogi or a yoga therapist, a healthcare professional or a patient looking for something more, you can engage this approach easily in your own daily life. Here is a simple life application suggestion.

### Engage a "transformational yoga practice" every day

- Integrate your yoga and meditation with your life—don't separate it out.

- Use your *daily life* as a practice, as well as your daily yoga. Use both as tools for awareness. When you engage a yoga posture do so with a curious and present-centered focus. Do the same in daily life. Every event is an opportunity to learn and look within.

- Be clear every morning how you want to show up in your life that day— who do you want to be?—and pick one small area of opportunity to practice that in life every day. This is a great practice that I engage every day of my life by simply placing one hand on my chest and asking sincerely within, "How do I want to show up in life today?"

- Be real—beware of premature transcendence—engage the *muck*. This is particularly important for yoga professionals. Beware of the need to show up to your clients and students as "more enlightened" than you really are. Be humble and own up to the actions you take that are not yet in keeping with the consciousness to which you aspire.

- Practice daily but take a vacation occasionally and don't take yourself too seriously. This last part is important. There is no rush. If you need to take a break, do it. One of my senior teachers would often sit down with a good horror movie after delivering a yoga therapy training. It was her way of "letting down."

- Change it up and be open to other vehicles of practice—learn what *serves* you (which is not necessarily what you "like"). This doesn't mean shop around all over the place and go to the next new thing. It means being very real and curious about what really serves your life now.

- Connect and engage with yourself—who are you?—what are you creating in your life?—accept it—learn from it. Admit you are a seeker and keep seeking.

- Use inner dialogue and introspection without self-absorption—be mindful of all others you meet. Learn from others by being curious about their life journey as well as your own.

- Stop *doing* yoga. Start *engaging* it, as a moment-to-moment experience, not part of a "to do" list. This puts yoga into a whole different place in your life. Don't make it a chore. Value it as a gift.

- Validate and affirm yourself and others daily for being human and sometimes struggling—it's part of the ride.

- Act and follow through on your insights and trust your gut more. Insight without action does not go anywhere. Be sure to follow each new awareness with life application in some way, no matter how small.

- Enjoy this ride we call life—it's either a daring adventure or nothing.

## Conclusion

Setting up the conditions for transformation to occur is something that you, as either yoga therapist, health practitioner, teacher, or individual, can support, in your own or another's life. The conditions that "give rise" to the potential for transformation include presence, awareness, engagement with what is, and a willingness to be open, to enquire, and to learn. Transformational change demands a present-centered focus rather than looking prematurely to the future or nostalgically to the past for answers to immediate issues. The process of transformation also demands the capacity to trust one's own unique experience. It involves as much of a letting go as it does "doing" anything—a willingness to stay in the unknown and to allow the emergence of insight and wisdom rather than engaging that innate desire to "fix it now."

A transformational experience of yoga leaves the receiver changed and empowered. It also leaves them open to more. The door to continuing growth is often opened very wide by an initial transformational experience. In the longer run, this results in the emergence of the kind of human being with qualities similar to those of people you admire. For me, people like the Dalai Lama, a magnetic, compassionate, kind, authentic, and generous-of-spirit person. More importantly, a state of equanimity enables you, the transformed individual, to live comfortably in the chaos of life as it is.

The teachers and teachings can point the way, but each one of us must walk our own path, on our own unique journey of life.

## Chapter 12

# Pain, Addiction, and Yoga

Tracey Sondik

Addiction is a serious concern in working with people in pain. The opioid crisis and issues of addiction are coming to public and healthcare attention as a significant issue for those suffering from pain. Yoga has been used to work with populations of addiction. This chapter will look at understanding addiction, how it relates to pain and how yoga can be utilized for working with people with addictions. The yamas and niyamas will also be a focus in this chapter.

## Opioid crisis

The excessive use of alcohol, tobacco, and other substances has become a public health crisis in the US and across the world. In the US alone, 20.2 million adults (8.4%) had a substance use disorder according to the 2014 National Survey on Drug Use and Health.[1] Alcohol and tobacco represent two of the most common substance use disorders, followed by cannabis, stimulants, hallucinogens, and the alarming increase in misuse of opioids.

Over the past two decades, the misuse of and addiction to opioids has become a worldwide epidemic, impacting the health, social, and economic systems that cut across all different demographic and cultural societies. Opioids are a class of drugs that act on the opioid receptors on nerve cells in the brain and nervous system to produce pleasurable effects and relieve pain. Examples of these drugs are heroin and prescription pain relievers such as morphine, Percocet, Vicodin and OxyContin. Opioids, whether prescribed or not, can be highly addictive for a variety of reasons. Addiction is a complex phenomenon that depends on numerous factors that will be described later in the chapter.[2]

Opioids act by attaching to opioid receptors in the brain, which are specific proteins found on nerve cells in the brain, spinal cord, and other organs in the body. Once they attach to these opioid receptors, they can produce a sense of wellbeing (or euphoria in the case of heroin) and decrease the perception of pain.[3] Many people report significant relief from opioid prescriptions. When taken as directed by their physician and monitored over time, opioids can be effective, especially when used for a short amount of time.[4] However, with repeated usage of opioid drugs (prescription or heroin), the production of the body's natural endogenous opioids is inhibited and there can be significant discomfort when the drug is discontinued.[5] People may feel as much or more discomfort and pain than they originally did prior to taking the medication, so discontinuing them does not appear to be a viable solution.

There has been an alarming trend from prescription opioid use to heroin use seen in communities across the US, particularly in young people, leading to what many public health authorities are describing as the "Opioid Crisis," an "opioid state of emergency," and a "national epidemic."[6]

Since the 1990s, prescription painkillers have been prescribed at increasingly alarming rates. Prescriptions for opioids went from an estimated 76 million in 1991 to nearly 207 million in 2013 in the US.[7] Between 1995 and 1996, prescriptions jumped from 3 million to 8 million in one year alone. The combination of new and powerful medications that went on the market in 1996 and a greater emphasis on pain assessment and management in the early 2000s based on the Joint Commission's standard that doctors must assess all patients' pain level, led to more and more prescriptions of opioids.[8]

The scope of the opioid crisis is enormous. There are an estimated 26.4–36 million people worldwide who are addicted to opioids.[9] In the US alone, there are estimated to be 11.8 million people that misused opioids including 11.5 million that misused prescription pain relievers and another 948,000 that misused heroin.[10] Even more alarming is the number of accidental deaths in the US due to drug overdose. In one year alone (2016), 20,000 deaths were related to prescription pain relievers and 12,990 overdose deaths related to heroin[11] (see Figure 12.1).

In 2016, 43 people died every day due to prescription pain relievers. Over 60 percent of those misusing opioids reported that the main reason they misused pain relievers was to relieve physical pain.[12]

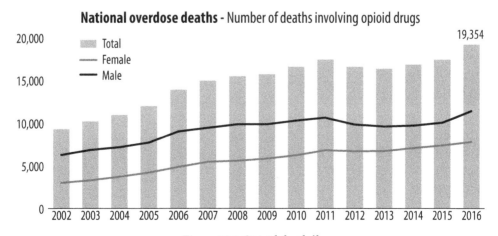

Figure 12.1 Opioid deaths[13]

To address this global crisis, organizations such as the Center for Disease Control (CDC) and the Federal Drug Administration are trying to take steps to combat the negative impact of opioid misuse and its potentially lethal consequences. In 2016, CDC created guidelines for prescribing opioids for chronic pain. Its recommendations include consideration for nonpharmacological options that may be more effective for treatment of chronic pain, including physical therapy, exercise therapy, and cognitive-behavioral psychotherapy.[14]

In April of 2017, the American College of Physicians provided clinical recommendations for back pain management and included among several recommendations:

> For patients with chronic low back pain, clinicians and patients should initially select nonpharmacologic treatment with exercise, multidisciplinary rehabilitation, acupuncture, mindfulness-based stress reduction, tai chi, **yoga**, motor control exercise, progressive relaxation, electromyography biofeedback, low-level laser therapy, operant therapy, cognitive behavioral therapy, or spinal manipulation.[15]

This represents a remarkable shift from pharmacological reliance for pain management to the use of complementary and alternative medicine (CAM). It also creates a larger paradigm shift for the addiction field in general as more and more people are willing to consider CAM interventions for physical, emotional, and spiritual relief from substance misuse. CAM interventions have become more and more popular for treatment of a variety of conditions including both mental health and substance use disorders. In 2008, the NIH National Center for Complementary and Alternative Medicine released initial findings on the use of CAM interventions in the US. According to this study, approximately 38 percent of adults used CAM treatments in 2008.[16] In 2017, the NIH released new data indicating significant increases in complementary health approaches for yoga, meditation, and chiropractors. The use of yoga increased from 9.5% to 14.3% over the past five years, meditation use increased from 4.1% to 14.2%, and the use of chiropractors from 9.1% to 10.3%.[17] These numbers continue to increase every year and are expected to rise with the new CDC and American College of Physician recommendations. Treatment for addiction using yoga, mindfulness, and other CAM interventions has now become mainstream in the addictions field.

## What is addiction?

According to the American Society of Addiction Medicine, the definition of addiction is:

> A primary, chronic disease of brain reward, motivation, memory and related circuitry. Dysfunction in these circuits leads to characteristic biological,

psychological, social and spiritual manifestations. This is reflected in an individual pathologically pursuing reward and/or relief by substance use and other behaviors. Addiction is characterized by inability to consistently abstain, impairment in behavioral control, craving, diminished recognition of significant problems with one's behaviors and interpersonal relationships, and a dysfunctional emotional response. Like other chronic diseases, addiction often involves cycles of relapse and remission. Without treatment or engagement in recovery activities, addiction is progressive and can result in disability or premature death.[18]

In 2013, the American Psychiatric Association (APA) published the DSM-5,[19] which included significant changes to the diagnostic classification of what was previously described as "substance dependence" and "substance abuse." Instead, a single diagnosis was introduced, "substance use disorder," to better match the symptoms that people experience. The term "dependence" was eliminated, as it was often confused with "addiction" and dependence can be a normal body response to a substance that is not in fact an "addiction." The diagnosis can be described as mild, moderate, or severe depending on the level of severity based on how many of the following 11 criteria the person meets.[20]

- Taking the substance in larger amounts or for longer than you're meant to.

- Wanting to cut down or stop using the substance but not managing to.

- Spending a lot of time getting, using, or recovering from use of the substance.

- Cravings and urges to use the substance.

- Not managing to do what you should at work, home, or school because of substance use.

- Continuing to use, even when it causes problems in relationships.

- Giving up important social, occupational, or recreational activities because of substance use.

- Using substances again and again, even when it puts you in danger.

- Continuing to use, even when you know you have a physical or psychological problem that could have been caused or made worse by the substance.

- Needing more of the substance to get the effect you want (tolerance).

- Development of withdrawal symptoms, which can be relieved by taking more of the substance.

There are many theories why people use substances and why ultimately some become addicted. Research has shown that a combination of factors, including biological deficits in the circuits of reward, genetic predisposition, environmental and interpersonal experiences, and culture, all play a role in how addiction may develop in individuals who already have "biological vulnerabilities."[21] Psychological theories of addiction have also examined the role of substance use as a form of self-medication. This theory suggests that substance use is a way to relieve distressing physical symptoms, including chronic pain, and emotional symptoms, including stress, depression and anxiety, or physical symptoms.[22] There is a strong link between substance use and mental health issues, as the number of people with co-occurring mental health and substance use disorder in the US is 7.9 million, making up nearly 40 percent of all those suffering from a substance use disorder.[23] Researchers are now beginning to understand the impact of early trauma and other adverse childhood experiences on substance use disorders. The Adverse Childhood Experiences (ACE) study completed in 1998 provided compelling data that adolescents and children who experience adverse events in childhood, including the categories of abuse, neglect, growing up with household members who have addictions, mental illness, or have committed crimes, and parental discord, are at increased risk to develop a wide range of medical, psychiatric, and alcohol and drug abuse problems.[24] The data from the ACE's study has been carefully analyzed to distill risk factors for substance dependence.[25] The findings indicate that children exposed to particular extreme adverse events including sexual abuse, physical abuse, or witnessing a violent crime were significantly more likely to suffer from some type of substance abuse dependence. In addition, there was a cumulative effect of adverse experiences in childhood. The more repeated and chronic the traumatic events were, the higher the risk for developing dependence on alcohol, cocaine, and/or opioids. The rate is nearly double for suffering repeated traumatic events versus a single event.[26]

New and innovative approaches for substance abuse treatment and prevention now include the study of environmental, genetic, and psychiatric factors, along with early childhood adverse experiences, to understand the full spectrum of substance use disorders. This compelling data from the ACE study has turned the focus toward early intervention for at-risk children to prevent the cumulative impact of trauma.[27]

## Models of recovery

The term "recovery" has grown in terms of popularity and importance when considering how to address the growing crisis of addiction, particularly with the opioid epidemic. There are several definitions for recovery that go beyond simply abstaining from use. Experts agree that recovery includes both remission from the symptoms of substance use disorder and positive life-enhancing changes that impact the whole person.[28]

Remission can occur when someone completely stops the substance use or reduces the intake to a safer level. In serious substance use disorders, which are often more chronic in nature, it can take several years and multiple episodes of treatment before it is sustained. The Substance Abuse and Mental Health Services Administration (SAMHSA) defines recovery as "a process of change through which individuals improve their health and wellness, live in a self-directed life, and strive to reach their full potential."[29] There are many negative stereotypes around addicts as "hopeless" with the adage "Once an addict, always an addict." People may be hesitant to seek help because of the pessimistic view around recovery that still affects many due to how the media portrays the "addict." However, the latest statistics around recovery show that more than 50 percent of those in treatment were able to achieve sustained remission that lasted at least one year.[30] Further, relapse does not necessarily mean that the treatment failed. Successful treatment for more serious substance use disorders requires continued evaluation, modification of interventions, and utilization of a multi-modal approach. Similar to other chronic illnesses such as diabetes, asthma, and hypertension, the relapse rate for substance use disorders ranges from 40 to 60 percent.[31] Lapses in drug use can indicate the need for return to treatment or adjustment or finding alternative treatment options for the individual. Just like a patient struggling to lower their blood pressure, the person suffering with addiction needs ongoing care to find the right combination of interventions.

There are many different paths and models to recovery depending on the type of substance use disorder, the individual's psychological and physical health, and access to healthcare. Based on evidenced-based practices, effective substance use treatment should consider the following principles.

- "Addiction is a complex but treatable disease that affects brain function and behavior.

- No single treatment is appropriate for everyone.

- Treatment needs to be readily available.

- Effective treatment attends to multiple needs of the individual, not just their drug abuse.

- Remaining in treatment for an adequate period of time is critical (at least three months).

- Behavioral therapies including individual, family, or group counseling are the most commonly used forms of drug abuse treatment along with peer support programs during and following treatment such as Alcoholics Anonymous (AA) and Narcotics Anonymous (NA).

- Medications are an important element of treatment for many patients, especially when combined with counseling and other behavioral therapies."[32]

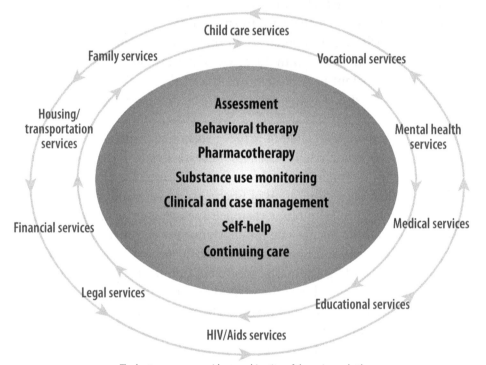

The best programs provide a combination of therapies and other services to meet a patient's needs.

*Figure 12.2 Components of comprehensive and holistic substance abuse treatments*[33]

Source: National Institute on Drug Abuse; National Institutes of Health; US Department of Health and Human Services.

There is a growing body of research supporting yoga and other mindfulness-based interventions as important complementary mind/body adjunctive approaches for the treatment of substance use disorders. Yoga can be an important addition to a comprehensive substance abuse treatment system, as described in Figure 12.2, which is aimed at treating the whole person. The evidence is encouraging, as a recent review found that seven out of eight randomized control trials demonstrated that yoga can be effective for alcohol, drug, and tobacco addiction.[34]

Proposed mechanisms of action for yoga and its positive impact for addiction recovery include the reduction of depression and anxiety, decreased stress levels, improved mental control and reduced impulsivity and addictive behaviors, and improved life satisfaction.[35] There is also growing empirical support that yoga can have a positive impact on several key components of recovery, including prevention of substance use, early addiction treatment, and remission.[36] Yoga can play a positive role in increasing life satisfaction, promoting personal development, and increasing overall emotional stability; all key factors in maintaining remission.[37] A recent pilot study using yoga as an adjunct treatment for alcohol use found that not only did the group practicing yoga reduce their drinking, but also yoga was embraced as part of an overall healthier lifestyle.[38]

## Conceptual framework for yoga and recovery

The underlying mechanisms for yoga and how it can be beneficial for recovery from addiction is a growing area of interest for researchers. Ancient yoga philosophy can provide a helpful conceptual framework to begin to understand how yoga can be an important part of recovery. Yoga addresses recovery with a mind/body/spirit connection that is often overlooked in more traditional behavioral approaches to substance treatment. Most of the current yoga research related to addiction recovery does not portray yoga as a whole lifestyle, rather it focuses on primarily the physical practice of asana and pranayama. However, it is important to note that yoga can and often does include meditation, breathing, nutrition, lifestyle philosophy, and body cleansing.

> To the pure of heart comes also a quiet spirit, one-pointed thought, the victory over sensuality, and fitness to behold the soul.

Yoga Sutra 11.41[39]

The philosophy of yoga and Patanjali's eight limbs, as outlined in Chapter 4 of this book, can develop a fuller appreciation for why yoga can have a positive impact across all stages of substance use recovery.

The most well-researched components of the eight limbs of yoga on addiction are asana, pranayama, and meditation. Asana or yoga postures have been shown to improve mood and overall wellbeing in people with addictions, much like traditional aerobic exercise, having a positive effect on the nervous, respiratory, and endocrine systems that release anti-depression hormones such as serotonin and dopamine.[40] Pranayama or breathing exercises involve learning how to regulate breath, develop conscious deep breathing, and utilize breath as an anchor to still the mind, and they have been shown to be effective with those recovering from substances including tobacco and other substance use disorders.[41] Meditation has been shown to be helpful with addiction as a way to improve attentional control, change a person's relationship with their thoughts, and produce increased levels of alertness and relaxation.[42] Mindfulness meditation can disrupt the experience of craving and provide a positive replacement behavior for dealing with urges rather than using the substance.[43] The cycle of addiction can be interrupted when the cues for addictive behaviors are present by applying ancient methods of pranayama and meditation. Cravings can be reduced through concentration and meditation practice along with withdrawal from the senses. Asana can help to shift mood into a more positive state, which may reduce the power of cravings and help to sustain ongoing recovery.

> *Whether these ever-present characteristics or forms are manifest or subtle, they are composed of the primary elements called the three gunas.*
>
> Yoga Sutra 4.13[44]

Yoga philosophy also provides a framework for both understanding the root causes for addiction and the development of a path of recovery. In Chapter 4 of this book, the authors outlined the three gunas as described in the *Patanjali Yoga Sutras* as tamas, rajas, and sattva. All three gunas are present in all beings and cannot be eliminated. However, they can be increased or decreased through lifestyle practices, including yoga. Addiction can be seen as a tamasic state with substances creating a lack of motivation, energy, or enthusiasm for life. Recovery can be seen as moving from an addictive state of tamas (inertia), through the fiery action of rajas (activity, fear), and eventually moving toward a more sattvic state, which can produce feelings of peacefulness and balance.

> *When one rises above the three gunas that originate in the body; one is freed from birth, old age, disease, and death; and attains enlightenment.*
>
> Bhagavad Gita 14.20[45]

Other limbs of the yoga path including the yamas and niyamas can be important tools on the path of recovery, particularly how they parallel the 12-step self-help model that has been an important part of many recovery models. The 12 steps were first published in 1938, and written by Bill Wilson, who founded Alcoholics Anonymous (AA) along with Bob Smith. AA was formulated as a support group that didn't just emphasize abstinence, but also focused on prayer, meditation, self-honesty, making amends for one's mistakes and harms, and placing trust in a higher power. Both the yoga path and the 12-step program encourage introspection and development of a spiritual practice that can be a vital component to maintaining recovery.[46] Table 12.1 shows the intersection of yoga philosophy and the 12-step recovery model.[47]

Table 12.1 Intersection of yoga and self-help

| 12-step | Yama/Niyamas | Gunas |
|---|---|---|
| **1.** We admitted that we are powerless over our addiction, that our lives had become unmanageable. | Satya—acknowledgement of one's personal truth is essential to recovery. | Tamas—inactive. |
| **2.** We came to believe that a power greater than our selves could restore us to sanity. | Brahmacharya—understanding that overindulgence in addictive behaviors can cause imbalance and cultivating self-restraint can restore balance. Santosha—through the practices of prayer, yoga, and meditation, we can learn to be more content and less reactive. | Tamas—inactive. |
| **3.** We made a decision to turn our will and our lives over to the care of God as we understood God. | Ishvara pranidhana —through the practice of surrender, we become more relaxed and at ease. | Tamas—inactive. |
| **4.** We made a searching and fearless moral inventory of ourselves. | Svadhyaya—thorough a personal commitment to self-study, we examine our behavior honestly. | Rajas—active. |
| **5.** We admitted to ourselves, to God, and to another human being the exact nature of our wrongs. | Satya—acknowledging and speaking the truth. Ahimsa—we intend to live our lives non-violently once we have been able to apologize for our wrongdoing. | Rajas—active. |
| **6.** We became entirely ready to have God remove all these defects of character. | Saucha—practicing purity in the body, mind, and spirit can begin to replace destructive patterns of behavior. | Rajas—active. |
| **7.** We humbly asked God to remove our shortcomings. | Tapas—practicing self-discipline to purify our old patterns of behavior. | Rajas—active. |
| **8.** We made a list of everyone we had harmed and became willing to make amends to them all. | Satya—acknowledging and speaking the truth including the persons we have caused harm to. Asteya—non-stealing or returning back what was not ours both on the physical and psychological dimension. | Rajas—active. |
| **9.** We made direct amends to all persons we had harmed except when to do so would injure them or others. | Ahimsa—committing to non-harming. Tapas—strong self-discipline to promote forgiveness and prepare to heal and move forward. Asteya—non-stealing/returning back what is not ours. | Rajas—active. |

| 10. We continued to take personal inventory and when we were wrong promptly admitted it. | Svadyaya—recovery becomes a lifelong journey of self-study and reflection including our behaviors and how they impact others.<br><br>Tapas—strong self-discipline to maintain a practice. | Sattva—pure. |
|---|---|---|
| 11. We sought through prayer and meditation to improve our conscious contact with God as we understood God. | Isvara pranidhana—daily devotion to practices such as yoga, meditation, prayer, and 12 steps to maintain our spiritual connection.<br><br>Pratyahara—ability to focus within and control over the senses using the power of the mind.<br><br>Dharana—one-pointed concentration.<br><br>Dhyana—uninterrupted concentration/meditation.<br><br>Samadhi—ultimate tranquility. | Sattva—pure. |
| 12. Having had a spiritual awakening as a result of these steps, we tried to carry this message to other addicts and to practice these principles in all of our affairs. | Aparigraha—as we experience our spiritual awakening, there is freedom from clinging and possessiveness and a sense of purpose to share practices with others.<br><br>Tapas—strong self-discipline to continue spiritual practice.<br><br>Santosha—contentment through self-discovery. | Sattva—pure. |

*Source: The 12-Step Restorative Yoga Workbook*[48]

## Integrative models of yoga for addiction

### Yoga/lifestyle approach

Yoga or a yoga lifestyle approach is well recognized as complementary or adjunctive therapy for substance abuse treatment, including alcohol, smoking cessation, and opioids.[49] While yoga can be effective in all phases of substance abuse recovery (once the person has medically stabilized and is out of acute withdrawals), it has been shown to be especially effective at two distinct periods during the recovery process. The first period includes the early stabilization phase following detoxification from the substance and the other period is during the recovery maintenance (relapse prevention) phase, which usually takes place three months or longer after stabilization occurs. During the early stabilization phase, research studies show that yoga can reduce the heart rate and blood pressure related to sympathetic nervous system arousal, which is vital during early recovery.[50] Regular yoga during the relapse prevention phase can reduce stress levels, improve mood, and help with coping skills to manage cravings.[51]

## Regular yoga in substance use recovery

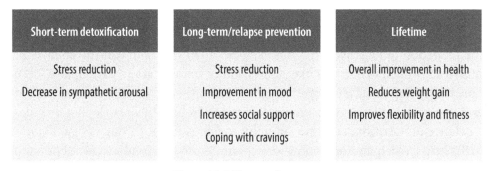

| Short-term detoxification | Long-term/relapse prevention | Lifetime |
|---|---|---|
| Stress reduction | Stress reduction | Overall improvement in health |
| Decrease in sympathetic arousal | Improvement in mood | Reduces weight gain |
| | Increases social support | Improves flexibility and fitness |
| | Coping with cravings | |

*Figure 12.3 Yoga and recovery*

Source: Sarkar, S. and Varshney, M. (2017) "Yoga and substance use disorders:
A narrative review." *Asian Journal of Psychiatry 25*, 191–196.

There are several mindfulness-based integrative models of recovery for substance use that include yoga as part of a broader treatment. Mindfulness-based interventions (MBIs) for substance use disorders are now widely utilized as part of a comprehensive integrative recovery approach. Current research suggests that MBIs can reduce the use of several different substances, including alcohol, cocaine, amphetamines, marijuana, cigarettes, and opiates.[52] Mindfulness meditation comes from the Eastern traditions of Buddhism and yoga and has been used for thousands of years. In 1979, a young researcher named Jon Kabat-Zinn, at the University of Massachusetts Medical School, created the Stress Reduction Clinic and offered an eight-week-long outpatient course called Mindfulness-Based Stress Reduction (MBSR) to help patients cope with stress and chronic pain.

The program is based on intensive training in formal and informal meditation, which helps participants cultivate mindfulness. Mindfulness, as defined in MBSR, is "the awareness that emerges through paying attention on purpose, in the present moment, and nonjudgmentally to the unfolding experience moment by moment."[53] Rather than focusing on curing participants, the focus of MBSR is "coming to terms with things as they are" and discovering how to attend and accept their present-moment experience. MBSR includes the body scan, seated meditation, and yoga. MBSR and other MBIs have been shown to be effective in substance abuse recovery, especially in the early stages when the present moment can be experienced as stressful, painful, or unpleasant to those suffering from addiction.[54] Mindfulness can teach participants to develop a different relationship with thoughts, feelings, and sensations by simply observing them nonjudgmentally.[55] Acceptance of the present moment, an important component of 12-step programs, is also the cornerstone of MBIs. Coping strategies for dealing with urges are also built into MBIs, as participants are able to notice cravings for drugs and alcohol and watch how the cravings can subside through the use of meditation, thus weakening the association between the urge to use drugs and the actual response.

Another way that MBIs can help participants in early recovery is through the reduction of negative emotions.[56] Rather than trying to control, change, or push away difficult emotions like anxiety, anger, or depression, participants learn how to develop an accepting attitude and learn that all emotions are transient and will pass. MBIs can be an important part of a healthy lifestyle that includes a balance of nutrition, self-care, and physical movement through yoga. Finally, MBIs help participants learn how to focus and train the mind to pay attention to one thing. This is extremely important in early recovery and people often struggle with feeling overwhelmed by different thoughts, feelings, and sensations. With regular practice over time, participants are able to improve their attention and cognitive capacity by focusing on an object of attention, primarily the breath and physical sensations of the body.[57] MBSR can be adapted for substance abuse relapse prevention by adding specific components around cravings, coping skills, and increasing self-efficacy to maintain recovery. Mindfulness-Based Relapse Prevention (MBRP) has two primary outcomes: to develop increased awareness of thoughts, feelings, and sensations through the development of mindfulness practice; and to utilize these new mindfulness skills to cope more effectively with triggers and high-risk situations.[58] Yoga is a staple in the MBRP. It can be substituted for other forms of meditation when a participant is too lethargic, agitated, or distracted to do other forms of meditation offered.[59] Mindfulness-Oriented Recovery Enhancement (MORE) is another MBI modified for substance abuse recovery using mindfulness meditation practices combined with cognitive restructuring, which is a cognitive-behavioral technique to challenge negative thoughts and increase emotion regulation capacity.[60]

## Example of integrative yoga treatment
I would like to highlight an example of an integrative yoga program that helps clients with substance use disorders and mental health challenges across the continuum of recovery.

Located in an urban city of Hartford, CT, the Toivo Center (which is Finnish for "Hope") is a mind/body-focused wellness center where people can engage in expert-facilitated yoga classes and workshops, which include asana (including adaptive chair practices), pranayama, and meditation. Other classes such as fitness and strength training, creative writing, expressive art, walk/run groups, nutrition workshops, drum circles, and other holistic practices are also offered. It is funded in part by the State of Connecticut Department of Mental Health and Addiction services along with other private donors. What is particularly unique about this program is that Toivo staff provide services to persons in recovery at all stages of their journey. Yoga and wellness coaches from Toivo also travel throughout the state to inpatient substance abuse programs, psychiatric facilities, and other clinics to offer yoga, meditation, and other healing arts programs to participants in early recovery who may not ordinarily have access to CAM modalities. They even lead weekly yoga classes at a maximum-security institute for forensic psychiatric patients, some of whom have severe substance abuse issues and may never have been exposed to yoga. As participants continue their healing journey, they can continue to attend Toivo programs in the community by going to the community center, which is centrally located in the city of Hartford, CT. The accessible location and low cost make it affordable for participants. Yoga can remain an important component of their lives and become part of a healthy lifestyle along with establishing a substance-free recovery support network.

Toivo represents a celebration of human experience in all of its forms and a belief in the unfathomable power of looking within for direction. We believe that no one should be denied the benefits of yoga, meditation or any of our offerings based on socioeconomic standing, psychiatric history and/or experiences with addiction.[61]

The use of opioids to treat chronic pain has led to an alarming increase in the number of people suffering from addiction. While there is a greater understanding of the multiple factors that lead to addiction in some individuals, there have been few effective long-term solutions to this growing crisis. People are now looking for help outside the traditional medical model to address their persistent pain and addiction. A new paradigm for addiction recovery has emerged that combines traditional yoga philosophy and practices (asana, pranayama, meditation) and Western psychological treatments. Promising research over the past two decades continues to demonstrate the effectiveness of yoga as part of a holistic treatment approach for persistent pain and addiction.

*Chapter 13*

# Pain, A Loss to Be Grieved

Antonio Sausys

*"Dad, how much pain can a heart take?"—asked I.*

*"All of it"—he answered. "All of it, my son."*

Perhaps research results can contest my dad's statement, for they indicate that when dealing with extremely stressful circumstances, even if emotionally induced, the heart muscle in the left ventricle enlarges and compromises the heart's ability to pump life-sustaining blood through the body, potentially causing pain or even death. What poets and romantics referred to as "the broken heart" in the past, science may today name as stress-induced cardiomyopathy.

Yoga, on the other hand, can contest that while dying of a broken heart attack can indeed be seen as an ultimate ending, it may also be the continuation of a cycle of reincarnation, learning more effective skills of resilience to cope with an aching heart. In any event, pain can disrupt the balanced state of health and, at the same time, signal the need to return to it. We are certainly attached to our health being balanced and stable, we count on it for normal functioning, and when we lose that balanced state, we grieve. Then pain is, without a doubt, a loss to be grieved.

Pain and grief are intimately related. Pain is, in fact, one of the most important symptoms of grief, whether physical or emotional. For that reason, it is important to understand how these two processes are related and the implications of their interconnection.

## Grief, what is it?

It is commonly acknowledged in the field of thanatology that grief is the normal reaction to the loss of things or people we are attached to. We seem to live as if the things we are attached to are always going to be there. When faced with their disappearance we feel awkward, clueless, confused, overwhelmed, and in pain. Some incorrectly consider the process of bereavement to be an illness, rather than a normal part of the human condition that seeks outlet and expression. The fact that grief is normal does not make it any easier to go through.

People experience grief in different ways and each culture relates to grief uniquely.

These cultural differences also affect the opinions, views, and beliefs of Western psychologists and clinicians, who often assume very contradictory views to those of the sadhus and swamis of yoga. Regrettably, Western culture tends to sweep grief under the rug by ignoring it entirely or compartmentalizing it. Only minimal attention to grief is allowed, effectively preventing us from understanding its nature.

## Pain: a primary loss that triggers multiple secondary losses

Traditionally, we think of grief as being the range of emotional and psychological responses experienced after the death of someone we love. But death is not the only type of loss that elicits grief. Some might feel grief over the loss of a prized possession, a pet, a job, a dream, or their youth. In fact, people can grieve the loss of perceived invincibility after breaking a bone, the discontinuation of a regularly scheduled TV show, or a favorite brand of sneakers.[1] The reason why these losses can cause grief is because we can develop attachment to virtually anything, not just to life or the permanence of it, therefore non-death-related losses are indeed a valid cause for grief. Attachment, in general, correlates the presence of something or someone with an individual's comfort, happiness, or safety. The individual's wellbeing depends on the presence and continued availability of the object of attachment.

As living beings, our proper survival depends on the normal functions of our physical and mental systems. When a stimulus harms the normal functions, it creates damage threatening the stability of our lives. The International Association for the Study of Pain (IASP) defines pain as "an unpleasant sensory and emotional experience associated to real or potential damage."[2] This unpleasant feeling can result from tissue damage, resulting in physical pain, or from the damage caused to the connective psychic matrix that ensures the integrity of the self, resulting in psychological pain. In any case, the integrative balance of physical or psychological life is ruptured or lost. This loss can then be considered as a primary loss, one that causes grief due to our natural attachment to such balance.

Pain cannot be eradicated completely; controlling its existence is not in the human realm of possibilities. One could think that hypothetically an individual suffering from both alexithymia—a personality construct characterized by the subclinical inability to identify and describe emotions in the self—and congenital insensitivity to pain (CIPA)—a rare genetic disorder that makes an individual unable to feel pain—could not feel pain at all. Yet, no known cases of both have been identified. The fact that we cannot control the existence of pain is yet another aspect that turns pain into a loss to be grieved, for most of us are attached to control, particularly control over unpleasant feelings. It is worth mentioning though that pain is a special kind of loss, an ambiguous one. The term "ambiguous loss," coined by researcher Pauline Boss, refers to losses that occur without closure or understanding, either because there is physical absence and psychological presence—like in a missing person case—or because there is physical presence and psychological absence—like in losing the connection with a family member to Alzheimer's disease.[3] The term can also refer to a psychological loss that can happen personally in terms of one losing sense of who they are. The deep changes in the personality that chronic pain can cause in an individual can lead to a situation of loss as the one Boss described. The difference between regular grief and grief from an ambiguous loss is that the latter prevents closure, often resulting in "disenfranchised grief"—grief that is not recognized by society. It is common to hear chronic pain sufferers say they feel misunderstood, isolated, and weary of disclosing their condition. Feeling that one is unable to do what most people can do, play the roles most people can play, and carrying stigmatizing labels as "the downer" or "the party pooper" can itself be a source of disenfranchised grief. Different cultures have rituals to process grief and support the grievers—such as the Jewish Yahrtzeit, the Mexican "Day of the Dead," or the "Memorial Day" in the US. In the case of pain though, no rituals support the sufferers. On the contrary, pain is used as a ritualistic self-sacrificial tool to, through developing courage and strength, invoke the favors of the gods. To not be able to take one's own pain can, in that case, be even more stigmatizing.

In the field of grief, two types of losses are acknowledged: the initial loss, the one that occurs first, is usually referred to as the *primary loss*, while the losses that occur as a result of this underlying primary loss are known as *secondary losses*. Primary losses are more easily identified, while the secondary ones can be more subtle and perhaps unacknowledged with regard to their profound emotional intensity. They too cause grief and can bring on tremendous sorrow and repeatedly reignite the pain that was experienced from the primary loss.

Pain, considered as a primary loss, elicits the appearance of several secondary losses. Recognizing them is important for it can help understand how they ultimately influence the subjective experience of pain. Many of these secondary losses will appear independently of whether they are caused by acute or chronic pain. It is fair to say that the more prolonged in time the experience of pain is, the deeper and more involved these losses will be. Perhaps the most evident is the "loss of the ideal of a pain-free life." We all know that, like loss, pain will happen simply because it is a normal feature of life. Yet, it is somehow met with surprise each time it appears because, somewhere buried in our beliefs, we think that we are supposed to live without it. It immediately calls our attention, interrupting the continuity of the experience being had. Often pain restricts the use of the painful area, challenging the functions associated to it, causing "loss of functionality." Not being able to perform the usual functions we are accustomed to—named the "loss of the familiar"—can affect an individual's livelihood—"loss of income or status"—possibly causing "loss of quality of life." Consequently, the possibility of achieving our goals may be shattered—"loss of dreams"—and the continuity of our view of ourselves may be challenged, causing "loss of self-image." Should this loss be deep enough, it can spark "loss of identity," both in the mind and/or the body. This cascade of losses can certainly increase pain and must be acknowledged as a contributing factor in the way an individual experiences pain.

I have found that inviting individuals to fill out a "loss chart" helps them identify losses that they may have not recognized before and understand the multilayered nature of their experience. The chart I have filled out below for the purpose of understanding is similar to the one I present them with—blank of course—asking them to "name the primary loss they are working with, then find at least three secondary losses associated with it."

Table 13.1 Pain's loss chart

| Primary loss | Secondary losses |
| --- | --- |
| Pain | Loss of the ideal of a pain-free life |
| | Loss of functionality |
| | Loss of the familiar |
| | Loss of income |
| | Loss of status |
| | Loss of quality of life |
| | Loss of dreams |
| | Loss of self-image |
| | Loss of body identity |
| | Loss of psychological identity |

The combined effects of our losses, big and small, major and minor, accumulate in our bodies. The judgment that some losses are trivial, and are therefore unimportant to consider, can exacerbate feelings of confusion, isolation, and shame, which happen to also be common consequences of pain.

## Symptoms of grief—pain is an important one

No two individuals grieve in the same way; similarly, each individual feels pain in a unique way. Yet, there is some consistency in the emotional, physical, and mental symptoms associated with both the grieving process and the experience of pain.

Some of the most commonly acknowledged symptoms of grief can be seen in Table 13.2 (adapted with permission from Howard Lunche).[4]

**Table 13.2 Symptoms of grief**

| Physical | Emotional | Mental |
|---|---|---|
| • Pain<br>• Feeling of tightness in the throat<br>• Feeling of tightness in the chest<br>• Alterations of the breathing patterns (shortness of breath—frequent sighing)<br>• Fatigue, exhaustion, low energy<br>• Sleep patterns disruption (insomnia or excessive sleep)<br>• Eating patterns disruptions (overeating or anorexia)<br>• Alterations of the cardiac rhythms (bradycardia, tachycardia, arrhythmia)<br>• Digestive system upset<br>• Generalized tension<br>• Restlessness, irritability<br>• Increased sensitivity to stimuli<br>• Dry mouth | • Shock, numbness<br>• Sadness<br>• Anger<br>• Guilt, regret<br>• Anxiety<br>• Emptiness<br>• Sorrow for the one who died<br>• Loneliness, longing, yearning<br>• Resentment<br>• "More I should have done"<br>• Fear<br>• Insecurity<br>• Feeling helpless, out of control<br>• Diminished self-concern<br>• "Don't care," "What does it matter?"<br>• Depression<br>• Desire to join the deceased<br>• Suicidal feelings<br>• Feelings of betrayal, disloyalty<br>• "Emotional roller coaster"<br>• Relief | • Negative anticipatory thinking<br>• Disbelief<br>• Confusion<br>• Disorientation<br>• Absentmindedness<br>• Forgetfulness<br>• Poor concentration<br>• Distraction<br>• Difficulty focusing and attending<br>• Low motivation<br>• Expecting to see the deceased<br>• Expecting the deceased to call<br>• Needing to tell and retell the story surrounding the loss<br>• Dreams or images of the deceased<br>• Denial<br>• Thinking about other deaths and losses |
| Social | Behavioral | Spiritual |
| • Withdrawing from social activities<br>• Being isolated by others<br>• Diminished desire for<br>• Coping with labels such as "widowed," "single," etc.<br>• Hiding grief by "taking care of others"<br>• Losing friends, making new friends | • Crying (sometimes unexpectedly)<br>• Searching for the deceased<br>• Carrying special objects<br>• Going to the grave site<br>• Making and keeping an altar<br>• Keeping belongings intact<br>• Looking at photos or videos of the deceased<br>• Listening to audio recordings of the deceased<br>• Talking to the deceased<br>• Avoiding situations that arouse grief<br>• Changes in daily routine<br>• "Staying busy"<br>• Assuming mannerisms of the deceased | • Questions about God: asking questions about God, like: Why would God allow this?<br>• Asking questions about the deceased, such as: Where are they now? Are they OK? Can they see me? Will I see them again? What will happen when I die?<br>• Sensing the deceased's presence<br>• Hearing, smelling, or seeing the deceased<br>• Having death affirm or challenge beliefs<br>• Experiencing awe, wonder, mystery<br>• Reflecting on personal finitude<br>• Feeling the need to continue the relationship with the deceased |

After reviewing this chart, it is not difficult to understand why people grieving believe they are ill! The similarity between the symptoms of grief and the symptoms of pain, particularly chronic pain, is remarkable. Whether pain arises from an initial injury, such as a back sprain, or an ongoing cause, such as illness, or even when there is no clear cause, pain as a primary loss causes grief that sparks similar symptoms to those related to chronic pain. For instance, both share fatigue, sleep disturbance, decreased appetite, and mood changes. The secondary losses related to pain can also add to the joint list of symptoms. Chronic pain may limit a person's movements, which can reduce flexibility, strength, and stamina. Subsequently, this difficulty in carrying out important and enjoyable activities can lead to disability and despair.

The intensity that these symptoms present themselves with is determined by the nature of the relationship with what or who is lost. In general terms, the deeper, more interdependent, and involved the relationship is, the more intense the symptoms will be. Another important determining factor relates to the circumstances around the loss itself. In this regard, the more unexpected, complicated, and traumatic the circumstances, the stronger the symptoms will be. William Worden called these factors the "mediators of grief."[5] They may as well be "mediators of pain," for they can influence the intensity of it in similar ways. For instance, if pain is related to an experience that does not involve survival—such as tying one's shoelaces—versus one that does—being able to feed oneself—the intensity of the pain may vary. The same would apply if pain were related to a predictable consequence of a non-traumatic experience—such as experiencing pain in the legs after a steep climb—versus the sudden pain of having a finger severed in a work-related accident.

Pain and grief are intimately related basic human experiences that enter into a particular feedback loop that perpetuates each other's appearance. Pain—physical or emotional—is itself a symptom of grief that results in a loss that prompts a grieving process. Their relationship is also evidenced in the fact that they share a similar common neurological path. Physical and emotional pains have similar neuronal signatures: activation of the anterior insula and the anterior cingulate. Recent studies regarding grief also showed activation of similar areas: the anterior cingulate cortex (ACC), posterior cingulate cortex (PCC), prefrontal cortex (PFC), insula, and amygdala.[6]

Currently, there is not enough measurable scientific data on grief, and further research is still needed. Western psychology usually views the body as an afterthought, proclaiming that the grieving process happens mainly in our minds. More recent research in the areas of psychology, immunology, and endocrinology reveals data that shows how emotional processes like grief affect more than just our mental functioning. Psychophysiology shows how life-changing events influence virtually every area of a person's physical and mental constitution, from thought patterns to emotional wellbeing, immune function, and overall health. Western science is just now discovering and documenting connections formulated ages ago from the meditative observations of practicing yogis. This integrated view of the human being and its processes and mechanisms is crucial to changing the outlook on pain's management and regulation. It is also a key component of yoga therapy.

## The influence of the individual's involvement

While true that many are the points where Western medicine and Eastern philosophy differ, many are the ones where the two meet, as well. One of them relates to the value of practice. In the 20th century, our brains were thought to develop within a critical period and that once we had passed it, we were basically stuck in those ways, forever hardwired, fixed in form and function. These beliefs have been challenged by findings that reveal that many functions of the brain remain plastic even into late adulthood.[7] An individual can consciously and profoundly affect both the brain's physical anatomy and functional organization in response to experience—the brain can and does change. New connections between nervous cells are formed as we engage in different activities that are subsequently strengthened through repetition, wiring them together. The more we repeat these activities, the more permanent the connections become.[8] Although this process is automatic, we can in fact enhance a sought-after result by increasing conscious practice. Given that pain has a strong subjective component, by learning new ways to connect with it, and practicing new ways of addressing it, we can become much more suited to manage it.

Coincidentally, two core yogic principles ensure success in spiritual development: abhyasa and vairagya. The first one can be translated as "practice"—having an attitude of persistent effort to attain and maintain a state of stable tranquility. The second translates as "non-attachment": learning to let go of the many attachments, aversions, fears, and false identities that are clouding the true Self. The latter is core to grief counseling, for grief is the price we pay for attachment. To make our wellbeing depend on the existence of anything is a sure ticket to suffering because all things are impermanent. Abhyasa is core to pain management because it proposes addressing tranquility while in pain. If an individual can cultivate a strong conviction, a persistent effort to choose actions, speech, and thoughts that lead in the direction of a stable tranquility, they may drastically change the experience of pain itself.

It is clear that both neuroplasticity and yoga honor the value of practice. Yoga is, in my opinion, the most complete and comprehensive manual offering practices to make the most of neuroplasticity; it is neuroplasticity in action! It offers techniques to be practiced by the individual, versus receiving manipulations from a technician, or depending on addictive painkillers. Empowering individuals to take matters in their own hands increases their self-efficacy and is effective in changing their perception of pain by rehearsing, through practice, new ways to tap into internal resources.

And why do we need practice? It is for the same reason that people in modern-day India sat in yogic postures 6000 years ago practicing meditation—because the desire to resolve suffering is universal. We all need coping mechanisms. We all need treatments that soothe our restless minds and our aching bodies but, above all, we need the knowledge that can be gained simply by basking in one's inner silence.[9]

Reducing suffering is a key intention of grief counseling and therapy. Leaders in the field have noted specific elements of grieving, suggesting they need to be addressed in order to fulfill a normal process. Of all thinkers, J. William Worden[10] offers the model I find best suited to the yogic ideal of practice. In his model, he names these elements "tasks," a term that clearly denotes the dynamism the process really involves. They are:

1. To accept the reality of the loss.

2. To process the pain of grief.

3. To adjust to the new environment.

4. To find an enduring connection with who or what is lost as one embarks in a new life.

Regarding the second task, Worden states, "It is necessary to acknowledge and work through this pain or it can manifest itself through physical symptoms or some form of aberrant behavior."[11] This task is of special significance to our discussion and it indicates that through conscious work and dedicated practice one can reduce pain. If so, what are some of the practices that can assist one in doing so?

## Balancing emotional reactivity to pain through eye gazing

Pain is deeply related to emotional life both as an emotion itself and as a constitutive component of certain feelings. It sparks emotions and is influenced by them; something evidenced at a cellular level by its relationship with the endocrine system. Severe pain has an effect on the endocrine system, which can lead to the production of hormones from the adrenals, gonads, and thyroid, including the activation of the hypothalamic pituitary adrenal (HPA) axis. Prolonged activation of this stress response can lead to detrimental health effects on many systems of the body.[12]

There is a group of yogic cleansing techniques used to release emotions, thoughts, or physical experiences trapped in the body-mind; they are called shatkarma. Eye gazing (tratak in Sanskrit) is the sixth and last shatkarma included in the old *Hatha Yoga Pradipika*, one of three classic texts on Hatha yoga, alongside the *Gheranda Samhita* and *Shiva Samhita*. The technique is thought of as being useful to help balance the pineal gland. Because of its involvement in regulating the functions of the other endocrine glands, this is a good way to bring the endocrine system into balance in its entirety. Balancing the pineal gland may also help to regulate the sleeping cycle, which is affected both in grief and pain.

The pineal gland reacts to light registered through the optic nerves, which makes eye gazing, or tratak, a plausible way to impact the function of this gland. This impact on the pineal gland helps to regulate stress by influencing the fight-or-flight reaction, modulates the immune system, decreases insomnia, relaxes the anxious mind, improves memory, and helps to develop good concentration and strong willpower.[13]

## EYE GAZING (TRATAK)

- Sit comfortably and extend your right arm with your thumb pointing up and the thumbnail facing you. If you need support for the arm, you may bend the right knee and use your knee to support the arm, and add a bolster or similar to reach the desired height.

- Locate a distant object (at least ten feet away) at eye level as a focal point, and while keeping your elbow straight, place your thumbnail within the line of vision between your eyes and the distant object of focus. The object being focused on should be relatively small, such as a doorknob or a drawn black dot.

- Focus on your thumbnail for one minute.

- Shift your focus to the distant object for one minute.

- Shift back to your thumbnail.

- Repeat the process of switching the focus three times (six times in total). Avoid blinking throughout the exercise if you can.

Suggested time: Including one minute of focus and three switches between focal points, the practice takes six minutes. For improving sleep, it can be practiced half an hour before going to bed and then again half an hour after you have woken up.

Precautions: Always avoid unnecessary strain and be tolerant of different experiences such as seeing two thumbs or two distant focal points—these experiences change with time.

Contraindications: Those suffering from glaucoma should be sensitive to pain and modify the practice as needed, by reducing the time focusing or the number of changes between focal points.[14]

Source: *Yoga for Grief Relief*, Antonio Sausys

Because current understanding of pain focuses on its subjective nature, adding imagery or conducive thoughts to this exercise can alter the nature of the experience of pain. I suggest substituting the distant focal point for a symbol or image that represents a "pain-free state" to the individual. This modification can help the individual in pain shift focus and possibly lessen the concentration on the painful experience.

## Pratipaksha bhavana—visiting the opposites to self-reassess pain

Feelings are intimately related to thoughts and thoughts are related to circumstances. They mutually influence each other in different and intricate ways in what is one more example of the core principle of yoga that expresses the interconnectedness of all existing things.

Reality adopts a dual presentation—day and night, hot and cold, movement and stillness. In an individual's life there is health and sickness, youth and old age, birth and death. Our minds function in a dual way and tend to perceive these opposites as completely different, somehow unrelated or disjointed. In fact, it is almost impossible for the mind to know one if it does not know the other. Yoga's pursuit is oneness, non-duality, ultimately realizing that the opposites are extreme sides of one continuum. Noise is the presence of sound; silence is the absence of sound—opposites in one continuum: sound. Whether a situation is perceived as noisy or silent depends on where the cursor of awareness is placed in the continuum of sound. Any change in such placement promotes a change in awareness. Patanjali, one of yoga's great wise men who wrote the Yoga Sutras—a collection of aphorisms or words of wisdom—brilliantly expressed this principle. Offering advice on how to combat the painful consequences of experiencing negative thoughts, or thoughts that move away from the integration of all existing things, he wrote, "*Vitarka badhane pratipaksha bhavana*,"[15] the equivalent of "When disturbed by negative thoughts, opposite and positive thoughts should be thought of." Some have associated this concept to "positive thinking." The mind is too intelligent to accept this; the ultimate intention of the practice is not substitution, but reassessment of awareness by moving towards the opposite side of what one is experiencing.

A deeper reassessment can be accomplished if we swing our awareness in both ways, visiting both opposites voluntarily, versus as prompted by life's occurrences, which are out of our control. If we are feeling cold, by imagining we are extremely cold, then imagining we are extremely hot, we change our assessment of how cold we are. This type of oscillation is crucial in yoga practice. This is why we do a forward bend, then a backbend; we bend to the right, then to the left; we practice, then we relax. Because pain is a subjective experience, one can modify its perception by resetting the awareness of it through practicing pratipaksha bhavana.

## "VISITING THE OPPOSITES"—PRATIPAKSHA BHAVANA

Adopt a position that you can assume for some time. Avoid moving as possible and go with your awareness to the pain you feel.

- Feel your pain as clearly as you are able to.

- Next, imagine it slowly starting to grow.

- Feel it growing until all you are is your pain, and nothing but your pain.

- Now feel it starting to decrease.

- Feel it continuously decreasing until it returns to the initial intensity you started with.

- Imagine it continuing to decrease until it disappears completely.

- Remain as a witness of your feeling for a moment and see how your pain feels now.

You may imagine the pain as a ball and work with its size, or as sound and work changing its intensity, or simply as a feeling and work directly with your perception. Work with any associated dimension of the pain that is easier for you or that you feel more connected with.

## Pain as a messenger—the meta-communication of pain

In different versions of the creation myth according to Hinduism, it is believed that the God Prajapati, who lived in eternal bliss and peace, desired change, something that occurs not in a permanent state of equilibrium. To accomplish it, he self-sacrificed himself and defragmented—all his potential became the sun, the planets, the elements of our bodies, the universe as we know it. With this came pain and suffering so to regain Prajapati's oneness, to achieve again the state of pure bliss and peace, one must conquer pain. In this context, pain was the result of falling out of integration and is, as well, a way back to it.

*Grief can be the garden of compassion. If you keep your heart open through everything, your pain can become your greatest ally in your life's search for love and wisdom.*

Rumi

So, what wisdom piece can be made available by using pain as an ally? According to yoga philosophy, all existing things are integrated and work as a unit. Ignoring that integration—acting as if that was not the truth—is the main cause of illness, conflict, and ultimately pain and suffering. This truism coincides with the standard definition of pain, which results from real or perceived damage—or rupture of the integrated functionality of anything, including our psychological fabric. This universe functions as a whole—this is why acting in opposition to that prevents normal function. Then, pain is a "call back to integration," a reminder of how the universe works and why it is important to adhere to that. Nothing forces us to bring our awareness back to ourselves as pain does; it interrupts our outward engagement and it stops us in our tracks. According to Buddhist teachings, when an individual is born, his eyes see; they do not need to go to school for differentiation between day sight and night sight. We come to this life equipped with all the information we need to live a connected life. Rumi expressed it beautifully when he wrote: "We are not a drop of the ocean, we are all the ocean in a drop." Tapping into the universal knowledge can then be attained by tapping into ourselves—for we contain all the knowledge of the universe.

Swami Satyananda offered a tool to connect with that aspect of ourselves that holds the universal knowledge: antar mouna. *Antar* means "inner," *mouna* means "silence." Antar mouna is a technique for withdrawal of the mind from the sense objects. It is a five-step technique to assist one in de-identifying from the outside reality—what is being experienced—to tap into "the one experiencing the reality." The concept being addressed is that when a mirror reflects a car, it does not become the car, instead, it remains a mirror. This differentiation may be very useful when dealing with pain, for it can help us understand that we are not our pain, but the one experiencing it.[16]

## THE FIRST STEP OF ANTAR MOUNA

- Hear all sounds, identifying loud ones and soft ones, distant ones, and those that are close by, known ones and unknown ones…

- Now feel your ears…the outer ear, its temperature, its shape, and continue trying to feel the middle, and even the inner ear.

- Now feel You, the witness of the sounds…not the sounds, not the ears, but You the witness of all sounds…

Consider the following adapted version for pain:

- Feel your pain, identifying when it is strong, when it weakens, what aspects are known to you, what aspects are not known…

- Now feel the actual part of your body in pain…its shape, its temperature, its surface, how it feels as you go deeper into your body…

- Now feel You, the witness of your pain…not the pain itself, not the part of the body that is in pain, but You the observer, the witness of the pain…

Pain's intense power to bring the attention within prevents us from being distracted outside—a place our awareness is engaged with most of the time. Practices such as antar mouna, or pratipaksha bhavana, provide an integration of the wholeness of the individual. Tapping into grief's core teaching—that all things are impermanent—we reunite with this universal spiritual law of existence. Doing so helps us connect with that wisdom needed for proper functioning.

## How to address pain's message

Pain is not just about how it feels, but also how it makes us feel. And it is these unpleasant feelings that cause the suffering we humans associate with pain.

Because of its unpleasant nature, pain is often regarded as something that needs to be conquered, avoided, or at least controlled. The dialogue we establish with pain is often confrontational and hostile. Imagine if this was the attitude towards someone who knocks on your door to let you know your house is burning and that you must exit immediately! To distance oneself from pain completely accomplishes the opposite of what the meta message of pain is; it contradicts integration. What if we can "get" the message, rather than oppose it? When Worden explained a general roadmap for healthy grieving, he proposed "processing the pain of grief"[17] as the second task to be accomplished. Processing feelings implies four basic steps, which are also applicable to processing pain. They are:

1. naming

2. identifying

3. managing and regulating

4. remaining functional.

Naming relates to finding the appropriate name for the feeling we are processing. An individual can be angry at their sadness, and while both feelings are true, naming sadness as the core feeling helps one stay focused in the work.

Similarly, finding the right name to characterize pain can help one address it. Identifying—has to do with finding physical, mental, and behavioral correlates associated with the onset of a feeling or of pain, transiting through it or its aftermath. Managing—learning how to address the feeling according to its nature and expression, and regulating—implementing regulation tactics is an important aspect of processing both feelings and pain, with the purpose of remaining functional in life. When grieving, until we are able to process pain, pain itself takes center stage, deviating the individual from the completeness of the full process of grief.

To relate with pain's message, one can also explore the possible connections between the place where pain manifests and certain emotional and psychic correlates. Because of the interconnectedness of all existing things, the universe's information is represented in all its parts. There is then a relationship between the state of an individual's skin and the way the individual relates to "boundaries." Someone's neck pain may be a call to improve the relationship between the emotional self, represented in the upper chest, and the mental reality, represented in the head. This correlation becomes even more clear in the absence of our ability to assign pain to such things as physical imbalances represented, for example, in spinal misalignment or a herniated disk. What possible psychological connotations may relate to a painful area or place in the body, what aspects of spiritual wisdom are expressed in those areas?

One can also tap into pain's message by analyzing what actions, thoughts, or speech may reduce or eliminate pain. When exploring these correlates, I have encountered people who express that "an accident is sometimes just an accident, OK?!" I must disagree; nothing is "just" something because nothing is isolated from the rest of existence. It would be like saying that a tree is "just" a tree, and not part of the forest or related to the oxygen we breathe. The trees and us are one; so are our bodies, minds, and spirits. Pain may be an indication that we have fallen out of the integration. Returning to it, hearing the message expressed by the mind or the body, can reduce or mediate pain. The call to self-observance and to relate more intimately with the self is evidenced in the fact that, physically, it is when we are in pain that we decide to take actions to change. Mentally and emotionally, it is not until our protective body armor—formed of tension and rigidity—hurts, that we seek therapy. That which is formed as a result of pain is challenged by it; the road in is the road out—the two are opposite sides of one continuum.

## Knowing the truth

It is often recognized that while pain is unavoidable, suffering—resulting from the mental and emotional responses to pain—is avoidable. The fact that pain is not avoidable is, in my opinion, a consequence of "the greatest cosmic joke"—the fact that we contain all the knowledge of the universe, yet we have forgotten it. We must remember it, and pain is there to remind us of that need. When describing the causes of human suffering, the Sadhu Patanjali mentioned five essential ones: ignorance of the Truth; egoism—or the false identification with the mind and the body only; attachment—depending on the permanence of things for our wellbeing; aversion—counting on the things we don't like not happening; and fearing death.

There is an order in the universe, and contradicting it causes pain in one way or another. Grief and its extreme pain are a direct result of having sustained the belief that who or what we were attached to was permanent. Practicing "detached attachment"—generating new attachments, yet fiercely remembering that who or what we are attached to will inevitably disappear, reduces future suffering.

In the case of pain, it is valid to ask ourselves what part of the integrations has not been acknowledged, and what actions would re-establish such integration so suffering is eased.

The very wisdom pain calls us to acknowledge can offer helpful tips for pain management. One is expressed in the metaphor that "when a mirror reflects a car, it does not become the car, it stays a mirror." We are not our pain, but the ones feeling it. What other parts of ourselves can we relate to that are not the pain we are feeling?

Another one relates to the impermanence of all existing things. Our pain, too, shall pass. Either because it will eventually stop or because we may learn to live with it and access the other aspects of our being where pain is not the focus. Certainly, regarding pain, we have more questions than answers, and that, too, is part of the order of the Universe, for by asking ourselves these questions we tap into the knowledge we need.

## Chapter 14

# Compassion in Pain Care

SHELLY PROSKO

As healthcare practitioners, part of our role is to provide care for those suffering. One might assume that *compassionate* care is inherently part of any healthcare provider's role, including caring for people in pain. Surely we do not need an entire chapter dedicated to this topic. After all, compassion is the heart of caring[1] and should be a natural response to those suffering, shouldn't it? However, research shows that the capacity to provide compassionate care varies, depending on a wide variety of factors.[2] Numerous health surveys and reports conclude that compassion is lacking in healthcare and many would argue there is a growing compassion deficit in some parts of the world.[3]

This chapter will outline the value of compassionate care for the person in pain provided by the healthcare practitioner, as well as the value of cultivating self-compassion in both the person in pain and the healthcare practitioner.

Yoga offers a valuable and accessible framework from which to enhance and support compassionate pain care. How yoga can be integrated into models of compassion and self-compassion will be described as a worthy contribution to the biopsychosocial approach in pain care.

## What is compassion?

Let's explore the meaning of compassion before elaborating on compassion in pain care. There is no one agreed-upon definition of compassion, leaving interpretations to consider. *Extending kindness towards another* is a simplistic definition of compassion. In *The Oxford Handbook of Compassion Science*, many of the leading compassion researchers present evidence that compassion can be described as an emotion, a motivation, a trait, an attitude, and can even include a behavioral component.[4] The working definition most widely used throughout the handbook is taken from Goetz *et al.*, which states that compassion includes two components: 1) the awareness of pain and suffering and 2) the desire and motivation to relieve the suffering.[5]

It is important to note that this awareness of pain and suffering along with the motivation to alleviate it also applies to oneself. Another definition highlights this, stating that compassion is "a sensitivity to suffering in self and others with a commitment to try to alleviate and prevent it."[6]

## What is self-compassion?

Self-compassion researcher Kristin Neff describes self-compassion simply as "compassion directed inward."[7] She describes three elements of self-compassion as mindfulness, common humanity and kindness, which are outlined in more depth below.[8]

- **Mindfulness**: First we must be fully present and aware to be able to observe, acknowledge and accept that we are experiencing pain or suffering in the moment, without judgment. Sometimes if we make a mistake or an unhealthy decision, we do not even realize we are feeling angry, guilty, shameful or critical towards ourselves. Often we want to fix, avoid or resist the pain or unpleasantness and make it go away. However, in order to alleviate pain or suffering, the first step is to become aware, and then to acknowledge and accept that we are indeed suffering. Neff also discusses over-identification when one ruminates or catastrophizes about a narrative. She suggests replacing over-identifying with mindfulness.

- **Common humanity**: When we can acknowledge that the experience of pain or feelings that accompany suffering are experiences shared by others, we realize that we are not alone in our suffering. Feelings of shame or guilt for saying something we wish we had not said, doing something we did not want to do or not doing something we think we should have done, making poor choices or reacting to someone in a way of which we were not proud can all be examples of experiences about which we can remind ourselves that we are not alone or isolated. Others share these experiences with us. We are not the only ones who struggle. Neff reminds us that when we fail or make mistakes, this is not what separates us from one another, but what unites us.[9]

- **Kindness**: This element of self-compassion is about extending kindness, comfort, support and a sense of love towards oneself, amidst the suffering. Often we judge ourselves and self-criticize because we think that may help us change our behavior, or it might be the only strategy we have ever used when we make a mistake. However, evidence suggests that people are more likely to change behavior or try again after making a mistake if they offer self-kindness and support, in a non-judgmental way, rather than self-criticizing.[10] Neff suggests that the motivation to change behavior through self-criticism comes from a place of fear, whereas the motivation to change behavior through kindness and compassion comes from a place of love and a desire to want to alleviate our own suffering.[11] Behavior change coming from a place of self-compassion may result in a more sustainable and steadfast joy; one that promotes the healing journey and eudaimonic wellbeing as described in Chapter 15.

## Measuring compassion

The lack of consensus on the definition of compassion makes it challenging to accurately study, measure and determine its effects as a trait or as a practice. There are, however, several compassion scales that are commonly used in compassion research. Strauss *et al.* conducted a systematic review that included nine self-reported measures of compassion. Two were self-compassion scales and seven were scales that measured compassion for others.[12] The overall validity, reliability and interpretability of all the measures were found to be lacking in strength. However, the authors suggested that part of the weaknesses found may be because the definition of compassion they used may have differed from the definitions on which the scales were based. Some of the scales showed greater strength and may have clinical usefulness for measuring components of compassion that could be relevant to pain care for both the patient and practitioner. The authors concluded that future research is warranted to develop more robust compassion questionnaires to better measure compassion and its effectiveness.[13]

## Compassion for the person in pain: The value in pain care

Compelling evidence shows that providing compassion in healthcare can enhance quality of care, improve patient outcomes and patient satisfaction, strengthen therapeutic alliance, improve management of people with chronic illness, maintain wellbeing of the health professional, reduce chances of professional burnout and even reduce medical costs, and rates of malpractice claims and medical errors.[14]

Research also shows that compassion as a personal trait of the healthcare provider correlates with a variety of positive health outcomes such as improved physical, mental and emotional wellbeing, lowered stress response and reduced anxiety.[15] We may think that compassion is a trait we all inherently possess, particularly those who choose to work in a profession that provides care. As such, there would be no need to train compassion specifically. However, research shows that our capacity for compassion can vary and that the determinants of compassion are extremely complex and can depend on context.[16] Gilbert and Mascaro outline and explore *inhibitors* to compassion that include a number of fears, blocks and resistances to compassion.[17] Such inhibitors may influence one's ability to provide compassionate care to people in pain.

Even though compassion is discussed as an important part of healthcare, evidence suggests that compassionate care may be lacking in healthcare delivery.[18] Many organizations recognize and promote the importance of patient-centered care, as defined by the Institute of Medicine, in which the person's wishes, preferences and needs are addressed.[19] Even so, patient-centered care including genuine concern and respect often falls short of including compassionate care.[20]

Compassionate care may also lead to improved self-care by people in pain. An eye-opening study from Arman and Hok showed that women suffering from persistent pain were only able to take successful steps towards active self-care once they were able to experience loving and compassionate care from healthcare providers. The women reported feeling welcomed, listened to, worthy and whole. The authors concluded: "Self care needs to be more than advice, education and training for people with complex suffering. The journey to health begins when the sufferer experiences what it is to be cared for."[21]

Some researchers caution us not to put all the blame on healthcare providers for the lack of compassionate care, as there are also organizational barriers and external factors that can make the environment challenging to provide compassionate care.[22]

It appears that compassionate pain care might be valuable for both the person in pain and the healthcare practitioner, but is compassion trainable?

## Can we train ourselves to increase compassion?

Growing research shows that compassion appears to be a trainable trait and that we can participate in certain mindfulness and compassion meditation practices to enhance our compassionate response.[23] It has been shown that compassion-focused training can result in physiological changes that promote compassionate responses towards others.[24] Singer and Bolz[25] and Seppala et al.[26] have outlined several compassion-focused training programs that are available, some which have been used in compassion outcome research. Seppala et al. conducted a study in 2014 to explore the effects of a commonly used compassion-focused training tool, loving-kindness meditation,[27] on healthcare provider compassion, resilience and patient care. The authors concluded that "loving-kindness meditation may provide a viable, practical and time-effective solution for preventing burnout and promoting resilience in healthcare providers and for improving quality of care in patients."[28]

Joan Halifax, Zen Buddhist teacher, anthropologist and ecologist, holds a different view. She states we cannot directly train compassion, but we can prime ourselves for compassion by training the components of compassion.[29] Halifax suggests that the definition of compassion as a feeling of caring for one's suffering and the motivation to relieve it is limiting because compassion is an emergent process that arises from an interaction of processes that are not, by nature, compassionate processes.[30] She posits that if an individual practices these elements or processes, it can provide an opportunity for compassion to emerge from the interaction between the living and changing organisms (us) and the environment.

Halifax's heuristic model of enactive compassion is a framework that informs her compassion-focused training program for healthcare professionals.[31] The model consists of six domains: attentional, affective, intentional, insight, embodiment and engaged. Let's briefly review each domain and its applicability and relevance to pain care by using examples of how a practitioner might incorporate each domain in clinical practice.

- **Attentional**: The first trainable domain of compassion is concentration or focused attention. The ability to sustain steady attention requires non-elaborative thinking and non-judgment to whatever may arise. This type of cognitive control experienced in mindfulness meditation training may result in improved discernment, fewer judgments on the other person and potentially acknowledging another's suffering more readily.[32] Research also suggests that people improve their ability to perform tasks that demand attention after meditation training.[33] An example of how the healthcare provider might put this into immediate practice is to continually attempt to be fully present during a therapeutic session and stay in the experience of whatever arises. Pay full attention to the patient and moment without allowing the mind to wander or elaborate with a story. This may include checking in with our own breath or any physical sensations that arise within our own body as an anchor to stay present. One can also train this attentional domain by performing mindfulness awareness practices focusing on the breath, body, thoughts, emotions and subtle energy as a separate personal practice outside the therapeutic interaction.

- **Affective**: The emotional or affective domain includes the capacity to be aware of and regulate our emotions in addition to cultivating positive emotions such as kindness. Halifax describes kindness as an affective process extending tenderness and concern.[34] Research shows that these positive and prosocial emotions can help with discernment and decision-making skills, while negative emotions may have the opposite effect and reduce discernment skills.[35] Loving-kindness meditation (LKM) has been shown to be an effective practice for increasing compassionate responses.[36] Interoceptive awareness practices have been shown to increase our ability to be present and aware of our own bodily sensations, and may improve the accuracy with which we perceive our own emotions and the emotions of others.[37] The more clearly aware we are of our emotions, the better chance we may have at regulating them. The more clearly aware we are of another individual's emotions, the better chance we have at responding appropriately and meeting their needs. It has also been shown that we have greater stress resiliency when we are able to self-regulate our emotions.[38] All of these abilities are key factors in providing compassionate responses in pain care.

- **Intentional**: Those who write about or practice intention setting often claim it can be a powerful practice that influences process and outcomes. As outlined thus far, compassion is not compassion unless it includes the motivation to relieve suffering.[39] Therefore, setting and maintaining the *intention* to help reduce suffering is fundamental for compassion[40] and distinguishes compassion from empathy.[41] One may feel empathy without a desire or motivation to help reduce the suffering of the individual. Conversely, one may offer a compassionate response with or without feeling empathy. As healthcare providers, we can address this domain by setting a clear intention at the beginning of each patient interaction. When we set and follow an intention and continue to visit it throughout the therapeutic interaction, it can keep us focused on the underlying purpose of the interaction, which can influence our thoughts, language, voice, body language and actions. This in turn can influence the progression in the desired direction that can create the reality or outcome that is based on mutual values between us and the person in pain (without being attached to the therapeutic outcome). Taylor illustrates the following simple and practical example of how a therapist can practice intention setting in the clinic:[42] set these three intentions during handwashing in between patients: 1) Be fully present and care for myself first; 2) Be completely present for the person in pain; 3) Recall the key purpose and intent of the interaction: *to help reduce suffering of this person in pain.* You may even repeat the phrase silently to yourself "I am here to serve." Many people find intention setting incredibly powerful. Give it a try and experience the outcome.

- **Insight**: If we engage in practices to address the above domains, this can help us gain greater clarity and insight into the suffering of the person in pain. It may enhance our perspective-taking skills so that we are better able to discern and progress towards the truth of the current reality, and positively influence our clinical decision making, critical thinking skills and ability to provide compassionate responses.[43] Gilbert and Mascaro claim that "working with a calm and insightful mind that allows us to bring our reflective wisdom to bear on situations is a common focus of compassion training. This is not only to help us stay 'in the moment', but over time to create the physiological conditions that help us orientate ourselves to a future of commitment to a compassionate self-identity."[44] Halifax also reminds us to maintain a sense of "therapeutic humility" and not be attached to the outcome that is beyond our control. Since humans are complex organisms, it makes sense to apply the theory of complexity to the therapeutic interaction and think of the interaction as a complex and emergent process, as Taylor discusses in Chapter 3, where outcomes are unpredictable and not prestatable and therefore we must be open to the emergence of numerous outcomes or possibilities.[45]

- **Embodiment**: The subjective experience of being in your body-mind, within the context of the environment around you, can be described as embodiment. As previously mentioned, the more we are in tune with our own current physiological states, the better chance we may have at self-regulation and being attuned to the state of others around us.[46] This in turn may give rise to a more accurate understanding of the needs of the person in pain and therefore an improved ability to connect and provide the compassionate care required. As the healthcare provider, one way to enhance the embodied experience during the therapeutic interaction is to maintain the felt sense of being in your body while being present with and attentive to the person and current situation. In other words, dividing your attention between awareness of what is happening in your body and what is happening with the patient and the environment around you. Bringing your awareness to your breath or physical sensations can serve as a tangible portal to embodiment.

- **Engaged**: "Service is not possible unless it is rooted in love and compassion. The best way to find yourself is to lose yourself in the service of others" (Mahatma Gandhi).[47]

  The final domain of Halifax's model of enactive compassion is essentially "compassion in action." Skillful use of the above domains results in the emergence of a compassionate response that is ethical, value based, practical and based on a partnership between therapist and the person in pain. The compassionate response will also be informed by best practices and the therapist's experience and insights. It may include offering strategies, giving advice, taking part in helping the person in pain set goals and make plans, active listening, recommending practices, offering compassionate inquiry,[48] asking a motivational open-ended question or allowing space and time for the person to reflect and experience.

  Behavioral neuroscientist and psychologist Stephen Porges emphasizes that compassion must also include "respecting the individual's capacity to experience their own pain."[49] From a neurobiological perspective, if we rush to try to fix the person's pain, without validating their pain experience, it may trigger the person's physiological defense mechanisms, which include activation of the sympathetic nervous system and "withdrawal of vagal influences."[50] This could then negatively influence the person's pain and therefore unintentionally not be compassionate care. This is where we can ask: How can I best serve? What can I learn? What does this person need to succeed? Gilbert and Mascaro state, "compassionate intention is to be backed up with commitment to acquire wisdom for action."[51] The engaged domain can also include self-compassion in action or self-care practices. Ending the interaction can be signified with an exhale and handwashing to acknowledge that your work is complete. This allows you to progress to the next therapeutic interaction with clarity and a fresh perspective, allowing compassion to emerge once again.[52]

It is important to note that these six domains work in conjunction with one another and are only described separately for ease of explanation. Each domain is influenced by the others and is dependent on the ever-changing context of the person and the environment. Table 14.1 summarizes examples of how healthcare practitioners can cultivate compassion by addressing the six domains of Halifax's model within the therapeutic interaction and parallels each domain to yoga concepts and practices.

Table 14.1 Examples of how healthcare practitioners cultivate compassion by training six domains of Halifax's Heuristic Model of Enactive Compassion[53] including parallels to yoga concepts and practice

| Domain of Halifax's Heuristic Model of Enactive Compassion | Examples: during therapeutic interaction | Yoga concepts and practices |
|---|---|---|
| Attentional | • Be fully present and attentive during therapeutic interaction without allowing the mind to wander or elaborate with story.<br>• Check in with your breath or physical sensations arising within your body as an anchor to stay present. | • Dharana, dhyana.<br>• Perform mindfulness awareness practices focusing on breath, body, thoughts, emotions and subtle energy as separate personal practice outside therapy session: kosha scan.[54]<br>• Jnana and Kriya yoga, and practice of drishti (single-focused attention) specifically train attention. |

| Affective | • Be aware of and regulate emotions.<br>• Cultivate kindness, concern and other prosocial/positive emotions.<br>• Listen to understand, not to fix nor to judge. | • Bhakti and Kriya yoga include compassion practices.<br>• Meditation as personal practice outside therapy session: pratyahara includes interoceptive awareness practices and LKM.[55] |
|---|---|---|
| Intentional | • Set three intentions during handwashing in between patients: 1) Be fully present and care for myself first, 2) Be completely present for the person in pain, 3) Recall key purpose and intent of interaction: to help reduce suffering of this person in pain.[56]<br>• Repeat phrase silently to self: "I am here to serve." | • Sankalpa—intention practice.<br>• Visualization prior to movement practice or any action. |
| Insight | • Engaging in above domains leads to insight.<br>• Practice therapeutic humility.<br>• Open to emergence of numerous outcomes.[57] | • Practice concepts of aparigraha, santosha, ishvara pranidhana. |
| Embodiment | • Maintain felt sense of being in your body during therapeutic interaction.<br>• Bring awareness to your breath or physical sensations—can serve as a tangible portal to embodiment. | • Asana, pranayama, pratyahara as personal practices, outside of therapy session. |
| Engaged | • Cultivation of above domains results in emergence of an ethical, value-based, mutually agreeable and practical compassionate response—compassion in action.<br>• May include offering advice, strategies, listening, allowing space and time for patient reflection, respecting and validating patient's experience.<br>• How can I best serve? What can I learn? What does this person need to succeed?<br>• Exhalation at end of session acknowledging your work is done—this allows you to progress to the next therapeutic interaction with clarity and a fresh perspective.[58] | • Yoga as "Skill in Action."[59]<br>• Karma and Kriya yoga. |

*Adapted from: Halifax, J. (2012) "A heuristic model of enactive compassion."*
*Current Opinion in Supportive and Palliative Care 6, 228–235.*

In summary, compassion and its domains appear to be skills, and as such are trainable. Compassionate care for the person in pain from the healthcare practitioner is valuable for both the person in pain and the healthcare practitioner. The practitioner will also experience personal health benefits of compassion training, including a protective effect on professional burnout. Now, how does yoga fit in?

## Yoga and compassion

In Yoga Sutra 1.33, Patanjali refers to compassion as *karuna*, one of the four attitudes towards those who are suffering.[60] The word karuna is derived from the Sanskrit term *kara* meaning "to do," which also implies that "taking action" to alleviate suffering is an essential part of compassion.

Interestingly, we find commonalities to yoga philosophy and practice in Neff's self-compassion elements and Halifax's domains of compassion. This is not surprising, given that yoga seeks to decrease suffering and can be understood as an experiential process in which emergence of compassion takes place, as described in Chapter 4 of this book.

Let's take a look at the common factors in yoga and in the above models.

## Yoga and Neff's three elements of self-compassion

- **Mindfulness**: In yoga, self-realization is an overarching concept where mindful awareness is the driving force behind all teachings. We see the concept of awareness specifically addressed in the limb of pratyahara as an interoceptive awareness practice, as discussed in Chapters 4 and 9 of this book. We also see similar concepts addressed in the yamas and niyamas of Chapter 4: satya (truthfulness of the situation), santosha (acceptance of the situation) and svadhyaya (mindful inner exploration and self-inquiry of one's present state). Mindfulness is also an aspect of meditation in yoga.

- **Common humanity**: The essence of yoga includes connection to self and others with a sense of being whole, complete and united. The word yoga can be translated as "union" or "to yolk." In Chapter 4, we discuss that through yoga practice, "the individual can realize a state of underlying connection or unity from which equanimity and qualities such as compassion emerge." In Chapter 15, Sullivan discusses the negative health effects of perceived social isolation and loneliness and the value of yoga practices for people in pain to enhance social connection and connection to meaning, purpose and something larger than oneself.

The Yoga *Upanishads* text[61] shares a teaching that we are all whole, complete and connected because we are of the same essence. These teachings give us an opportunity to hold the mirror up to ourselves when we interact with others. What we see in others is also within us and in this we can seek and find refuge within the grounds of compassion. It reminds us that we are all more the same than different. Our imperfections are a part of who we are and offer great truths and insights into life and living as humans together here on earth. Connection to something beyond self allows one to learn the compassionate skill of surrender. This is known as ishvara pranidhana in yoga.

- **Kindness**: Ahimsa (the first yama of the first limb of Raja yoga as outlined in Chapter 4) is described as non-harming or kindness to all, including kindness towards oneself. In Yoga Sutra 1.33, kindness is another one of the four attitudes recommended towards those who are suffering, which can include kindness towards oneself.[62]

## Yoga and Halifax's six domains of enactive compassion

- **Attentional**: This domain is similar to the sixth and seventh limbs of Raja yoga, dharana (concentration) and dhyana (meditation), as discussed in Chapter 4. Yoga Sutra 1.2 *chitta vritti nirodhah* commonly translates yoga as "the restraint of the modifications of the mind-stuff"[63] or to calm the fluctuations of the mind without distraction. Yoga Sutras 1.34–1.36 state that one can focus his or her attention on the breath, physical sensations or subtle energetic sensations within the body in order to help focus the mind and calm these fluctuations of "mind-stuff."[64] Jnana and Kriya yoga and the practice of drishti (single-focused attention) specifically train attention.

- **Affective**: Emotional awareness and emotional regulation are aspects of yoga. Interoceptive awareness practices can be translated as pratyahara, the fifth limb of Raja yoga, which is discussed in Chapters 4 and 9. Loving-kindness and other meditative practices that cultivate positive emotions such as kindness, love and gratitude can be included in the sixth and seventh limbs of Raja yoga, dharana and dhyana. Bhakti and Kriya yoga also include compassion practices.

- **Intentional**: It is a common yoga teaching that *where our intention goes, the energy follows* and that all action first begins with a thought, then manifests into word and then translates into action.[65] Practitioners of classic yoga asana visualized the movement entering into and exiting out of asana, prior to performing it. This would set a clear intention for

conscious movement and allow the intention to create reality. In yoga, a
sankalpa is a personal vow and commitment that is consciously made and
repeated often to support and hold us to our values, honoring our deepest
intentions. Sankalpa is a call to action that reminds us of our true nature
and guides our choices.[66]

- **Insight**: Yoga Sutra 3.17: "An object, the word for it, and the idea evoked
  by it all tend to be confused with each other. Total attentiveness paid to the
  differences between these brings a true understanding of the utterance of
  all living beings."[67]

  In yoga, we can relate Halifax's concept of therapeutic humility to
  aparigraha, non-possessiveness or non-grasping of things, ideas or beliefs.
  This can be illustrated by the concept of neither grasping nor clinging to
  the need of "fixing" the person in pain nor attaching to the idea that there
  is one solution to a problem (linear thinking).

  We can also see the relevance of santosha (contentment and acceptance)
  and ishvara pranidhana (letting go, surrendering) where acceptance of and
  surrendering to the current situation and outcome can be part of acquiring
  insight and contribute to compassionate pain care.

- **Embodiment**: Yoga asana is a practice of embodiment. It teaches us to
  acknowledge and embrace our body and mind each time we practice. We
  notice and accept that our experiences change from moment to moment.
  Asana teaches us to explore what is currently happening in the body,
  mind and emotions by being fully present during the practice. We become
  more attuned in our body with continued inquiry, and eventually our
  interoception and proprioception are enhanced. Like asana, pratyahara
  and pranayama can be regularly practiced by the health provider outside
  of the therapeutic interaction to help cultivate and enhance the embodied
  experience. As a result, embodiment may be more readily accessed and
  experienced during the therapeutic interaction.

- **Engaged**: The engaged domain is inherently a part of yoga. The *Bhagavad
  Gita* describes yoga as "Skill in Action."[68] Karuna, kriya and karma are
  relevant to this domain. Recall that the Sanskrit word for compassion,
  karuna, means "to do" and implies that action to alleviate the suffering
  is part of compassion. The word kriya is a Sanskrit verb that means to
  act with conscious volition. Compassion becomes a kriya by consciously
  setting the intention to respond and act with mindfulness, care,
  kindness and concern for another. The path of Karma yoga, as outlined in
  Chapter 4, includes action or selfless service, without expecting anything
  in return.

In summary, yoga not only allows us to practice and become more skilled in domains of compassion, it is also inherently a compassionate practice.

Yoga teaches us to accept and embrace the present moment and to hold the space of acceptance of our suffering or suffering of another with complete awareness and full recognition. Yoga reminds us to remember our true nature with a deeper recognition of who we really are and to recognize the impermanence of the experience of suffering, then to take conscious action (a kriya) to eliminate, decrease and avoid future suffering.

Based on the similarities between what contemporary compassion science scholars are learning and sharing about compassion and the practices and philosophy of yoga, it is apparent that yoga can be used as a framework to both inform and provide compassionate pain care.

## Self-compassion in the patient: The value in pain care

I believe that people in pain would benefit tremendously from cultivating self-compassion and should be a part of compassionate pain care. This belief is based on working with people in pain and listening to their stories, anecdotal evidence from my colleagues who work with people in pain, and the growing evidence surrounding the health benefits of self-compassion both in the general population and in the persistent pain population.

We know that emotional and psychological health can be influenced when pain persists. Anger towards self and others, frustration, self-blame, shame, self-criticism, anxiety and fear are just a few of the emotions and attitudes that people with persistent pain commonly experience.[69] Growing research shows self-compassion can counteract many of these tendencies in the general population. In healthy populations, people with higher levels of self-compassion are shown to have greater physical and psychological wellbeing, motivation, life satisfaction, emotional resiliency, adaptive coping strategies and health-promoting behaviors, ability to cope with failure, feelings of social connectedness, healthier physiological responses to stress and reduced negative affect including lower levels of rumination, anxiety, depression, body shame and fear of failure.[70]

But what about self-compassion as it relates to people with persistent pain?

### Research on self-compassion and persistent pain

Preliminary research shows that people suffering from persistent pain who have higher levels of self-compassion showed greater pain self-efficacy, higher positive affect, decreased pain catastrophizing, lower levels of pain disability and reduced negative affect.[71] Purdie and Morley conducted a vignette study with 60 chronic pain patients and showed that "higher levels of self-compassion were associated with significantly lower negative affect and lower reported likelihood of avoidance, catastrophizing and rumination."[72] Evidence also shows that self-compassion is associated with increased pain acceptance and reduced levels of depression, anxiety and stress in a sample group of people with persistent pain.[73] It is worth noting this association of self-compassion and increased pain acceptance, as there is a growing body of research that supports the value of pain acceptance for people suffering from persistent pain. Reported benefits of pain acceptance include less depression, anxiety and physical and psychological disability, and may be associated with higher quality of life and behavior change.[74] Acceptance is closely related to mindfulness, the first element in Neff's description of self-compassion. Mindfulness includes being aware of the present moment and acknowledging the fact that one is experiencing a moment of pain and suffering. In yoga, satya (truthfulness) is one of the yamas, as discussed in Chapter 4. The idea of resisting or avoiding the truth about what is happening in the present moment is believed to lead to further resistance, tension and suffering. However, when the person in pain embraces acknowledgement of the truth about the pain experience, it can result in a clearer understanding of what is required to create change, allowing more possibility for less pain and suffering. We have evidence that self-regulation through mindfulness meditation, an aspect of yoga, modulates the pain.[75]

So far, we have only discussed the research surrounding self-compassion as a trait in relationship to persistent pain. To date, there are only two studies available that explore self-compassion as a therapeutic intervention for people with pain. Chapin et al. conducted a study that included 12 chronic pain patients who participated in a standardized nine-week Compassion Cultivation Training course. This included guided mindfulness compassion meditations and group discussions during a weekly two-hour class setting. The compassion meditations were also recorded for home practice and homework was provided, such as writing a compassion letter to oneself. Results showed a significant reduction in pain severity and anger and an increase in pain acceptance.[76] Carson et al. studied the effects of an eight-week LKM program on 43 people with persistent low back pain. This program included weekly 90-minute group sessions consisting of guided LKM, group discussions and activities, as well as encouragement of patients to perform daily loving-kindness behaviors independently. Results showed a reduction in pain intensity, psychological distress and anger.[77]

The exact mechanisms behind the positive results of compassion training for people in pain are unknown. Growing research suggests that compassion practices activate brain regions responsible for engaging the endogenous opioid system.[78] Compassion training also seems to improve positive affect through up-regulation of the social affiliation system instead of downregulating negative affect, a different mechanism than cognitive reappraisal during emotional regulation practices.[79]

Compassion training may allow the person in pain to respond to their own challenges and difficulties with kindness and compassion rather than shame, blame or anger, leading to healthier behaviors, improved stress management strategies and resiliency.[80]

More rigorous research is needed to show that self-compassion training is appropriate and effective for people in pain as a treatment intervention. Adverse side effects of self-compassion training are currently unknown.

### Example: self-compassion yoga practices for the person in pain

Listening to stories from people in pain reveals that many have a tendency to feel guilty for a variety of things such as not being able to follow through with instructions given by a health provider or not being able to participate in certain activities or contribute to household or family responsibilities. Some report feeling shameful for not being healthier, not responding favorably to treatments or not being able to focus or concentrate like they think they should.

In Chapter 1 of this book, Belton suggests that extending kindness to oneself can be difficult for people in pain at a time when feelings of shame, guilt, anger, grief, sadness, despair, purposelessness, hopelessness and worthlessness might be prevalent. Belton has reported that people in pain, including herself, may not "feel like ourselves anymore, and we perhaps may not like who we've become very much."[81] She describes her struggle with self-compassion as a person living with persistent pain:

> I was quite angry and upset with myself for a long time, beating myself up constantly for not being able to figure it out, for not doing this pain thing right, for not getting better when I was supposed to. I beat myself for being in pain at all, for not handling it better. Handling it like I should have.[82]

In Chapter 1, she goes on to state:

> During the worst years of my pain, I felt guilty taking time to take care of myself. It felt selfish. I found it much easier to care for others, even at the expense of my own wellbeing. It took some time for me to recognize that I was of value, that I was worthy of care. That I deserved kindness and compassion, just the same as anyone who is struggling with pain or is suffering. That we are all deserving of kindness and compassion—of care.

Belton reports that mindfulness meditation helped her be less reactive and more accepting of where she is in the moment. At the same time, she remained curious and open to possibilities including a new narrative, which changed her pain experience.

Here is a brief example using yoga practices to cultivate self-compassion in a moment of suffering, using Neff's three elements of self-compassion as a framework.[83]

A person in pain is feeling frustrated and angry because his pain flared up with what he describes as a minimal amount of yardwork that he feels he should be able to do easily and quickly. He feels guilty and thinks he is incompetent and useless because he cannot complete the "simple" project he promised his wife. He feels ashamed of not knowing how to manage his pain, considering all the time, effort and money he has spent on therapy.

1. **Mindfulness**: Notice, acknowledge and accept that you are in a moment of suffering. Briefly perform a kosha scan[84] where you intentionally notice the characteristics of all five koshas: notice the general state of your thoughts and emotions; become aware of the breath (notice the quality of the breath (smooth or rigid), the rate, depth, length of inhale/exhale, sound, sensation of breath at the nostrils including temperature of the breath); notice the general state of the body (physical sensations, temperature, tension); notice your overall energetic state; and finally, see if you can get a felt sense of connection to your "true self," or a sense of your spirit. Notice any judgments or elaborative stories that the mind is creating. Watch and observe the characteristics within each kosha without trying to change anything.

2. **Common humanity**: Recognize that other people have shared this experience also. You are not alone. This acknowledgement may provide some comfort. Try repeating this mantra in silence or chanting it three times out loud: *Loka Samasta Sukhino Bhavantu*. The words mean "May the whole world attain peace and harmony." The purpose of the chant is to create a greater sense of belonging and capacity for love to all sentient beings, bring a feeling of harmonious connection to humanity.[85]

3. **Kindness**: Take this opportunity to extend kindness towards yourself. You can practice karuna mudra, a yoga hand mudra conveying a gesture of compassion:[86] Cup the hands and place them in an asymmetrical prayer position with pads of the left fingers touching the base of the right fingers. As you breathe in, imagine the breath is softening the area around your heart (front, sides and back) and repeat silently to yourself, "It's OK." As you breathe out, take your time and imagine letting go of any tension around the heart and repeat, "This is enough," in a

tone that is patient, soothing and forgiving. Repeat this for a few slow breaths and stop when you feel ready. You can choose a different mantra or affirmation that provides you with a sense of kindness and love towards yourself.

In summary, there is value in practicing self-compassion, with preliminary research supporting positive effects for people living in pain. I propose that self-compassion practices have a promising role to play in providing novel, safe and effective complementary pain reduction and management strategies as part of a biopsychosocial approach to pain care.

## Self-compassion in the healthcare practitioner: The value in pain care

So far, we have discussed the value of healthcare practitioners providing compassionate care and the value of people in pain cultivating self-compassion.

I also believe it is immensely valuable for healthcare providers to cultivate self-compassion. First, consider the evidence surrounding the numerous positive physical and psychological health benefits of self-compassion as mentioned previously in this chapter, including increased emotional resiliency and healthier physiological responses to stress. Second, preliminary research suggests that self-compassion practices may help reduce the chances of clinician burnout and empathic distress fatigue.[87] Third, increased self-compassion has been shown to be linked to an increase in concern for others.[88] This may enhance the therapeutic relationship between the healthcare provider and the person in pain, improving patient outcomes and quality of care.[89]

I believe that healthcare providers appreciate the importance of and have the best intentions and desire to provide compassionate care. However, evidence suggests there can be barriers to providing compassionate care. Whether it is lack of support from our organization, long hours, overwhelming workload and paperwork, shortage of time with patients, unmanaged stress at work and home or feelings of inadequacy and guilt for not providing the care we intended, these can all contribute to a reduced capacity to offer compassionate responses and potentially lead to burnout and empathic distress.[90] A state of professional burnout may be characterized by a state of autonomic nervous system (ANS) dysregulation. Porges suggests that this ANS dysregulation can lead to a reduced capacity in a person to both express and receive compassion, which includes giving and receiving self-compassion.[91] Although we may not always have the resources to address the challenges of the organizational or external support, there are things we can do to attend to our own state and internal support system, particularly if there is a deficit in our inner resources. Neff suggests that self-compassion "appears to provide the emotional resources needed to care for others" that "mitigates caregiver fatigue."[92]

### How do we train self-compassion in the healthcare practitioner?

There are many ways to cultivate self-compassion. Yoga, a system that is inherently compassionate, and other systems have been mentioned above. Formal training programs, practicing simple techniques or embracing opportunities throughout the day are practice options. LKM has been shown to increase self-compassion[93] even after one single ten-minute practice.[94] Shapiro *et al.* studied a group of healthcare professionals that underwent a Mindfulness-Based Stress Reduction (MBSR) program, finding an increase in self-compassion and reduction in stress levels.[95] The Mindful Self-Compassion program by Neff and Germer includes numerous compassionate meditations, and their research showed that participants of the program demonstrated increased compassion towards self and others as well as increased life satisfaction.[96] However, recall that current research measures of compassion do not show strong reliability and validity. As such, we must view all reported effects with this in mind.

### Example: self-compassion yoga practices for the healthcare provider

Here is a practical example of how you, the healthcare provider, may use yoga to cultivate self-compassion in a moment of suffering, using Neff's three elements of self-compassion[97] as a framework.

Imagine a time when you may have experienced an interaction with a patient in which you felt frustrated, irritated, angry or indifferent towards the person. You were not fully present, and your mind was on other things that you considered more of a priority at the time. As a result, you acted impatiently, aloof, and were somewhat abrupt during the session. After the session, you felt a sense of guilt or shame for experiencing such negative feelings and behaving in a way that was not in line with your values. Perhaps you remained angry and felt hopeless because you did not have enough time to spend with the person or the resources to offer. Perhaps you noticed that you were blaming yourself or others for not helping, fixing or curing the person's pain.

1. **Mindfulness**: Pause, take a moment to bring awareness to breath and body. Acknowledge and accept: "OK, I did not choose well. I am aware that I feel guilty, ashamed and angry. This is a challenging moment for me right now." The Resurrection Breath[98] can be practiced, as described in the box below.

### The Resurrection Breath[99]

The Resurrection Breath can serve as a reminder to begin again and return to focus on this present moment. If we are present in each passing moment, we realize that all is changing. Remaining present with *what is* helps us to move through changing experiences with greater ease rather than getting caught up in the past or projecting into the future.

**Technique**: Begin with inhaling through the nose with the head at center. Turn the head over the left shoulder as you double exhale out the mouth making a "haa haa" sound with light force. This breath is symbolic of leaving the past behind. Then, as you inhale, bring the head back to center. Turning the head over the right shoulder, exhale by gently blowing out through pursed lips. This breath is symbolic of extending the future from grasp. Inhaling, return the head to center position having established a ritual of a new beginning. Exhaling, bow your chin to heart center and allow yourself to connect to the present moment with greater focus and clarity on the now.

2. **Common humanity**: You can offer self-talk such as, "I'm human. I'm not the only one this happens to. I made a poor choice, as many people would do in this situation. Our lives are a practice." Bring your hands to your heart, one on top of the other, and repeat the phrase silently to yourself: "I am not alone in my suffering."

3. **Kindness**: What would you say to a close loved one who made a similar mistake? Offer that same advice to yourself. Remind yourself that you have another chance to practice a different response next time. In meditation practice, we talk about "beginning again" each time the mind wanders. Sharon Salzberg, meditation teacher, suggests that each time our mind wanders, it actually provides us with an opportunity to be different. It provides us with the opportunity to bring kindness and compassion into our meditation practice. She states that nothing is ruined. We simply begin again.[100] We can use this same concept and practice during the moment after we made a choice of which we are not proud, or a mistake we made. Forgive yourself and offer compassionate self-talk, reminding yourself that you have a chance to "begin again" at this moment.

## Compassion fatigue: can too much compassion lead to burnout?

As healthcare professionals, we are exposed to people's pain, suffering and stories on a daily basis and are expected to listen compassionately and provide quality care; yet, we have no formal education or training in compassion or advice on how to provide ongoing compassionate care without burnout. Some believe that being too compassionate or empathetic over prolonged periods of time may lead to burnout and compassion fatigue.[101] The belief is that avoiding empathy or limiting compassion may help protect against professional burnout and compassion fatigue. However, the concept of "compassion fatigue" is debated among compassion science researchers.[102] The literature suggests that excessive empathy contributes to burnout and exhaustion, and not excessive compassion.[103] Empathy can be described as the capacity to share the feelings that another person is experiencing, whether the emotions are positive or negative. One can have different empathic reactions or responses to an individual's pain and suffering, such as empathic concern or empathic distress.[104] Empathic distress, also known as personal distress,[105] includes sharing and being overwhelmed by the negative emotions that the person suffering or in pain is experiencing. If we over-identify with another's distress, it can lead to empathic distress and personal discomfort and result in a reduction of our ability to provide a compassionate response.[106] Compassion, on the other hand, is recognizing one's suffering *with* the motivation to relieve it.[107] Empathy or empathic responses do not always lead to compassion.[108] Furthermore, empathy is neither necessary nor sufficient for compassion.[109] Evidence shows that empathy and compassion differ neurobiologically.[110] When exposed to another person's distress, fMRI studies show that compassion results in activation of brain regions that are associated with positive affect, love and prosocial affiliation; whereas empathy activates regions of the brain related to the *empathy* for *pain* network and is associated with negative affect. Enhancing compassion can "counteract the potential detrimental effects of empathizing too much with the suffering of others"[111] and "empathy can lead to burnout" but "compassion can help foster resilience."[112] As mentioned, the Seppala *et al.* study suggested compassion-focused training (LKM) may be useful to help promote resilience and prevent burnout in healthcare providers.[113] Considering all the above, it makes sense that Klimecki and Singer in 2011 redefined compassion fatigue as "empathic distress fatigue."[114]

Perhaps professional burnout is more related to the practitioner's unrelenting desire to "fix" or "cure" patients with a focus on *doing* something *to* someone to *fix* them, rather than being the facilitator of the person's own processes of healing and recovery. The approach of being the facilitator of the patient's own internal resources and processes to empower them to progress towards improved pain self-care, health and wellbeing might buffer against professional burnout. Yoga therapy, offering a framework for this empowered process, can be an effective approach to compassionate pain care.

## Compassionate pain care

This chapter has focused on exploring the value of the healthcare practitioner cultivating compassionate care for the person in pain and the value of both the healthcare practitioner and the person in pain cultivating self-compassion. These can be part of compassionate pain care as informed by Gilbert's three orientations of compassion—compassion for others, compassion from others and self-compassion[115]—and may serve as a useful starting point for making a difference in the quality of pain care. However, a more comprehensive compassionate pain care plan may be important to consider, as compassionate healthcare is complex and depends on many interdependent factors.[116] As such, it may require systems-based thinking and approaches to create significant change towards more compassionate pain care. For example, in addition to the components discussed in this chapter, the plan may also include the following: close family and friends practicing compassion towards self and others, including the person in pain; the values of the healthcare organization and its leaders being in line with compassionate care (this includes not only patient-centered care, but also a commitment to providing and supporting an environment where compassion can be cultivated by both the healthcare provider and the person in pain); and, finally, enhancing public awareness and understanding from the community at large surrounding the importance, health benefits and practices of compassion for self and others, including people in pain. See Table 14.2 for an overview of a potential model for compassionate pain care.

Table 14.2 Model of comprehensive compassionate pain care

| Compassionate pain care |
| --- |
| • Healthcare practitioner cultivates compassionate care for the person in pain. |
| • Healthcare practitioner and the person in pain cultivate self-compassion. |
| • Close family and friends cultivate compassion towards self and others, including the person in pain. |
| • Support and values of the healthcare organization, including its leaders, are in line with compassionate care; includes commitment to providing and supporting an environment where compassion can be cultivated by both the healthcare provider and the person in pain. |
| • Public awareness and understanding from the community at large surrounding importance, health benefits and practices of compassion for self and others, including people in pain. |

## Conclusion

People who live with persistent pain come to us often in desperation to be heard, seen, believed, understood, supported and helped. As healthcare practitioners, we do our best to help by using our knowledge and experience within the confines of the system, but can we do better?

This chapter shows us the value of compassion in pain care, which consists of compassion for the patient by the healthcare practitioner and self-compassion in both the patient and the practitioner. Although the research is not yet clear on *how* important or essential compassion is in pain care, growing research and a myriad of therapeutic experiences support that there may be benefits of training compassion, including self-compassion, for the person in pain and for us practitioners. Compassionate pain care includes our capacity to gain a deeper understanding of the patient's lived experience of pain and suffering and our ability to discern and have the courage to respond in a way that best serves the person in pain and our self, within the context of the situation. This includes providing a safe space for the person and listening patiently to their story so we can learn what the unique compassionate response might look like.

Compassionate care also means having the skills to facilitate self-compassion in our patients and in ourselves. This is no small task.

As professionals we do not yet have a guiding path to help us become more compassionate and to then share this with our patients. Yoga offers this path and provides many different techniques to enhance compassion, and even love, in ourselves and for others. As healthcare professionals, we may feel confused or uncomfortable with the thought of "loving" our patients and may believe it sounds odd, inappropriate or not within our standards of practice. However, consider this definition of love from biologist Humberto Maturana: love is "the act of allowing another to be a legitimate other."[117] Based on this definition, I suggest that we can indeed develop *loving relationships* with our patients. When Joletta Belton asked leading pain researcher Lorimer Moseley what the most important piece of advice would be for people in pain, he responded, "To love and be loved."[118] I believe love and compassion (and their neurobiological link) may be the most overlooked missing pieces in providing the kind of comprehensive pain care that people in pain require in order to thrive and live with ease. Compassionate pain care, in all its forms as described in this chapter, can be a way to love or to "allow another to be a legitimate other," including ourselves. The practice of yoga helps us experience that there is little difference between self-compassion and self-love or compassionate care and loving another. Yoga therapy provides a unique framework for this compassionate approach to pain care and offers many accessible, safe and effective practices that enhance compassion and this loving relationship, benefitting both the person in pain and those of us who help people in pain.

## Chapter 15

# Connection, Meaningful Relationship, and Purpose in Life

## Social and Existential Concerns in Pain Care

### Marlysa Sullivan

## Introduction

Social and existential concerns arising from living with chronic, persistent pain can have a significant impact on the health and wellbeing of an individual.[1] Changes in the ability to participate in previously meaningful and enjoyable occupational or recreational activities can drastically alter or diminish a person's quality of life. People in pain may find themselves questioning their core beliefs or values as they experience a challenge to their self-concept, social roles, life goals, or expectations. This predicament of change to one's way of interacting with life, including oneself, calls for the identification of intervention strategies that can focus on issues such as the transformation of self-identity, social relationships, and purpose in life.

The focus of this chapter will be on the following three primary themes that arise from the social and existential concerns of the person living with pain: connection, meaningful relationships, and purpose in life. The lived, or subjective, experience of the person living with pain will be emphasized. In addition, the relevance of these themes to adverse health outcomes, and specifically to pain, will be discussed. Spirituality and eudaimonic wellbeing are two streams of research that will be used to consider restoring a sense of wellbeing to the individual living with chronic pain. Finally, a look at the philosophy and practices of yoga therapy will address how this practice represents a much-needed therapy to help with the social and existential concerns of the person living with pain.

## Understanding how these themes impact health, wellbeing, and pain

### Connection

The loss of connection that may arise from the experience of chronic pain can include an isolation from oneself (including from one's sense of identity, self-concept, and one's own body) as well as from others (including social roles, social relationships, occupation, and leisure activities).[2] The loss of both an integrated internal and external identity can have profound implications leading to an existential crisis of sorts. The way in which people in pain understand themselves and how they fit into the world changes. There comes a need to recreate both the sense of internal cohesion and self-identity, and how they fit into and understand their place in the world and in relationships.

Occupational and recreational activities that were once enjoyed and may have formed the basis of a person's self-concept may become inaccessible. The person in pain has to resolve the longing for a past identity (both internal and external) with their current state and capabilities.[3]

Edwards *et al.*[4] explored this existential challenge for those living with chronic pain and found the loss of connection extended from that with one's own self to one's place or role in the world. People in pain have described a diminished connection with or decreased awareness of their body, including a rejection, distancing, or separation from the body or body part in pain.[5] In addition, the painful body part was seen as a threat or an "assault on the self" that took over all aspects of the person's life—resulting in feelings of powerlessness, isolation, being entrapped, exclusion, and alienation.[6] The loss of social roles and identity was described as a discrepancy between the past and current self with a longing for the past self.[7] People described this "unraveling" of self-identity as a loss of personal integrity and value, autonomy, and self-efficacy.[8]

An important part of working with people in pain is helping them to reconnect to their own body, self-identity, or self-concept, as well as to their social world and worldly engagement. It is imperative to help foster opportunities for a re-identification of personal values and goals, and a new way of living and interacting with the world. Through these experiences, the person may find a sense of agency, self-worth, and ultimately an integrated sense of both internal and external identity.

### Meaningful relationships

While having meaningful relationships can be part of the theme of connection, it also warrants its own separate category, as it has profound benefits on the wellbeing of the person.

Meaningful relationships, with an emphasis on the *quality* of those connections, has significant and important effects on the overall health of individuals and on pain. Research demonstrates differences in health effects between objective and subjective—or perceived—social isolation.[9] Objective isolation refers to a decrease in the *actual* number, proximity, or frequency of relationships. Perceived isolation refers to *feeling* isolated with an absence of meaningful relationships, irrespective of the number, proximity, or frequency of social interactions.

The negative health effects of social isolation have been found to be related to this domain of perceived social isolation rather than objective isolation. Perceived social isolation predicts negative health outcomes independent of the objective features of social interactions such as marital status, living arrangements, proximity, number, frequency, or amount of time spent with others.[10] Studies that have controlled for social support, social network size, and frequency of social activity have corroborated that it is the perception of social isolation that is a risk factor for negative effects on health, including mortality and morbidity.[11] It is important to reiterate that the presence of others is not sufficient to address the subjective experience of isolation, as it is the quality and not quantity of interactions that predicts positive effects for health and wellbeing.[12]

The following list presents a look at the research on the overall health effects of perceived social isolation.

- It is a risk factor for broad-based mortality and morbidity, including high blood pressure, metabolic syndrome, cognitive decline, and Alzheimer's disease.[13]

- It affects and is affected by functional limitation and depressive symptoms.[14]

- It upregulates the conserved transcriptional response to adversity (CTRA) gene expression profile indicative of increased inflammatory processes and diminished immunity. This CTRA profile is considered part of an underlying factor in the promotion of many chronic conditions such as cardiovascular and neurodegenerative diseases, and cancer.[15]

- The influence of social support has been found to help mediate the negative health effects of early trauma on adverse health outcomes later in life.[16]

The following list presents a look at the research on the effect of perceived social isolation on pain.

- Greater perceived social isolation has been found to be related to lower level of physical function and greater disability in those with chronic pain, including low back pain and rheumatoid arthritis.[17]

- Perceived social isolation has been found to predict the amount that pain interferes with life activities for those living with chronic pain.[18]

- Lowered perception of social support is associated with greater distress and severity of pain and decreased adjustment to chronic pain.[19]

- Social support has been shown to help improve pain behavior, disease activity, and anxiety for the chronic pain patient.[20]

- There is a greater perception of social isolation in those living with chronic pain as reported in low back pain, chronic pelvic pain, and endometriosis populations.[21]

- Social distress and pain distress have a reciprocal relationship—experiences that heighten distress in one domain (social or pain) create more potential for distress in the other.[22]

## Purpose and meaning in life

*In some way, suffering ceases to be suffering at the moment it finds meaning...*

Viktor Frankl[23]

Living with chronic pain can necessitate a re-evaluation of expectation, goals, and even beliefs around meaning or purpose in life. The person may become less able to engage in those activities that provided meaning and purpose such that a need to re-assess one's identity, values, and life goals may become evident.[24] The divide between what once offered meaning and what is now accessible or available deepens, which may lead to a disillusionment with life. This diminishment of meaning makes it imperative for the person to undertake a process of rediscovery for renewed meaning and purpose in life.[25]

The following list presents a look at the research on the relationship between meaning and purpose in life and overall health.

- The presence of meaning and purpose has been found to be predictive of all-cause mortality with higher purpose associated with lower risk of mortality.[26]

- A higher purpose in life:

  - predicts a reduced risk for a number of diseases such as Alzheimer's, mild cognitive impairment, stroke, and myocardial infarction[27]

  - is associated with better cognitive function and may offer a protective influence for the risk of cognitive impairment and Alzheimer's even in the presence of organic pathology in the brain[28]

  - is associated with lower levels of salivary cortisol in the morning and throughout the day.[29]

- The effect on the CTRA profile (mentioned above as the gene expression profile associated with increased inflammatory processes and diminished immunity and associated with chronic conditions) is as follows.

  - Higher meaning and purpose in life is associated with downregulation of this gene expression profile.[30]

  - It is particularly noteworthy that the effect of purpose and meaning on the CTRA profile is stronger than that of perceived isolation, thereby presenting a potentially significant intervention to counter the negative health effects of such isolation.[31]

The following list presents a look at the research on the relationship of meaning and purpose to pain.

- The presence of meaning in life predicted wellbeing in those with chronic pain conditions such as low back pain, arthritis, neck pain, and headaches.[32]

- Lower meaning was associated with both lower wellbeing and lower acceptance of the condition, while higher meaning was related to both higher levels of wellbeing and acceptance of the condition.[33]

- Higher presence of meaning predicted patient functioning and was associated with more optimal adjustment to chronic pain including fewer depressive symptoms, lower pain intensity, less pain medication use, and greater life satisfaction.[34]

As illustrated thus far, the themes of connection, meaningful relationship, and purpose in life contribute to optimal physiological and mental health, as well as improved function. As such, it is essential to address these social and existential concerns for the person living with chronic or persistent pain.

The practitioner can support the client in pain by facilitating a transformative process of rediscovery. The client can learn how to reconnect to their own body, redefine their self-identity, form meaningful relationships, and find renewed meaning or purpose in life. This active approach to care enables a foundation for the client to explore their own meaning and to reform their personal and social identity.[35] Yoga therapy, as discussed throughout this book and later in this chapter, offers a philosophical foundation for this transformative work, as well as various practices that can be suited to the individual.

Both spirituality and eudaimonic wellbeing (defined and discussed below) offer complementary and thought-provoking avenues of research to assist in the mitigation of the negative health outcomes discussed thus far. In addition, they point to approaches that can help the person recover and recreate a sense of connection, meaningful relationships, and purpose in life.

## Spirituality as a methodology for fostering connection, meaningful relationships, and purpose

Distinctions between the concepts of religion and spirituality can be captured by the three themes focused on in this chapter.

### Connection

Spirituality usually involves a sense of connectedness or unity that extends from an internal resourcing to an external transcendent entity or energy.[36]

### Meaningful relationships

Spiritual wisdoms often support the development of positive, meaningful social connection and relationships through the teaching of virtues, positive emotional states, and encouragement of prosocial behavior. Positive emotional states encouraged by spiritual teachings include: love, hope, optimism, wellbeing, awe, and joy. Virtues and prosocial attributes emphasized include: forgiveness, honesty, gratefulness, patience, humility, and compassion. These positive psychological states, virtues, and prosocial behaviors provide a foundation from which meaningful social connection, relationships, social support, and community may be formed.[37]

### Purpose in life

Spirituality includes a search for both meaning and purpose, as well as providing such meaning to life.[38] Spiritual teachings often communicate a worldview through which a reappraisal of negative events, such as pain, can occur. Through meaning-making the individual can re-interpret their circumstance such that the pain becomes an opportunity for personal growth and transformation rather than a threat to one's identity.[39] Yoga therapy emphasizes that this shift in worldview and reappraisal of events, while facilitated by the yoga therapist or yoga practice, comes from within the person.

## More on the relationship between spirituality and pain

Research has demonstrated that spirituality can provide a valuable coping resource that improves the quality of life in chronic pain conditions such as irritable bowel syndrome and musculoskeletal pain syndromes.[40] Spiritual coping strategies have been shown to improve pain tolerance, leading to greater functioning and participation in life activities in conditions such as: arthritis, chronic pain, sickle cell disease, migraine, and headache.[41] Spirituality is also associated with decreased level of perceived pain.[42]

Spiritual coping strategies can help facilitate connection, meaningful relationships, and purpose in life as follows. Prayer serves to connect the individual to a sense of internal resource or to something greater than oneself and has been found to reduce pain intensity and promote greater psychological wellbeing and positive affect.[43] The creation of meaningful relationships can be found within the spiritual community and includes seeking spiritual support in adverse experiences such as pain.[44] Spirituality encourages a positive reappraisal of life circumstances, providing an opportunity for personal growth and a redefining of purpose in life. For example adversity, such as pain, can be reconsidered in its capacity to help the individual cultivate positive psychological and prosocial attributes such as compassion.[45]

As many chronic pain patients use spiritual forms of coping, it is important for clinicians to be aware of and sensitive to both the spiritual concerns of the patient and their integration into care.[46]

## Eudaimonia

Another stream of research important to this discussion of cultivating connection, meaningful relationships, and purpose is that of eudaimonic wellbeing.

Aristotle taught that everything had a final purpose, end, or goal.[47] Eudaimonia described this ultimate purpose, or aim, of a human life, which was to flourish, live well, or live "excellently." Two types of happiness were described by Aristotle, with one leading to this goal of eudaimonia. Hedonic happiness referred to transitory experiences such as pleasure or comfort, which may or may not promote long-term flourishing or wellbeing in life.[48] Eudaimonic happiness, while not always related to short-term pleasure or comfort, signified a steadfast type of happiness or wellbeing that may be more accurately conceptualized as flourishing.[49]

In research, eudaimonia has been related to constructs such as personal growth, personal development, meaning, and purpose in life and is differentiated from the subjective pleasure, or transitory relaxed happiness, of hedonia.[50]

Another noteworthy topic relevant to the discussion of yoga that stems from Aristotle's teachings on eudaimonia are the virtue ethics. The virtue ethics included principles such as courage, humility, and patience. These ethical principles were meant to be explored such that the individual could live in alignment with these values for the fulfillment of an "excellent," or flourishing life.[51] To achieve eudaimonia was to live in alignment with the virtues as they fostered the "excellence of the person."[52] Aristotle's methodology of working with the virtues can be applied to the ethical principles (yamas and niyamas) of yoga and may help in the development of positive psychological and prosocial attributes.

## EXPERIENCE: THE GOLDEN MEAN AND YAMAS AND NIYAMAS
### Finding the excess and deficiency

- Choose a yama or niyama. It could be non-harming, contentment, truth, forgiveness, courage, humility, patience.

- Each ethical principle can be understood along a spectrum of meaning. On one end is having an excess of that virtue, on another is its deficiency, and in the middle is the "golden mean" taught by Aristotle.

- Take a moment to write the excess and deficiency of the principle you chose.

  - For example: Truth

    » Excess: You decide what you think is the truth, irrespective of understanding another's perspective or feelings.

    » Deficiency: You never speak your truth or perspective, you constantly doubt what you consider the truth.

- What is the "golden mean" of truth?

  - Each virtue has a spectrum from excess to deficiency. The golden mean is the balanced position in the middle.

  - For truth: What is the balance between speaking "your truth," your perspective, feeling, and needs and the consideration for others' perspectives, other "truths," other ways of seeing and understanding?

  - Write about the golden mean of the virtue you chose.

- What is your nature or tendency?

  - Do you tend to stick to your perspective regardless of other input or views?

  - Do you tend to not stick to your perspective at the expense of your own needs, values, ideals?

- Can you contemplate and explore the golden mean of this virtue and interact with the world and others from that balanced virtue?

## Eudaimonic wellbeing as a methodology for fostering connection, meaningful relationships, and purpose

The two types of wellbeing (hedonic and eudaimonic) have been found to have distinct health effects with specific measurement tools created to discern the difference.[53] Hedonic wellbeing is assessed through the measurements of subjective happiness, pleasure, feeling good, or positive affect.[54] Eudaimonic wellbeing is evaluated through measurements of optimal functioning, flourishing, and purpose in life.[55]

A well-established measurement tool for eudaimonic wellbeing describes six scales that differentiate it from hedonic wellbeing.[56] The six scales look at: autonomy, environmental mastery, personal growth, positive relations with others, purpose in life, and self-acceptance.[57] These scales relate to the themes in this chapter of connection, meaningful relationships, and purpose as follows.

### Connection

Self-acceptance, autonomy, and environmental mastery relate to our theme of connection to oneself and with life. Self-acceptance includes the capacity to be aware of one's strengths and weaknesses and to create positive evaluations of oneself and one's life.[58] Autonomy includes a sense of self-determination and personal conviction, as well as the capability to live in accordance with one's values.[59] Self-acceptance and autonomy both facilitate a strong, integrated self-concept with greater awareness of one's values, beliefs, needs, strengths, and limitations. This self-knowledge helps the individual to live in alignment and in connection with a deeper sense of self through which greater confidence, self-esteem, agency, and self-efficacy can be realized.

Environmental mastery includes the ability to navigate and meet the demands of one's surroundings. As an individual finds they can effectively manage their life situations, they may learn to connect with and engage more positively with the surrounding world.[60]

### Meaningful relationships

The measure of positive relations with others includes having close and valued connection and relationships with others.[61] As mentioned earlier, exploring the presence of meaningful relationships is important, as it is the quality of relationships that impacts and predicts wellbeing—not the quantity or number of interactions with others.[62]

## Meaning and purpose

The two measures of personal growth and purpose in life both correlate to this theme. In personal growth the person is able to see themselves as learning and growing over time. They are able to explore their own personal gifts and see life circumstances as an opportunity for transformation and personal development— including the experience of pain. The purpose-in-life scale investigates to what extent people feel their life is meaningful and purposeful.[63]

## Health effects of eudaimonic wellbeing

The following list presents a look at the research on the effect of eudaimonic wellbeing on overall health.

- The effect on the CTRA profile (its upregulation was mentioned before as being associated with increased inflammatory processes and diminished immunity) is as follows.

  - Meaning and purpose in life has been found to downregulate this gene profile, thereby helping regulate inflammatory and immune processes.[64]

  - Eudaimonic wellbeing has been found to have a stronger effect on CTRA expression than perceived social isolation and therefore may compensate for its adverse health effects.[65]

  - Five of the six scales for eudaimonic wellbeing predicted the down-regulation of CTRA gene expression independent of demographics and other health variables. These included: purpose in life, environmental mastery, self-acceptance, autonomy, positive relations with others.[66]

  - Hedonic and eudaimonic wellbeing may have similar affective outcomes but demonstrate different effects on CTRA expression. Eudaimonic wellbeing is associated with a downregulation of this profile, while hedonic wellbeing its upregulation.[67]

- Higher eudaimonic wellbeing is associated with:

  - decreased levels of salivary cortisol, proinflammatory cytokines, and lessened cardiovascular disease risk, while hedonic wellbeing has minimal effect on these biomarkers.[68]

  - less amygdala activation and more engagement of higher cortical structures in reference to negative stimuli and sustained activation of reward circuitry in response to positive stimuli.[69]

- The absence of eudaimonic wellbeing was found to increase the probability of all-cause mortality, independent of factors such as age, gender, race, physical inactivity, and conditions such as cardiovascular disease, cancer, or stroke.[70]

The following list presents a look at the research on eudaimonic wellbeing specific to pain:

- Research demonstrates that individuals with fibromyalgia (FM) have a lower sense of eudaimonic wellbeing than healthy controls and people with rheumatoid arthritis (RA).[71]

  - Individuals with FM scored lower on four of the six scales of eudaimonic wellbeing including: environmental mastery, purpose in life, positive relations with others, and self-acceptance.[72]

  - The scale of personal growth was lower in those with FM than healthy controls, but not RA.

  - Those with higher overall eudaimonic wellbeing experienced less disability and fatigue.

  - Eudaimonic wellbeing mediated the relationship between social network size and disability.[73]

- The presence of meaning predicted wellbeing in chronic pain conditions with higher meaning related to both greater patient functioning and optimal adjustment to chronic pain including fewer depressive symptoms, lower pain intensity, less pain medication use, and greater life satisfaction.[74]

The eudaimonic domains of purpose in life, self-acceptance, positive relations, and environmental mastery appear to be the most important domains to address when caring for people living with chronic pain.[75] They are also reflected in this chapter's focus on connection (to oneself through self-acceptance and with the world through environmental mastery), meaningful relationships, and purpose in life. Yoga therapy offers novel ways in which to integrate these domains into pain care.

## Yoga therapy, spirituality, and eudaimonia: shared foundations and effects

With the significant impact of these social and existential concerns on overall health and the pain experience, it is essential to identify appropriate and effective intervention strategies. What has been described thus far can be seen as a cycle of events influencing one another involving the following: loss of personal, interpersonal, and existential sense of connection; perceived social isolation; lack of meaningful relationships; loss of meaning and purpose; adverse health effects including the pain experience (see Figure 15.1).

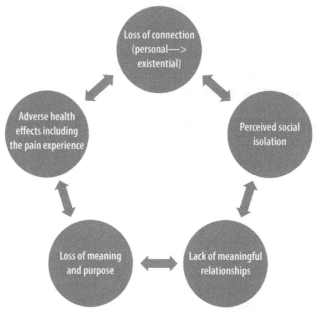

*Figure 15.1 Cycle of relationships between loss of connection, isolation, meaning and purpose, and adverse health effects*

Both spirituality and eudaimonic wellbeing have been described as strategies to improve connection, meaningful relationships, and purpose in life, as well as to help mitigate adverse health outcomes for the person living with pain.

The processes through which spirituality may improve health and wellbeing that are shared with yoga include: supporting personal and existential connection; development of prosocial and positive psychological attributes to support improved relationships with others; cultivation of a worldview for a positive reappraisal of life situations; and a like-minded community.[76] Yoga has also been shown to improve facets of eudaimonic wellbeing, including personal meaning, purpose in life, meaningful relationships, and acceptance of oneself.[77]

When yoga therapy is delivered in alignment with its philosophical foundations, it becomes a powerful methodology to realize the benefits of both spirituality and eudaimonic wellbeing for cultivating connection (existential, interpersonal, personal) and purpose in life (see Figure 15.2). These philosophical foundations will be discussed and related to the social and existential concerns for the person living with chronic or persistent pain below.

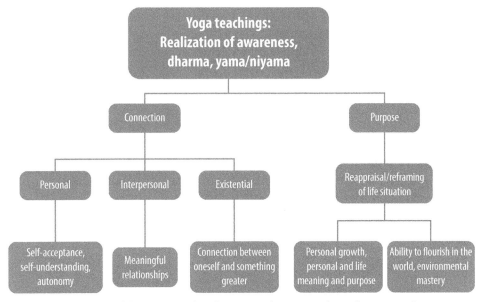

*Figure 15.2 Addressing social and existential concerns through yoga teachings*

Yoga philosophical foundations such as the realization of awareness, dharma, yama, and niyama can address the social and existential concerns of the person living with pain such that connection (personal, interpersonal, and existential) and purpose are fostered. Personal connection is cultivated through the development of self-acceptance, self-understanding, and autonomy. Social relationships may be improved through the understanding of connection or unity between people, as well as development of positive psychological and prosocial attributes. From a more existential sense, the person can realize the connection between themselves and something greater. Purpose is cultivated through a reappraisal of one's life situations such that adverse events can become opportunities for personal growth and renewal of personal and life meaning or purpose. From this the capacity to flourish and navigate the world more successfully may emerge.

## Connections between yoga and eudaimonia

The *Bhagavad Gita* teaches:

> The joy of lucidity at first seems like poison, but is in the end like ambrosia, from the calm of self-understanding. (18.37)[78]

Yoga teaches that underneath the constant fluctuations of the body, mind, and environment is a steadfast, abiding state of joy stemming from the realization of oneself as the equanimity of "awareness" within. The alleviation of suffering arises from the development of discriminative wisdom that enables the person to differentiate between that which is ever-changing (all phenomena of the body, mind, and environment) from that which is unchanging (underlying awareness).[79]

A recent explanatory framework for yoga therapy was proposed by a group of colleagues and myself whereby suffering can be alleviated in the experience of pain, illness, or disability by shifting the relationship and identification with the fluctuations of the body, mind, and environment[80] (see Figure 15.3). Yoga teaches that this connection to the steadfast joy of unchanging awareness can help to alleviate or mitigate suffering.

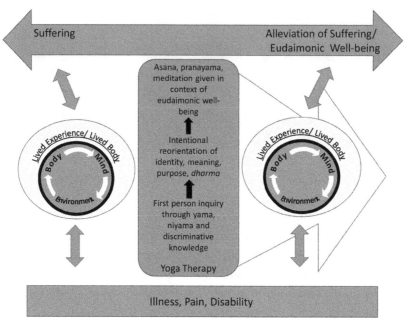

*Figure 15.3 Explanatory model for yoga therapy*

*Source*: Sullivan, M., Moonaz, S., Weber, K., Taylor, J.N., & Schmalzl, L. (2018) "Toward an Explanatory Framework for Yoga Therapy Informed by Philosophical and Ethical Perspectives." *Alternative Therapies in Health and Medicine 21*, 1, 38–47.

According to this framework, illness, pain, or disability can change the person's relationship to their body, mind, or environment to create an experience of suffering. Likewise, suffering can change the person's relationship to their body, mind, or environment to adversely affect their pain, or illness. Yoga therapy focused on ethical inquiry and discrimination can foster a reorientation of one's identity, meaning, and purpose. Concepts such as dharma are essential to this process. Practices of asana, pranayama, and meditation are provided within a context of supporting dharma and eudaimonic well-being. The relationship to the body, mind, and environment changes—even in the presence of pain, illness, or disability—such that suffering is alleviated and eudaimonic well-being realized.

The above quote from the *Bhagavad Gita* likens the joy that arises from understanding oneself as the equanimity of unchanging awareness to the "nectar of the gods." This joy is not a transitory nor insubstantial experience such as comfort or pleasure. Rather it is an enduring type of joy that can be present amidst disturbance—such as pain.

Both Aristotle and yoga teach this differentiation of a steadfast and abiding form of happiness or joy from that of transitory pleasurable experience. The virtue ethics taught by Aristotle offer a methodology of inquiry that helps to develop self-knowledge. Ethical inquiry thus forms a path for practical action towards the abiding "happiness" of eudaimonia. Similarly, the quote above demonstrates that yoga emphasizes that the joy of the realization of awareness stems from a path of self-understanding.

The practices of yoga can at times "seem like poison" as they ask the person to delay or put aside immediate gratification. However, the joy that results from realizing the self as "awareness" fosters a steadfast joy that can be present independent of outer circumstance—such as pain. In sum, the "happiness" of eudaimonia and the "joy" fostered through yoga is one of calmness or equanimity arising from self-understanding, is steadfast and abiding, and stems from disciplined work.

## Yoga therapy's methodology for facilitating connection and purpose for the person living with pain
### Existential connection

*The Self is the source of abiding joy... When one realizes the Self, in whom all life is one, changeless, nameless, formless, then one fears no more. Until we realize the unity of life, we live in fear.*

*Taittiriya Upanishad*[81]

*But where there is unity...this is the supreme goal of life, the supreme treasure, the supreme joy.*

*Brihadaranyaka Upanishad*[82]

*As a lump of salt thrown in water dissolves and cannot be taken out again, though wherever we taste the water it is salty, even so, beloved, the separate self dissolves in the sea of pure consciousness, infinite and immortal.*

*Brihadaranyaka Upanishad*[83]

The existential connection in yoga stems from the realization of underlying awareness of oneself as the same awareness in all. The above quotes illustrate the teachings of understanding the unity of life and the dissolution of the separate self that is the goal or intention of yoga. Yoga teaches that misperception of our separateness from life and from others creates fear or suffering. It is when we understand this connection between all and to something greater that abiding and supreme joy emerge.

As stated earlier, yoga teaches a process for the realization of this state of awareness and unity that is present underneath all of the shifting phenomena of the body, mind, and environment—regardless of circumstance or situation.[84] Yoga's capacity to facilitate transformative experiences including a sense of connection extending from oneself, others, and something greater has been described in the literature.[85]

This realization of the Self as a state of unity with all beings and with something greater has many potential positive effects. A broadening of one's perspective may occur which can help in the re-interpretation, reframing or redefinition of the pain experience. The person can potentially make meaning from the experience to facilitate personal growth and renewal of purpose, and to develop acceptance and connection with oneself and others. Experiencing a state of unity can also help either foster the emergence of or assist in the development of positive psychological and prosocial traits such as joy, peace, and compassion thus improving social relationships and healthy engagement with life.

When this teaching is incorporated as the intention of the various practices of yoga—such as movement, breath, and meditation as described throughout this book and in the example at the end of the chapter—the person may learn to understand adverse experiences, such as pain, in a different way. As the individual learns that this greater connection is accessible to them amidst their pain experience they can develop a broadening of perspective; the capacity to reframe and learn from experience; support positive qualities such as compassion or patience towards themselves and others; and find a purpose-filled life.

## Interpersonal connection

*Those who realize that all life is one are at home everywhere and see themselves in all beings.*

*Taittiriya Upanishad*[86]

*…seeing everything with an equal eye, he sees the Self in all creatures and all creatures in the Self.*

*Bhagavad Gita (6.29)*[87]

*…as long as there is separateness, one sees another as separate from oneself, hears another as separate from oneself, smells another as separate from oneself, speaks to another as separate from oneself, thinks of another as separate from oneself, knows another as separate from oneself. But when the*

*Self is realized as the indivisible unity of life, who can be seen by whom, who can be heard by whom, who can be smelled by whom, who can be spoken to by whom, who can be thought of by whom, who can be known by whom.*

*Brihadaranyaka Upanishad*[88]

Similar to the previous quotes, these excerpts describe an essential teaching in yoga to recognize the same self within all creatures and of the inseparability of life. The individual learns to no longer regard others as separate from oneself. Rather the person learns to see the commonality and shared experiences between themselves and others, which can help facilitate the development of meaningful, quality relationships. This point cannot be underscored enough, as it was mentioned earlier in this chapter that it is meaningful relationships that help to create the positive health effects of social connection. This realization of the inseparability between oneself and others is key to the building of meaningful social connection.

Through the realization of the connection between oneself and others, positive psychological and prosocial attributes or values—such as compassion, kindness, and patience—may be cultivated. To this point, practitioners have attributed to their yoga practice helping improve their relationships, including the development of greater patience, peacefulness, kindness, tolerance, and respect in their interactions.[89] In addition, greater compassion has been associated with yoga practice.[90]

The yoga teachings of yamas and niyamas (ethical principles) are crucial to this process as they encourage the inquiry into and practical application of positive psychological and prosocial traits such as non-harming or contentment.

Another way that yoga may help to decrease perceived social isolation and cultivate meaningful relationships is through participation in yoga classes. Individuals may find a like-minded community where they can meet new friends or share common activities with friends or partners through attending classes.[91]

Additionally, it is worth mentioning that yoga has been found to help mitigate the effect of perceived social isolation on CTRA gene expression, thereby helping to regulate inflammatory and immune processes.[92]

## Personal connection

The *Bhagavad Gita* teaches:

*But when a man finds delight within himself and feels inner joy and pure contentment in himself, there is nothing more to be done. (3.17)*[93]

*The man of discipline [yoga] has joy, delight, and light within; becoming the infinite spirit he finds the pure calm of infinity. (5.24)*[94]

Yoga teaches a process of self-inquiry and self-reflection that can help foster self-acceptance, autonomy, and personal growth. The individual is supported in an exploration of their habitual patterns of relationship and reaction to their body, mind, and the environment. Insight into the differentiation between these habitual patterns and underlying awareness is supported through both the philosophy and practices of yoga (including movement, breath, meditation, ethical principles) as described throughout this book and in the exercise at the end of this chapter. The individual is supported on a journey to ultimately realize the inner joy, pure contentment, and the "pure calm of infinity" described in the above quotes as their essential nature.

These yoga teachings and practices can help people in pain broaden their perspectives and reframe experiences such that adversity becomes an opportunity for personal growth. Ultimately, new ways of being in relationship to body sensations, the mind, and the environment are learned. The cultivation of qualities such as kindness, contentment, patience, and acceptance empower the person to reconnect to their body with the same attributes that serve to improve relationships with others. The yamas and niyamas such as non-harming, truthfulness, and contentment can be applied to oneself for greater self-compassion, self-acceptance, and self-care. To this end, yoga practitioners have described the practice as one that fosters personal growth and transformation including the development of greater insight, self-awareness, and positive coping mechanisms.[95]

It was mentioned earlier that pain can result in a distancing, rejection, or alienation from one's body.[96] Research has demonstrated that practicing yoga is correlated with greater body awareness—including interoceptive, proprioceptive, and vestibular processes.[97] The meditative movements of yoga in addition to other practices, as described in Chapter 9, can help facilitate this reconnection to the body.

## *Purpose and meaning in life*

> *Better to do one's own duty [dharma] imperfectly than to do another man's well; doing action intrinsic to his being, a man avoids guilt.*
>
> *Bhagavad Gita* (18.47)[98]

Yoga's philosophical concept of dharma helps to illuminate a way to understand and work with the idea of purpose in life. The word dharma has a complex meaning and is central to many yogic teachings, including the *Bhagavad Gita*.[99]

Richard Miller describes how the root of the word dharma comes from the Sanskrit word ṛta—to be in harmony with the totality of the universe. When our way of living is congruent with our dharma we are in harmony with the totality of the universe. We sense this feeling of harmony within ourselves as our alignment with universal harmony (Richard Miller, oral and written correspondence). Dharma can also be understood as those actions that sustain oneself and those around them (this concept is further described in Chapter 4).[100]

The above quote from the *Bhagavad Gita* emphasizes the necessity to understand one's own personal dharma. Harm may result to the individual and/or the world if the individual does not act in alignment with one's own dharma. Therefore, the individual is encouraged to explore the path of right action in each situation in life such that there is this sustenance, support, or congruence between oneself and others. This fosters personal, interpersonal, and environmental harmony. To satisfy dharma, it is paramount that one explores and understands their personal path of right action rather than adopting a path of action, or way of life, that is not their own.

As mentioned previously, living with chronic pain can create a shift in a person's values, meaning, and expectations. This can include a change in the ability to participate in occupational or recreational activities that were formerly enjoyed or that had provided a sense of identity or purpose. The individual may experience suffering due to this potential loss of purpose, meaningful engagement with others or with life, or the holding on to past ideals. The pain experience thus becomes an opportunity to rediscover or redefine one's values, meaning, and purpose.

The many practices of yoga including ethical principles, movement, breath, and meditation can be oriented towards this philosophical foundation of dharma. The ethical principles (yama and niyama) can become a process of self-inquiry and self-discovery such that the person is able to reappraise and reframe adverse circumstances, such as pain. This process may help clarify a renewed sense of purpose and meaning such that the person is able to discover and reorient towards a way of living that supports harmony with oneself, others, and the world within which they are situated.

The other practices of yoga such as movement, breath techniques, and meditation can also be utilized to help the individual access states of equanimity, contentment, or steadfast joy, reflecting the harmony of dharma or the connection to awareness. The individual thus learns to use these techniques of yoga to influence physiological and psychological states, to regulate the body and mind, to find states of equanimity, and to lessen or alleviate suffering. Through the integrated practices of yoga, the individual gains multiple tools and avenues for restoring a sense of inner and outer connection or harmony, as well as a renewed sense of purpose. To this point, yoga practitioners have reported the practice helping to facilitate such a greater sense of purpose and contribution to the greater good.[101]

## *Focusing on yama and niyama as ethical inquiry*

Yamas and niyamas are crucial for this process to support connection, meaningful relationships, and purpose in life. They offer principles for ethical inquiry that can be used to help the individual explore and create new values, meaning, and purpose. This self-reflective process may facilitate positive psychological and prosocial attributes such that a renewed sense of connection to oneself, others, and life is encouraged. In addition, the person may find the capacity to reframe experience as an opportunity for personal growth and ultimately find new ways to flourish in life.

The emphasis on ethical reflection shared by different wisdom traditions, such as Aristotle and yoga, draws attention to the importance of this teaching and practice. Aristotle highlights ethical reflection for the fulfillment of eudaimonia and yoga for the realization of dharma.[102] Both express that ethical principles such as kindness, forgiveness, generosity, and truthfulness lead the practitioner on a path of flourishing and harmony.[103]

The potential for this ethical inquiry through the practice of the yamas and niyamas to facilitate eudaimonic wellbeing has significant effects for mortality, physical and mental health, gene expression profile, pain intensity, pain adjustment including pain medication use, and the promotion of greater wellbeing.[104] Edwards *et al.*[105] wrote that working with the moral experience of pain can facilitate a reconnection to one's body, identity, meaning, values, expectations, and purpose such that the person learns to re-engage positively with themselves, others, and life.[106]

There are a limited number of studies that include the yamas and niyamas. One small study compared a yoga class that included the yamas and niyamas to a class without. Both groups improved in terms of depression, stress, hopefulness, and increased flexibility. However, only the class with the incorporation of the ethical principles found improvement in anxiety symptoms and decreased salivary cortisol.[107] In another study, postural yoga (defined as classes without philosophy nor yama/niyama) was correlated with improvement in body awareness and compassion. However, the improvement in body awareness was negatively related to altruism.[108]

The inclusion of yamas and niyamas may be an important focus of yoga practice in working with clients living with chronic or persistent pain to help shift, rediscover, or realign with their values, meaning, and purpose to foster a healthier engagement and connection to oneself, others, and life.

## A PRACTICE WITH THE YAMAS AND NIYAMAS

We will use truth and contentment as our beginning ethical principles and then bring in non-grasping.

Sit for a moment in a comfortable position with something to write with and on. Take a moment to contemplate the ideas of truth and contentment. Consider the following points and write anything that is important for you to write along the way.

- Is there a memory that arises, an image, a word for the concepts of truth and contentment?

- Is there a feeling in your body including a place in the body from which you can feel the image or concept of truth and of contentment?

- Strengthen both feelings in your body. That of contentment and of truth. Take time for each to be strengthened. Go back and forth between the two.

- Notice if there is a movement or posture that would help you to strengthen the feeling of truth and the feeling of contentment. Take time to strengthen both feelings in their respective postures.

   - Play and investigate postures such as a strong standing posture, a letting-go or restorative posture, a rhythmic moving posture.

- As you work with these concepts of truth and contentment and are able to feel them strongly, notice what else arises—feelings, emotions, beliefs, wants.

- Notice the tendency to grasp for something different than what you feel— to try and change the experience you are having. If pain arises, allow it— if discomfort arises, allow it—if other thoughts, emotions, ideas pull you away—allow it. Shift positions whenever you need.

   - What does it mean to be content with the present-moment experience? To stay connected to truth even amidst other arisings and fallings?

- What would it mean to relate to yourself from contentment and truth, in your relationships to others, in your life activities?

- Notice if you are left with a posture or movement and inner sensation that can remind you of truth and contentment—something that can become a practice for you to strengthen these ethical principles.

## Conclusion

Research has demonstrated the serious adverse health effects of decreased social and spiritual wellbeing such as perceived social isolation and diminished meaning or purpose in life for many populations, including people in pain. Yoga therapy offers a novel methodology to work with these social and existential concerns for pain care. Through these practices, the person suffering from chronic or persistent pain can find a renewed sense of personal, interpersonal, and existential connection and purpose in life.

# About the Contributors

### Neil Pearson, PT, MSc (RHBS), BA-BPHE, C-IAYT, ERYT500

Neil Pearson is a physiotherapist and clinical assistant professor at the University of British Columbia. He is an experienced yoga teacher, a yoga therapist and creator of the Pain Care Yoga training programs for health professionals and yoga therapists. Neil is founding chair of the Physiotherapy Pain Science Division in Canada, recipient of the Canadian Pain Society's Excellence in Interprofessional Pain Education award, author of a conversational patient education book and 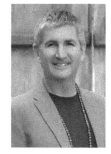 faculty in multiple yoga therapist training programs. Neil develops innovative resources, collaborates in research and serves as a mentor for health professionals and yoga practitioners seeking to enhance their therapeutic expertise.

### Shelly Prosko, PT, C-IAYT

Shelly Prosko is a physiotherapist, yoga therapist, educator and respected pioneer of PhysioYoga www.physioyoga.ca. She advocates for the integration of yoga into modern healthcare with a focus on enhancing care for people suffering from persistent pain, pelvic health conditions and professional burnout. She teaches at universities and yoga therapy schools, presents at international conferences, contributes to academic research, provides mentorship to health professionals and 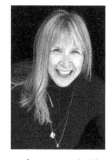 offers onsite and online continuing education courses on a variety of topics. Shelly maintains a clinical practice in Sylvan Lake, Canada and believes that cultivating meaningful connections, compassion and joy can be powerful contributors to recovery and wellbeing.

## Marlysa Sullivan, PT, C-IAYT

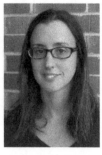

Marlysa Sullivan is a physical therapist and yoga therapist specializing in working with people living with chronic pain conditions. She is a professor at Maryland University of Integrative Health in the Masters of Science in Yoga Therapy program as well as Emory University where she teaches the integration of yoga into physical therapy practice. Her research interests focus on developing an explanatory and theoretical framework for yoga therapy to assist its utilization in both research and clinical contexts. She is actively involved in helping grow the profession of yoga therapy through international collaborations and teaching.

## Timothy McCall, MD

Timothy McCall is the bestselling author of *Yoga as Medicine*, and a co-editor and contributor to the medical textbook, *The Principles and Practice of Yoga in Health Care*. *Yoga Journal's* medical editor since 2002, Dr. McCall also serves on the editorial board of *The International Journal of Yoga Therapy*. He lives in Burlington, Vermont and lectures and teaches yoga therapy seminars around the world. His latest book is *Saving My Neck: A Doctor's East/West Journey Through Cancer*. See DrMcCall.com

## Joletta Belton

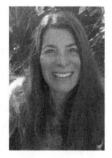

Joletta Belton is cofounder of the nonprofit organization the Endless Possibilities Initiative where their mission is to empower people living with pain to live well. They provide experiential learning retreats and workshops for people living with pain, as well as for healthcare professionals. Jo also has a blog, MyCuppaJo.com, where she shares her story through the lens of science in order to give hope to others living with pain and lend valuable insights into the lived experience of pain and recovery to health professionals.

### Matt Erb, PT

Matt Erb is a physical therapist with a focus on mind-body integrated care. He has specialization in chronic pain conditions including headache and migraine. He is a leader in translating the construct of integrative healthcare into rehabilitation therapy practice and is an advocate for equipping therapists to safely support and work with the whole-person experience. He has a deep appreciation for yoga, the wisdom traditions and indigenous teachings. Matt is faculty with The 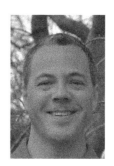 Center for Mind-Body Medicine, founder of Embody Your Mind and maintains a clinical practice in Tucson, AZ.

### Michael Lee, MA, Dip.Soc.Sci., C-IAYT

Michael Lee is the founder of Phoenix Rising Yoga Therapy, a leading-edge, yoga-based modality for psycho-emotional wellbeing, which is an IAYT accredited program. Michael's conference keynote presentations include the IYTA Conference in Singapore, IAYT Conference 2016, Yoga Journal Conferences, Family Therapy Networker, 2018 Yoga Australia, 2018 Japan Yoga Therapy Conference and Inaugural Global Consortium on Yoga Therapy in 2018. Michael is the 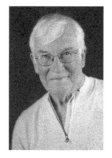 author of two books, *Phoenix Rising Yoga Therapy* and *Turn Stress Into Bliss*, and a contributing author in the APA-published text *Movement and Expressive Techniques in Clinical Practice* and the recently published *Yoga Therapy and Integrative Medicine: Where Ancient Science Meets Modern Medicine*. Michael also offers programs for psychotherapists and professionals wanting to apply a yoga-based embodied mindfulness approach to therapy and life change, and teaches in various locations around the world.

### Steffany Moonaz, PhD, C-IAYT

Steffany Moonaz is a yoga therapist and researcher in Baltimore, MD. She currently serves as director of clinical and academic research at the Maryland University of Integrative Health, which offers the only Masters of Science in Yoga Therapy in the United States. She is the founder and director of Yoga for Arthritis, which offers yoga programs and trainings for people with arthritis and the professionals who serve them. Her first book, *Yoga Therapy for Arthritis:* 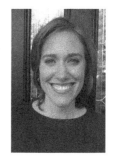 *A Whole Person Approach to Movement and Lifestyle*, was released by Singing Dragon in 2018.

### Lori Rubenstein Fazzio, PT, DPT, MAppSc, C-IAYT

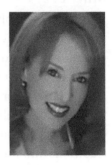

Dr. Lori Rubenstein Fazzio practices integrative physical therapy and yoga therapy in her private practice in Los Angeles, www.mosaicpt.com. She has been compassionately helping people with persistent pain since the 1980s and her expertise is frequently featured in news and magazine articles across the country. She is on faculty in the Yoga Studies graduate and extension programs at Loyola Marymount University and is a lifelong student and practitioner of yoga and compassionate care.

### Antonio Sausys, MA, IGT, CMT, C-IAYT

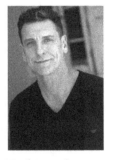

Antonio Sausys is a somatic psychologist and yoga therapist specializing in grief counseling and therapy. Antonio presents his work both nationally and internationally at schools and universities, leads retreats at ashrams, retreat centers and yoga studios and is a member of the World Yoga Council, the founder and executive director of Yoga for Health, the International Yoga Therapy Conference, and a TV host for YogiViews. He is the author of *Yoga for Grief Relief: Simple Practices for Transforming Your Grieving Mind and Body* (New Harbinger).

### Tracey Sondik, PsyD, C-IAYT, E-RYT-500

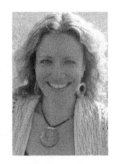

Tracey Sondik is a licensed clinical psychologist and certified C-IAYT yoga therapist with an expertise in neuropsychological assessment, trauma-informed therapies, positive behavioral support plans and integrative medicine including the use of yoga and mindfulness for mental health. She has authored several publications and book chapters around holistic behavioral treatment for mental health conditions. Tracey is an assistant clinical professor at Yale University Department of Psychiatry and adjunct faculty member at University of Hartford Graduate School of Professional Psychology in Hartford, CT and Maryland University of Integrative Health Master's of Science Yoga Therapy program in Laurel, MD.

## Matthew J. Taylor, PT, PhD, C-IAYT

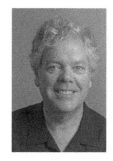

Matthew J. Taylor creates and shares resources to incorporate smart, safe yoga for yoga professionals and conventional medical professionals. His leadership in the field of yoga risk management, as well as being an expert legal witness, make him an expert in yoga safety and injuries. He was president of the International Association of Yoga Therapists when the professional development strategy was established and continues to serve in numerous capacities. His books, *Fostering Creativity in Rehabilitation* and *Yoga Therapy as a Creative Response to Pain*, and over 30 publications have been the vanguard in integrative rehabilitation.

# Endnotes

## CHAPTER 2

1   Cramer, H., Klose, P., Brinkhaus, B., Michalsen, A. and Dobos, G. (2017) "Effects of yoga on chronic neck pain: A systematic review and meta-analysis." *Clinical Rehabilitation 31*, 11, 1457–1465.

2   Yogitha, B., Nagarathna, R., John, E. and Nagendra, H. (2010) "Complimentary effect of yogic sound resonance relaxation technique in patients with common neck pain." *International Journal of Yoga 3*, 1, 18–25.

3   Cramer, H., Lauche, R., Haller, H. *et al.* (2013) "'I'm more in balance': A qualitative study of yoga for patients with chronic neck pain." *Journal of Alternative and Complementary Medicine 19*, 6, 536–542.

4   Saper, R. B., Sherman, K. J., Delitto, A. *et al.* (2014) "Yoga vs. physical therapy vs. education for chronic low back pain in predominantly minority populations: Study protocol for a randomized controlled trial. *Trials*. doi: 10.1186/1745-6215-15-67.

5   Saper, R. B., Boah, A. R., Keosaian, J. *et al.* (2013) "Comparing once- versus twice-weekly yoga classes for chronic low back pain in predominantly low income minorities: A randomized dosing trial." *Evidence-Based Complementary and Alternative Medicine*: ECAM 2013: 658030.

6   Sherman, K. J., Cherkin, D. C., Wellman, R. D., Cook, A. J., Hawkes, R. J., Delaney, K. and Deyo, R. A. (2011) "A randomized trial comparing yoga, stretching, and a self-care book for chronic low back pain." *Archives of Internal Medicine 171*, 22, 2019–2026.

7   Saper *et al.* (2013).

8   Keosaian, J. E., Lemaster, C. M., Dresner, D., Godersky, M. E. *et al.* (2016) "'We're all in this together': A qualitative study of predominantly low income minority participants in a yoga trial for chronic low back pain." *Complementary Therapies in Medicine 24*, 34–39.

9   Cramer, H., Lauche, R., Haller, H. and Dobos, G. (2013) "A systematic review and meta-analysis of yoga for low back pain." *Clinical Journal of Pain 29*, 5, 450–460.

10  Chang, D. G., Holt, J. A., Sklar, M. and Groessl, E. J. (2016) "Yoga as a treatment for chronic low back pain: A systematic review of the literature." *Journal of Orthopedics and Rheumatology 3*, 1, 1–8.

11  Chou, R., Qaseem, A., Snow, V. *et al.* (2007) "Diagnosis and treatment of low back pain: A joint clinical practice guideline from the American College of Physicians and the American Pain Society." *Annals of Internal Medicine 147*, 7, 478–491.

12  Kan, L., Zhang, J., Yang, Y. and Wang, P. (2016) "The effects of yoga on pain, mobility, and quality of life in patients with knee osteoarthritis: A systematic review." *Evidence-Based Complementary and Alternative Medicine*: ECAM 2016: 6016532.

13  Kolasinski, S. L., Garfinkel, M., Tsai, A. G., Matz, W., Van Dyke, A. and Schumacher, H. R. (2005) "Iyengar yoga for treating symptoms of osteoarthritis of the knees: A pilot study." *Journal of Alternative and Complementary Medicine 11*, 4, 689–693.

14  Cheung, C., Wyman, J. F., Resnick, B. and Savik, K. (2014) "Yoga for managing knee osteoarthritis in older women: a pilot randomized controlled trial." *BMC complementary and alternative medicine 14*, 1, 160.

15  Ebnezar, J., Nagarathna, R., Yogitha, B. and Nagendra, H. R. (2012) "Effects of an integrated approach of Hatha yoga therapy on functional disability, pain, and flexibility in osteoarthritis of the knee joint: A randomized controlled study." *Journal of Alternative and Complementary Medicine 18*, 5, 463–472.

16  Nambi, G. S. and Shah, A. A. (2013) "Additional effect of Iyengar yoga and EMG biofeedback on pain and functional disability in chronic unilateral knee osteoarthritis." *International Journal of Yoga 6*, 2, 123–127.

17  Ghasemi, G. A., Golkar, A. and Marandi, S. M. (2013) "Effects of Hata yoga on knee osteoarthritis." *International Journal of Preventive Medicine 4*, S1, S133–138.

18  Akyuz, G. and Kenis-Coskun, O. (2018) "The efficacy of tai chi and yoga in rheumatoid arthritis and spondyloarthropathies: A narrative biomedical review." *Rheumatology International 38*, 3, 321–330.

19  Bosch, P. R., Traustadóttir, T., Howard, P. and Matt, K. S. (2009) "Functional and physiological effects of yoga in women with rheumatoid arthritis: A pilot study." *Alternative Therapies in Health and Medicine 15*, 4, 24–31.

20  Singh, V. K., Bhandari, R. B. and Rana, B. B. (2011) "Effect of yogic package on rheumatoid arthritis."

*Indian Journal of Physiology and Pharmacology 55*, 4, 329–335.

21  Evans, S., Moieni, M., Lung, K., Tsao, J., Sternlieb, B., Taylor, M. and Zeltzer, L. (2013) "Impact of iyengar yoga on quality of life in young women with rheumatoid arthritis." *The Clinical Journal of Pain 29*, 11, 988.

22  Ward, L., Stebbings, S., Athens, J., Cherkin, D. and Baxter, G. D. (2017) "Yoga for the management of pain and sleep in rheumatoid arthritis: A pilot randomized controlled trial." *Musculoskeletal Care 16*, 1, 39–47.

23  Jerath, R., Barnes, V. A. and Crawford, M. W. (2014) "Mind-body response and neurophysiological changes during stress and meditation: Central role of homeostasis." *Journal of Biological Regulators and Homeostatic Agents 28*, 4, 545–554.

24  Akyuz and Kenis-Coskun (2018).

25  Ward, L., Stebbings, S., Cherkin, D. and Baxter, G. D. (2013) "Yoga for Functional Ability, Pain and Psychosocial Outcomes in Musculoskeletal Conditions: A Systematic Review and Meta-Analysis." *Musculoskeletal Care 11*, 4, 203–217.

26  Sherman, K. J., Cherkin, D. C., Erro, J., Miglioretti, D. L. and Deyo, R. A. (2005) "Comparing yoga, exercise, and a self-care book for chronic low back pain: a randomized, controlled trial." *Annals of Internal Medicine 143*, 12, 849-856.

27  Williams, K., Abildso, C., Steinberg, L., Doyle, E., Epstein, B., Smith, D., ... and Cooper, L. (2009) "Evaluation of the effectiveness and efficacy of Iyengar yoga therapy on chronic low back pain." *Spine 34*, 19, 2066.

28  Haaz, S. and Bartlett, S. J. (2011) "Yoga for arthritis: A scoping review." *Rheumatic Diseases Clinics of North America 37*, 1, 33–46; Bartlett, S. J., Moonaz, S. H., Mill, C., Bernatsky, S. and Bingham, C. O. (2013) "Yoga in rheumatic diseases." *Current Rheumatology Reports 15*, 12, 387.

29  Cramer, H., Lauche, R., Langhorst, J. and Dobos, G. (2013) "Yoga for rheumatic diseases: a systematic review." *Rheumatology 52*, 11, 2025-2030.

30  Page, M. J., O'Connor, D., Pitt, V. and Massy-Westropp, N. (2012) "Exercise and mobilisation interventions for carpal tunnel syndrome." *Cochrane Database of Systematic Reviews 6*, CD009899.

31  Moonaz, S. H., Bingham, C. O., Wissow, L. and Bartlett, S. J. (2015) "Yoga in sedentary adults with arthritis: Effects of a randomized controlled pragmatic trial." *Journal of Rheumatology 42*, 7, 1194–1202.

32  Middleton, K. R., Ward, M. M., Moonaz, S. H. *et al.* (2018) "Feasibility and assessment of outcome measures for yoga as self-care for minorities with arthritis: A pilot study." *Pilot and Feasibility Studies.* doi

33  Middleton, K. R., Magaña López, M., Moonaz, S. H. *et al.* (2017) "A qualitative approach exploring the acceptability of yoga for minorities living with arthritis: 'Where are the people who look like me'?" *Complementary Therapies in Medicine 31*, 82–89.

34  Langhorst, J., Klose, P., Dobos, G. J., Bernardy, K. and Häuser, W. (2013) "Efficacy and safety of meditative movement therapies in fibromyalgia syndrome: A systematic review and meta-analysis of randomized controlled trials." *Rheumatology International 33*, 1, 193–207.

35  Kim, S.-D. (2015) "Effects of yoga exercises for headaches: A systematic review of randomized controlled trials." *Journal of Physical Therapy Science 27*, 7, 2377–2380.

36  John, P. J., Sharma, N., Sharma, C. M. and Kankane, A. (2007) "Effectiveness of yoga therapy in the treatment of migraine without aura: a randomized controlled trial." *Headache: The Journal of Head and Face Pain 47*, 5, 654-661.

37  Kiran, K. G., Chalana, H. and Singh, H. (2016) "Physiological effect of rajyoga meditation on chronic tension headache and associated co-morbidities." *Pakistan Journal of Physiology 12*, 2, 22–25.

38  Doulatabad, S. N., Nooreyan, K., Doulatabad, A. N. and Noubandegani, Z. M. (2012) "The effects of pranayama, Hatha and Raja yoga on physical pain and the quality of life of women with multiple sclerosis." *African Journal of Traditional, Complementary, and Alternative Medicines 10*, 1, 49–52.

39  Salgado, B. C., Jones, M., Ilgun, S., McCord, G., Loper-Powers, M. and van Houten, P. (2013) "Effects of a 4-month Ananda yoga program on physical and mental health outcomes for persons with multiple sclerosis." *International Journal of Yoga Therapy 23*, 27–38.

40  Glassford, J. A. G. (2017) "The neuroinflammatory etiopathology of myalgic encephalomyelitis/chronic fatigue syndrome (ME/CFS)." *Frontiers in Physiology* doi: 10.3389/fphys.2017.00088.

41  Oka, T., Tanahashi, T., Chijiwa, T., Lkhagvasuren, B., Sudo, N. and Oka, K. (2014) "Isometric yoga improves the fatigue and pain of patients with chronic fatigue syndrome who are resistant to conventional therapy: A randomized, controlled trial. *BioPsychoSocial Medicine 8*, 1, 27.

42  Schumann, D., Anheyer, D., Lauche, R., Dobos, G., Langhorst, J. and Cramer, H. (2016) "Effect of yoga in the therapy of irritable bowel syndrome: A systematic review." *Clinical Gastroenterology and Hepatology: The Official Clinical Practice Journal of the American Gastroenterological Association 14*, 12, 1720–1731.

43  Evans, S., Lung, K. C., Seidman, L. C., Sternlieb, B., Zeltzer, L. K. and Tsao, J. C. (2014) "Iyengar yoga for adolescents and young adults with irritable bowel syndrome." *Journal of Pediatric Gastroenterology and Nutrition 59*, 2, 244–253.

44  Shahabi, L., Naliboff, B. D. and Shapiro, D. (2016) "Self-regulation evaluation of therapeutic yoga and walking for patients with irritable bowel syndrome: A pilot study." *Psychology, Health and Medicine 21*, 2, 176–188.

45 Kavuri, V., Selvan, P., Malamud, A., Raghuram, N. and Selvan, S. R. (2015) "Remedial yoga module remarkably improves symptoms in irritable bowel syndrome patients: A 12-week randomized controlled trial." *European Journal of Integrative Medicine 7*, 6, 595–608.

46 Gonçalves, A. V., Makuch, M. Y., Setubal, M. S., Barros, N. F. and Bahamondes, L. (2016) "A qualitative study on the practice of yoga for women with pain-associated endometriosis." *Journal of Alternative and Complementary Medicine 22*, 12, 977–982.

47 Gonçalves, A. V., Barros, N. F. and Bahamondes, L. (2017) "The practice of Hatha yoga for the treatment of pain associated with endometriosis." *Journal of Alternative and Complementary Medicine 23*, 1, 45–52.

48 Bruckenthal, P., Marino, M. A. and Snelling, L. (2016) "Complementary and integrative therapies for persistent pain management in older adults: A review." *Journal of Gerontological Nursing 42*, 12, 40–48; Miller, S., Gaylord, S., Buben, A. *et al.* (2017) "Literature review of research on chronic pain and yoga in military populations. *Medicines* doi: 10.3390/medicines4030064.

49 Bruckenthal, Marino, and Snelling (2016).

50 Miller (2017).

51 Peregoy, J. A., Clarke, T. C., Jones, L. I., Stussman, B. J. and Nahin, R. L. (2014) "Regional variation in use of complementary health approaches by US adults." *NCHS Data Brief 146*, 1–8.

52 Schmid, A. A., Miller, K. K., Van Puymbroeck, M. and DeBaun-Sprague, E. (2014) "Yoga leads to multiple physical improvements after stroke, a pilot study." *Complementary Therapies in Medicine 22*, 6, 994–1000; Ferrari, M. L., Thuraisingam, S., von Känel, R. and Egloff, N. (2015) "Expectations and effects of a single yoga session on pain perception." *International Journal of Yoga 8*, 2, 154–157.

53 AARP (2011) *AARP and National Center for Complementary and Alternative Medicine Survey Report: What People Aged 50 and Older Discuss with Their Health Care Providers.* Accessed on 3/12/18 at https://nccih.nih.gov/research/statistics/2010.

54 Nahin, R. L. (2017) "Severe pain in veterans: The effect of age and sex, and comparisons with the general population." *Journal of Pain: Official Journal of the American Pain Society 18*, 3, 247–254.

55 Toblin, R. L., Quartana, P. J., Riviere, L. A., Walper, K. C. and Hoge, C. W. (2014) "Chronic pain and opioid use in US soldiers after combat deployment." *JAMA Internal Medicine 174*, 8, 1400–1401.

56 Department of the Army (2015) *Health Promotion, Risk Reduction, and Suicide Prevention.* Pamphlet 600-24. Washington, DC: Department of the Army.

57 Groessl, E. J., Weingart, K. R., Aschbacher, K., Pada, L. and Baxi, S. (2008) "Yoga for veterans with chronic low-back pain." *Journal of Alternative and Complementary Medicine 14*, 9, 1123–1129; Groll, D., Charbonneau, D., Bélanger, S. and Senyshyn, S. (2016) "Yoga and Canadian Armed Forces members' well-being: An analysis based on select physiological and psychological measures." *Journal of Military, Veteran and Family Health 2*, 2; King, K., Gosian, J., Doherty, K. *et al.* (2014) "Implementing yoga therapy adapted for older veterans who are cancer survivors." *International Journal of Yoga Therapy 24*, 87–96.

58 Groessl, E. J., Liu, L., Chang, D. G. *et al.* (2017) "Yoga for military veterans with chronic low back pain: A randomized clinical trial." *American Journal of Preventive Medicine 53*, 5, 599–608.

59 Nahin (2017).

60 Miller (2017).

61 Büssing, A., Ostermann, T., Lüdtke, R. and Michalsen, A. (2012) "Effects of yoga interventions on pain and pain-associated disability: A meta-analysis." *J Pain 13*, 1, 1–9.

## CHAPTER 3

1 Siegler, R., DeLoache, J. and Eisenberg., N. (2003) *How Children Develop.* New York, NY: Worth Publishers.

2 Combs, A. (2010) *Consciousness Explained Better.* St. Paul, MN: Paragon House; Wilber, K. (2001) *A Theory of Everything: An Integral Vision for Business, Politics, Science and Spirituality.* Boulder, CO: Shambhala Publishers.

3 Random House (2018) Dictionary.com. Accessed on 11/1/19 at www.dictionary.com.

4 Ganeri, J. (2013) "Well-ordered science and Indian epistemic cultures" *ISIS 104*, 2, 348–359.

5 Ganeri (2013).

6 Chen, J. (2011) "History of pain theories." *Neuroscience Bulletin 27*, 5, 343–350.

7 Feuerstein, G. (1998) *The Yoga Tradition.* Prescott, AZ: Hohm Press.

8 Feuerstein, G. (1998) *The Yoga Tradition.* Prescott, AZ: Hohm Press.

9 Feuerstein (1998), p.212.

10 Butler, D. and Moseley, L. (2003) *Explain Pain.* Adelaide: Noigroup Publications.

11 Chen (2011).

12 Moseley, L. and Butler, D. (2017) *Explain Pain Supercharged.* Adelaide: Noigroup Publications.

13 Chen (2011).

14 Chen (2011).

15 Chen (2011).

16 Physiopedia (n.d.) "Theories of Pain." Accessed on 4/12/18 at www.physio-pedia.com/Theories_of_Pain.

17 Engel, G. L. (1977) "The need for a new medical model: A challenge for biomedicine." *Science 196*, 4286, 129–136.

18 Rabey, M. (2017) "A misty, multidimensional crystal ball." Accessed on 4/12/18 at www.bodyinmind.org/low-back-pain-prognosis.

19  Kelly, J. (2018) "Editor's picks: Clinical prediction rules: Use the babies and throw the bathwater?" Accessed on 4/12/18 at https://bodyinmind.org/editors-picks-clinical-prediction-rules.

20  Van de Velde, D., Eijkelkamp, A., Peersman, W. and De Vriendt, P. (2016) "How competent are healthcare professionals in working according to a bio-psycho-social model in healthcare?" The current status and validation of a scale. *PLoS One 11*, 10, e0164018.

21  Malfliet, A., Kregel, J., Meeus, M. *et al.* (2017) "Applying contemporary neuroscience in exercise interventions for chronic spinal pain: Treatment protocol." *Brazilian Journal of Physical Therapy 21*, 5, 378–387.

22  Malfliet (2017).

23  Mezirow, J. (2000) *Learning as Transformation*. San Francisco, CA: Josey-Bass Inc.

24  Elgelid, S. (2015) "Systemic Limits on Creativity from Academia or Professional Association." In: M. Taylor (ed.) *Fostering Creativity in Rehabilitation*. New York, NY: Nova Publishers. 3–34.

25  Senge, P. M., Scharmer, C. O., Jaworksi, J. and Flowers, B. S. (2004) *Presence: Human Purpose and the Field of the Future*. New York, NY: Doubleday Books.

26  Moseley and Butler (2017).

27  Capra, F. and Luisi, P. L. (2016) *The Systems View of Life: A Unifying Vision*. Cambridge: Cambridge University Press.

28  Barron, F. (1990) *No Rootless Flower: Towards an Ecology of Creativity*. Cresskill, NJ: Hampton Press.

29  Taylor, M. J. (ed.) (2015) *Fostering Creativity in Rehabilitation*. 1st edition. New York, NY: Nova Publishing.

30  Senge *et al.* (2004).

31  Moseley and Butler (2017), p.119.

32  Siegler, DeLoache and Eisenberg (2003).

33  Feuerstein (1998).

34  Walsh, R. (2015) "What is wisdom? Cross-cultural and cross-disciplinary syntheses." *Review of General Psychology 19*, 278–293.

35  Kauffman, S. A. (2016) *Humanity in a Creative Universe*. New York, NY: Oxford University Press.

36  Feuerstein (1998), p.295.

37  Kauffman (2016).

38  Walsh (2015).

39  Engel (1977), p.135.

## Chapter 4

1   Mallinson, J. and Singleton, M. (2017) *Roots of Yoga*. New York, NY: Penguin Classics.

2   Mallinson and Singleton (2017).

3   Mallinson and Singleton (2017).

4   Mallinson and Singleton (2017).

5   Easwaran, E. (2007) *The Upanishads*. Tomales, CA: The Blue Mountain Center of Meditation, p.91.

6   Mallinson and Singleton (2017), p.17.

7   Sargeant, W. and Chapple, C. K. (eds) (1984) *The Bhagavad Gītā*. Revised edition. Albany, NY: State University of New York Press, p.133.

8   Mallinson and Singleton (2017); Sargeant and Chapple (1984), p.135.

9   Mallinson and Singleton (2017), p.17.

10  Sargeant and Chapple (1984), p.294.

11  Stoler-Miller, B. (2004) *The Bhagavad-Gita*. New York, NY: Bantam Classics, p.66.

12  Smith, J. D. (ed.) (2009) *Mahābhārata*. London: Penguin, p.654.

13  Stoler-Miller, B. (1998) *Yoga: Discipline of Freedom*. New York, NY: Bantam Books, p.29.

14  Burley, M. (2012) *Classical Samkhya and Yoga: An Indian Metaphysics of Experience*. London: Routledge.

15  Miller, R. (2012) *The Samkhya Karika*. San Rafael, CA: Integrative Restoration Institute.

16  Stoler-Miller (1998).

17  Embree, A. T., Hay, S. N. and De Bary, W. T. (eds) (1988) *Sources of Indian Tradition*. 2nd edition. New York, NY: Columbia University Press; Fitzgerald, J. L. (2004) "Dharma and its translation in the Mahābhārata." *Journal of Indian Philosophy 32*, 5–6, 671– 685; Doniger, W. (2010) *The Hindus: An Alternative History*. New York, NY: Penguin Books; Sullivan, M. and Robertson, L. (in press) *Understanding Yoga Therapy: Applied Philosophy and Science for Health and Well-Being*. Routledge, Taylor and Francis Group.

18  Sullivan and Robertson.

19  Sullivan and Robertson.

20  Sullivan and Robertson.

21  www.iayt.org

22  Taylor, M. J. (2007) "What is yoga therapy? An IAYT definition." *Yoga Therapy in Practice* doi: 10.1155/2013/945895.

23  Taylor, M. J. (2018) *Yoga Therapy as a Creative Response to Pain*. London: Singing Dragon.

24  Craig, A. D. (2002) "How do you feel? Interoception: the sense of the physiological condition of the body." *Nature Reviews Neuroscience 3*, 8, 655–666.

25  Kriyananda, G. (1976) *The Spiritual Science of Kriya Yoga*. Chicago, IL: Temple of Kriya Yoga.

26  Mallinson and Singleton (2017); Flood, G. (2005) *The Tantric Body: The Secret Tradition of Hindu Religion*. London: IB Tauris; Wallis, C. D. and Ellik, E. (2012) *Tantra Illuminated: The Philosophy, History, and Practice of a Timeless Tradition*. The Woodlands, TX: Anusara Press.

27  Wallis and Ellik (2012), p.26.

# CHAPTER 5

1 Porges, S. (2009) "The polyvagal theory: New insights into adaptive reactions of the autonomic nervous system." *Cleve Clin J Med 76*, S2, S86–S90.

2 International Association for the Study of Pain (2017) "Terminology." Accessed on 4/12/18 at www.iasp-pain.org/terminology?navItemNumber=576.

3 International Association for the Study of Pain (2017).

4 International Association for the Study of Pain (2017).

5 Legrain, V., Ianetti, G., Plaghki, L. and Mouraux, A. (2011) "The pain matrix reloaded: A salience detection system for the body." *Progress in Neurobiology 93*, 1, 111–124.

6 Brascher, A., Becker, S., Hoeppli, M. and Schweinhardt, P. (2016) "Different brain circuitries mediating controllable and uncontrollable pain." *Journal of Neuroscience 36*, 18, 5013–5025; Jensen, M. and Karoly, P. (1991) "Control beliefs, coping efforts, and adjustment to chronic pain." *Journal of Consulting and Clinical Psychology 59*, 431–438.

7 Nijs, J., Malfliet, A., Ickmans, K., Baert, I. and Meeus, M. (2014) "Treatment of central sensitization in patients with 'unexplained' chronic pain: An update." *Expert Opinion on Pharmacotherapy 15*, 12, 1671–1683.

8 Ji, R., Chamessian, A. and Zhang, Y. (2016) "Pain regulation by non-neuronal cells and inflammation." *Science 4*, 354, 6312, 572–577.

9 Edwards, R., Dworkin, R., Sulivan, M., Turk, D. and Wasan, A. (2016) "The role of psychosocial processes in the development and maintenance of chronic pain." *Journal of Pain 17*, S9, T70–92.

10 Edwards *et al.* (2016).

11 Hannibal, K. and Bishop, M. (2014) "Chronic stress, cortisol dysfunction, and pain: A psycho-neuroendocrine rationale for stress management in pain rehabilitation." *Phys Ther 94*, 12, 1816–1825.

12 Cormier, S., Lavigne, G. L., Choinière, M. and Rainville, P. (2016) "Expectations predict chronic pain treatment outcomes." *Pain 157*, 2, 329–338.

13 Perl, E. (1996) "Cutaneous polymodal receptors: Characteristics and plasticity." *Prog Brain Res 113*, 21–37; Liu, X. and Zhou, L. (2015) "Long-term potentiation at spinal C-fiber synapses: A target for pathological pain." *Curr Pharm Des 21*, 7, 895–905.

14 Perl (1996).

15 Liu and Zhou (2015).

16 Abraira, V., Kuehn, E., Chirila, A. *et al.* (2017) "The cellular and synaptic architecture of the mechanosensory dorsal horn." *Cell 168*, 1–2, 295–310.e19.

17 Jensen, T. and Finnerup, N. (2014) "Allodynia and hyperalgesia in neuropathic pain: Clinical manifestations and mechanisms." *Lancet Neurol 13*, 9, 924–935.

18 Todd, A. (2017) "Identifying functional populations among the interneurons in laminae I–III of the spinal dorsalhorn. *Mol Pain 13*, 1744806917693003.

19 Todd (2017).

20 van den Broeke, E., van Rijn, C. M., Biurrun Manresa, J., Andersen, O. K., Arendt-Nielsen, L. and Wilder-Smith, O. H. (2010) "Neurophysiological correlates of nociceptive heterosynaptic long-term potentiation in humans." *J Neurophysiol 103*, 4, 2107–2113.

21 Todd (2017).

22 van den Broeke *et al.* (2010).

23 Colloca, L. and Benedetti, F. (2007) "Nocebo hyperalgesia: How anxiety is turned into pain." *Curr Opin Anaesthesiol 20*, 5, 435–439.

24 Ossipov, M., Morimura, K. and Porreca, F. (2014) "Descending pain modulation and chronification of pain." *Curr Opin Support Palliat Care 8*, 2, 143–151.

25 Taylor, B. and Westlund, K. (2017) "The noradrenergic locus coeruleus as a chronic pain generator." *Journal of Neuroscience Research 95*, 6, 1336–1346.

26 Lau, B. and Vaughan, C. (2014) "Descending modulation of pain: The GABA disinhibition hypothesis of analgesia." *Curr Opin Neurobiol 29*, 159–164; Lu, C., Yang, T., Zhao, H. *et al.* (2016) "Insular cortex is critical for the perception, modulation, and chronification of pain." *Neuroscience Bulletin 32*, 2, 191–201.

27 Lynch, J. (2009) "Native glycine receptor subtypes and their physiological roles." *Neuropharmacology 56*, 303–309.

28 Bannister, K. and Dickenson, A. (2017) "The plasticity of descending controls in pain: Translational probing." *Journal of Physiology 595*, 13, 4159–4166.

29 Bannister and Dickenson (2017).

30 Bannister and Dickenson (2017).

31 Ji, R. R., Berta, T. and Nedergaard, M. (2013) "Glia and pain: Is chronic pain a gliopathy?" *Pain 154*, S1, S10–28.

32 Ji, Berta and Nedergaard (2013).

33 Liu, X., Pang, R., Zhou, L., Wei, X. H. and Zang, Y. (2016) "Neuropathic pain: Sensory nerve injury or motor nerve injury?" *Adv Exp Med Biol 904*, 59–75.

34 Leung, A., Gregory, N. S., Allen, L. A. and Sluka, K. A. (2016) "Regular physical activity prevents chronic pain by altering resident muscle macrophage phenotype and increasing interleukin-10 in mice." *Pain 157*, 1, 70–79; James, G., Sluka, K. A., Blomster, L. *et al.* (2018) "Macrophage polarization contributes to local inflammation and structural change in the multifidus muscle after intervertebral disc injury." *European Spine Journal 27*, 8, 1744–1756.

35 Boadas-Vaello, P., Homs, J., Reina, F., Carrera, A. and Verdú, E. (2017) "Neuroplasticity of supraspinal structures associated with pathological pain." *Anatomical Record (Hoboken) 300*, 8, 1481–1501.

36 Koganemaru, S., Mikami, Y., Maezawa, H., Ikeda, S., Ikoma, K. and Mima, T. (2018) "Neurofeedback control of the human GABAergic system using non-invasive brain stimulation." *Neuroscience 1*, 380, 38–48.

37  Pagano, R., Fonoff, E., Dale, C., Ballester, G., Teixeira, M. J. and Britto, L. R. (2012) "Motor cortex stimulation inhibits thalamic sensory neurons and enhances activity of PAG neurons: Possible pathways for antinociception." *Pain 153*, 12, 2359–2369.

38  Lu, Yang and Zhao (2016).

39  Lu, Yang and Zhao (2016).

40  Lu, Yang and Zhao (2016).

41  Lazar, S., Kerr, C., Wasserman, R. *et al.* (2005) "Meditation experience is associated with increased cortical thickness." *Neuroreport 16*, 17, 1893–1897; Tsay, A., Allen, T., Proske, M. and Giummarra, M. (2015) "Sensing the body in chronic pain: A review of psychophysical studies implicating altered body representation." *Neuroscience and Biobehavioral Reviews 52*, 221–232.

42  Martenson, M. E., Cetas, J. S. and Heinricher, M. M. (2009) "A possible neural basis for stress-induced hyperalgesia." *Pain 142*, 3, 236–244.

43  Ossipov, Morimura and Porreca (2014).

44  Ossipov, Morimura and Porreca (2014).

45  Coombes, S. A. and Misra, G. (2016) "Pain and motor processing in the human cerebellum." *Pain 157*, 1, 117–127.

46  van der Meulen, M., Kamping, S. and Anton, F. (2017) "The role of cognitive reappraisal in placebo analgesia: An fMRI study." *Social Cognitive and Affective Neuroscience 12*, 7, 1128–1137; Seminowicz, D. A. and Moayedi, M. (2017) "The dorsolateral prefrontal cortex in acute and chronic pain." *Journal of Pain 18*, 9, 1027–1035.

47  Seminowicz and Moayedi (2017); Wiech, K., Kalisch, R., Weiskopf, N., Pleger, B., Stephan, K. E. and Dolan, R. J. (2006) "Anterolateral prefrontal cortex mediates the analgesic effect of expected and perceived control over pain." *Journal of Neuroscience 26*, 44, 11501–11509.

48  Seminowicz, D. A., Wideman, T., Naso, L. *et al.* (2011) "Effective treatment of chronic low back pain in humans reverses abnormal brain anatomy

and function." *Journal of Neuroscience 31*, 20, 7540–7550.

49  Alshuft, H. M., Condon, L. A., Dineen, R. A. and Auer, D. P. (2016) "Cerebral cortical thickness in chronic pain due to knee osteoarthritis: The effect of pain duration and pain sensitization." *PLoS One 11*, 9, e0161687; Coppieters, I., De Pauw, R., Caeyenberghs, K. *et al.* (2018) "Differences in white matter structure and cortical thickness between patients with traumatic and idiopathic chronic neck pain: Associations with cognition and pain modulation?" *Human Brain Mapping 39*, 4, 1721–1742.

50  Seminowicz *et al.* (2011).

51  Legrain *et al.* (2011).

52  Maurer, A., Lissounov, A., Knezevic, I., Candido, K. D. and Knezevic, N. N. (2016) "Pain and sex hormones: A review of current understanding." *Pain Management 6*, 3, 285–296.

53  Maurer, Lissounov, Knezevic, Candido and Knezevic (2016).

54  Dum, R. P., Levinthal, D. and Strick, P. (2016) "Motor, cognitive, and affective areas of the cerebral cortex influence the adrenal medulla." *PNAS 113*, 35, 9922–9927.

55  Porges, S. W. (2009) "The polyvagal theory: New insights into adaptive reactions of the autonomic nervous system." *Cleve Clin J Med 76*, S2, S86–90.

56  Strigo, I. A. and Craig, A. D. (2016) "Interoception, homeostatic emotions and sympathovagal balance." *Philos Trans R Soc Lond B Biol Sci.* doi: 10.1098/rstb.2016.0010.

57  Melzack, R. and Katz, J. (2013) "Neuromatrix model." *Wiley Interdisciplinary Reviews: Cognitive Science 4*, 1, 1–15.

58  Katz, J. and Rosenbloom, B. N. (2015) "The golden anniversary of Melzack and Wall's gate control theory of pain: Celebrating 50 years of pain research and management." *Pain Research and Management 20*, 6, 285–286.

## Chapter 6

1  Paton, J. F. R., Boscan, P., Pickering, A. E. and Nalivaiko, E. (2005) "The yin and yang of cardiac autonomic control: Vago-sympathetic interactions revisited." *Brain Research Reviews 49*, 3, 555–565.

2  Levy, M. N. (1971) "Brief reviews: Sympathetic-parasympathetic interactions in the heart. *Circulation Research 29*, 5, 437–445; Levy, M. N. and Martin, P. J. (1981) "Neural regulation of the heart beat." *Annual Review Physiology 43*, 1, 443–453.

3  Paton *et al.* (2005).

4  Tracy, L. M., Ioannou, L., Baker, K.S., Gibson, S. J., Georgiou-Karistianis, N. and Giummarra, M. J. (2016) "Meta-analytic evidence for decreased heart rate variability in chronic pain implicating parasympathetic nervous system dysregulation." *Pain 157*, 1, 7–29.

5  Gard, T., Noggle, J. J., Park, C. L., Vago, D. R. and Wilson, A. (2014) "Potential self-regulatory

mechanisms of yoga for psychological health." *Front Hum Neurosci* doi: 103389/fnhum.2014.0070.

6  Gard *et al.* (2014); Taylor, A. G., Goehler, L. E., Galper, D. I., Innes, K. E. and Bourguignon, C. (2010) "Top-down and bottom-up mechanisms in mind-body medicine: Development of an integrative framework for psychophysiological research." *EXPLORE. The Journal of Science and Healing 6*, 1, 29–41.

7  Gard *et al.* (2014).

8  Taylor *et al.* (2010); Muehsam, D., Lutgendorf, S., Mills, P. J. *et al.* (2017) "The embodied mind: A review on functional genomic and neurological correlates of mind-body therapies." *Neurosci Biobehav Rev 73*, 165–181; Schmalzl, L., Powers, C. and Henje Blom, E. (2015) "Neurophysiological and neurocognitive mechanisms underlying the effects of yoga-based practices: Towards a comprehensive

theoretical framework." *Front Hum Neurosci* doi: 10.3389/fnhum.2015.00235; Streeter, C. C., Gerbarg, P. L., Saper, R. B., Ciraulo, D. A. and Brown, R. P. (2012) "Effects of yoga on the autonomic nervous system, gamma-aminobutyric-acid, and allostasis in epilepsy, depression, and post-traumatic stress disorder." *Medical Hypotheses 78*, 5, 571–579.

9   Ernst, G. (2017) "Hidden signals: The history and methods of heart rate variability." *Frontiers in Public Health 5*.

10  Haase, L., Stewart, J. L., Youssef, B. *et al.* (2016) "When the brain does not adequately feel the body: Links between low resilience and interoception." *Biological Psychology 113*, 37–45; Resnick, B., Galik, E., Dorsey, S., Scheve, A. and Gutkin, S. (2011) "Reliability and validity testing of the physical resilience measure." *The Gerontologist 51*, 5, 643–652; Tugade, M. M. and Fredrickson, B. L. (2004) "Resilient individuals use positive emotions to bounce back from negative emotional experiences." *J Pers Soc Psychol 86*, 2, 320–333; Whitson, H. E., Duan-Porter, W., Schmader, K. E., Morey, M. C., Cohen, H. J. and Colón-Emeric, C. S. (2016) "Physical resilience in older adults: Systematic review and development of an emerging construct." *J Gerontol A Biol Sci Med Sci 71*, 4, 489–495.

11  Resnick *et al.* (2011); Tugade and Fredrickson (2004); Whitson *et al.* (2016).

12  Dale, L. P., Carroll, L. E., Galen, G., Hayes, J. A., Webb, K. W. and Porges, S. W. (2009) "Abuse history is related to autonomic regulation to mild exercise and psychological wellbeing." *Appl Psychophysiol Biofeedback 34*, 4, 299–308.

13  Resnick *et al.* (2011).

14  Tracy *et al.* (2016); Streeter *et al.* (2012); Koenig, J., Falvay, D., Clamor, A. *et al.* (2016) "Pneumogastric (vagus) nerve activity indexed by heart rate variability in chronic pain patients compared to healthy controls: A systematic review and meta-analysis." *Pain Physician 19*, 1, E55–78; Kolacz, J. and Porges, S. W. (2018) "Chronic diffuse pain and functional gastrointestinal disorders after traumatic stress: Pathophysiology through a polyvagal perspective. *Front Med* doi: 10.3389/fmed.2018.00145.

15  Kolacz and Porges (2018); Caceres, C. and Burns, J. W. (1997) "Cardiovascular reactivity to psychological stress may enhance subsequent pain sensitivity." *Pain 69*, 3, 237–244; Maletic, V. and Raison, C. L. (2009) "Neurobiology of depression, fibromyalgia and neuropathic pain." *Frontiers in Bioscience Landmark Edition 14*, 5291–5338; Yunus, M. B. (2007) "Role of central sensitization in symptoms beyond muscle pain, and the evaluation of a patient with widespread pain." *Best Practice and Research: Clinical Rheumatology 21*, 3, 481–497.

16  Barakat, A., Vogelzangs, N., Licht, C. M. M. *et al.* (2012) "Dysregulation of the autonomic nervous system is associated with pain intensity, not with the presence of chronic widespread pain." *Arthritis Care and Research 64*, 8, 1209–1216.

17  Staud R. (2008) "Heart rate variability as a biomarker of fibromyalgia syndrome." *Future Rheumatology 3*, 5, 475–483.

18  Kang, J. H., Kim, J. K., Hong, S. H., Lee, C. H. and Choi, B. Y. (2016) "Heart rate variability for quantification of autonomic dysfunction in fibromyalgia." *Annals of Rehabilitation Medicine 40*, 2, 301–309.

19  Tracy *et al.* (2016).

20  Benarroch, E. E. (2006) "Pain-autonomic interactions." *Neurological Sciences 27*, S2, S130–S133.

21  Benarroch (2006).

22  Porges, S. W. (2004) "Neuroception: A subconscious system for detecting threats and safety." *Zero Three 24*, 5, 19–24; Porges, S. W. (2011) *The Polyvagal Theory: Neurophysiological Foundations of Emotions, Attachment, Communication, and Self-Regulation*. 1st edition. New York, NY: W. W. Norton.

23  Koenig *et al.* (2016); Barakat *et al.* (2012); Frangos, E., Richards, E. A. and Bushnell, M. C. (2017) "Do the psychological effects of vagus nerve stimulation partially mediate vagal pain modulation?" *Neurobiology of Pain 1*, 37–45; Randich, A. and Gebhart, G. F. (1992) "Vagal afferent modulation of nociception." *Brain Research Reviews 17*, 2, 77–99.

24  Frangos, Richards and Bushnell (2017).

25  Bonaz, B., Sinniger, V. and Pellissier, S. (2016) "Anti-inflammatory properties of the vagus nerve: Potential therapeutic implications of vagus nerve stimulation: Anti-inflammatory effect of vagus nerve stimulation." *Journal of Physiology 594*, 20, 5781–5790; Yuan, H. and Silberstein, S. D. (2016) "Vagus nerve and vagus nerve stimulation, a comprehensive review: Part I: Headache." *Headache 56*, 1, 71–78.

26  Frangos, Richards and Bushnell (2017); Bushnell, M. C., Čeko, M. and Low, L. A. (2013) "Cognitive and emotional control of pain and its disruption in chronic pain." *Nat Rev Neurosci 14*, 7, 502–511.

27  Frangos, Richards and Bushnell (2017).

28  Streeter *et al.* (2012); Porges (2011); Park, G. and Thayer, J. F. (2014) "From the heart to the mind: Cardiac vagal tone modulates top-down and bottom-up visual perception and attention to emotional stimuli." *Front Psychol 5*, 278; Thayer, J. F. and Lane, R. D. (2000) "A model of neurovisceral integration in emotion regulation and dysregulation." *Journal of Affective Disorders 61*, 3, 201–216.

29  Tracy *et al* (2016); Muehsam *et al.* (2017); Koenig *et al.* (2016); Azam (2016); Meeus (2013); Staud R. (2008); Kang *et al.* (2016); Park and Thayer (2014); Thayer and Lane (2000); Adlan, A. M., Veldhuijzen van Zanten, J. J. C. S., Lip, G. Y. H., Paton, J. F. R., Kitas, G. D. and Fisher, J. P. (2017) "Cardiovascular autonomic regulation, inflammation and pain in rheumatoid arthritis." *Autonomic Neuroscience 208*, 137–145; Sowder, E., Gevirtz, R., Shapiro, W. and Ebert, C. (2010) "Restoration of vagal tone: A possible mechanism for functional abdominal pain." *Appl Psychophysiol Biofeedback 35*, 3, 199–206;

Tsuji, H., Venditti, F. J., Manders, E. S. *et al.* (1994) "Reduced heart rate variability and mortality risk in an elderly cohort: The Framingham Heart Study. *Circulation 90*, 2, 878–883.

30 Porges (2004); Porges (2011); Porges, S. W., Doussard-Roosevelt, J. A. and Maiti, A. K. (2008) "Vagal tone and the physiological regulation of emotion." *Monographs of the Society for Research in Child Development 59*, 2–3, 167–186; Porges, S. W. (2017) *The Oxford Handbook of Compassion Science* (Seppala E., ed.). New York, NY: Oxford University Press.

31 Ceunen, E., Vlaeyen, J. W. S. and Van Diest, I. (2016) "On the origin of interoception." *Front Psychol 7*, 743.

32 Haase *et al.* (2016); Porges (2011); Ceunen, Vlaeyen and Van Diest (2016); Craig, A. D. (2015) *How Do You Feel?: An Interoceptive Moment with Your Neurobiological Self.* Princeton, NJ: Princeton University Press; Farb, N., Daubenmier, J., Price, C. J. *et al.* (2015) "Interoception, contemplative practice, and health." *Front Psychol 6*, 763; Strigo, I. A. and Craig, A. D. (2016) "Interoception, homeostatic emotions and sympathovagal balance." *Philos Trans R Soc B Biol Sci 371*, 1708, 20160010.

33 Haase *et al.* (2016); Farb *et al.* (2015).

34 Muehsam *et al.* (2017); Porges (2004); Porges (2011).

35 Porges, S. W. (2003) "The polyvagal theory: Phylogenetic contributions to social behavior." *Physiol Behav 79*, 3, 503–513.

36 Porges (2011).

37 Taylor *et al.* (2010); Porges (2011); Porges (2003); Porges, S. W. (2009) "The polyvagal theory: New insights into adaptive reactions of the autonomic nervous system." *Cleve Clin J Med 76*, S2, S86–S90.

38 Porges (2003).

39 Porges (2011); Porges, S. W. (1998) "Love: An emergent property of the mammalian autonomic nervous system." *Psychoneuroendocrinology 23*, 8, 837–861.

40 Porges (2011); Porges (2017); Porges, S. W. and Carter, C. S. (2017) *Complementary and Integrative Treatments in Psychiatric Practice.* 1st edition. (Gerbarg, P. L., Muskin, P. R., Brown, R. P., American Psychiatric Association, eds.). Arlington, VA: American Psychiatric Association Publishing.

41 Porges (1998); Porges, S. W. (2007) "The polyvagal perspective." *Biological Psychology 74*, 2, 116–143.

42 Porges (2011); Porges (2017); Porges (2003); Porges (1998); Porges and Carter (2017).

43 Porges (2011); Porges, Doussard-Roosevelt and Maiti (2008); Porges (2003); Porges (2009); Porges (1998); Porges and Carter (2017).

44 Sowder *et al.* (2010); Kolacz, J. and Porges, S. W. (2018) "Pathophysiology of post traumatic chronic pain and functional gastrointestinal disorders: A polyvagal perspective." *Front Med 5*, 145.

45 Taylor *et al.* (2010); Streeter *et al.* (2012); Chu, I.-H., Wu, W.-L., Lin, I.-M., Chang, Y.-K., Lin, Y.-J. and Yang, P.-C. (2017) "Effects of yoga on heart rate variability and depressive symptoms in women: A randomized controlled trial." *J Altern Complement Med 23*, 4, 310–316; Khattab, K., Khattab, A. A., Ortak, J., Richardt, G. and Bonnemeier, H. (2007) "Iyengar yoga increases cardiac parasympathetic nervous modulation among healthy yoga practitioners." *Evidence-Based Complementary and Alternative Medicine 4*, 4, 511–517; Sarang, P. and Telles, S. (2006) "Effects of two yoga based relaxation techniques on heart rate variability (HRV)." *International Journal of Stress Management 13*, 4, 460–475; Telles, S., Sharma, S. K., Gupta, R. K., Bhardwaj, A. K. and Balkrishna, A. (2016) "Heart rate variability in chronic low back pain patients randomized to yoga or standard care." *BMC Complementary Alternative Medicine* doi: 10.1186/s12906-016-127-1; Tyagi, A. and Cohen, M. (2016) "Yoga and heart rate variability: A comprehensive review of the literature." *International Journal of Yoga 9*, 2, 97–113.

46 Cramer, H., Lauche, R., Haller, H., Langhorst, J., Dobos, G. and Berger, B. (2013) "'I'm more in balance': A qualitative study of yoga for patients with chronic neck pain." *J Altern Complement Med 19*, 6, 536–542; Fiori, F., Aglioti, S. M. and David, N. (2017) "Interactions between body and social awareness in yoga." *J Altern Complement Med 23*, 3, 227–233; Mehling, W. E., Wrubel, J., Daubenmier, J. J. *et al.* (2011) "Body awareness: A phenomenological inquiry into the common ground of mind-body therapies." *Philosophy, Ethics, and Humanities in Medicine* doi: 10.1186/1747-5341-6-6; Thomas, R., Quinlan, E., Kowalski, K., Spriggs, P. and Hamoline, R. (2014) "Beyond the body insights from an Iyengar yoga program for women with disability after breast cancer." *Holistic Nursing Practice 28*, 6, 353–361.

47 Dale, L. P., Carroll, L. E., Galen, G. C. *et al.* (2011) "Yoga practice may buffer the deleterious effects of abuse on women's self-concept and dysfunctional coping." *Journal of Aggression, Maltreatment and Trauma 20*, 1, 90–102.

48 Mackenzie, M. J., Carlson, L. E., Paskevich, D. M. *et al.* (2014) "Associations between attention, affect and cardiac activity in a single yoga session for female cancer survivors: An enactive neurophenomenology-based approach." *Conscious Cognition 27*, 129–146.

49 Fiori, Aglioti and David (2017); Ivtzan, I. and Papantoniou, A. (2014) "Yoga meets positive psychology: Examining the integration of hedonic (gratitude) and eudaimonic (meaning) wellbeing in relation to the extent of yoga practice." *J Bodyw Mov Ther 18*, 2, 183–189; Ross, A., Bevans, M., Friedmann, E., Williams, L. and Thomas, S. (2014) "'I am a nice person when I do yoga!!!': A qualitative analysis of how yoga affects relationships." *J Holist Nurs 32*, 2, 67–77.

50 Gard *et al.* (2014); Schmalzl, Powers and Henje Blom (2015); Streeter *et al.* (2012); Ross, A. and Thomas, S. (2010) "The health benefits of yoga and

exercise: A review of comparison studies." *J Altern Complement Med 16*, 1, 3–12.

51 Stoler-Miller, B. (2004) *The Bhagavad-Gita*. New York, NY: Bantam Classics.

52 Stoler-Miller (2004).

53 Kolacz and Porges (2018).

54 Sullivan, M. B., Erb, M., Schmalzl, L., Moonaz, S., Noggle Taylor, J. and Porges, S. W. (2018) "Yoga therapy and polyvagal theory: The convergence of traditional wisdom and contemporary neuroscience for self-regulation and resilience." *Front Hum Neurosci 12*, 67.

55 Gard *et al.* (2014); Schmalzl, Powers and Henje Blom (2015).

56 Goetz, J. L., Keltner, D. and Simon-Thomas, E. (2010) "Compassion: An evolutionary analysis and empirical review." *Psychological Bulletin 136*, 3, 351–374; Hofmann, S. G., Andreoli, G., Carpenter, J. K. and Curtiss, J. (2016) "Effect of Hatha yoga on anxiety: A meta-analysis: Yoga for anxiety." *Journal of Evidence-Based Medicine 9*, 3, 116–124; Neff, K. D. and McGehee, P. (2010) "Self-compassion and

psychological resilience among adolescents and young adults." *Self Identity 9*, 3, 225–240; Stellar, J. E., Cohen, A., Oveis, C. and Keltner, D. (2015) "Affective and physiological responses to the suffering of others: Compassion and vagal activity." *J Pers Soc Psychol 108*, 4, 572–585; Taylor, Z. E., Eisenberg, N. and Spinrad, T. L. (2015) "Respiratory sinus arrhythmia, effortful control, and parenting as predictors of children's sympathy across early childhood." *Developmental Psychology 51*, 1, 17–25.

57 Porges (2011); Raghuraj, P. and Telles, S. (2008) "Immediate effect of specific nostril manipulating yoga breathing practices on autonomic and respiratory variables." *Appl Psychophysiol Biofeedback 33*, 2, 65–75; Telles, S., Singh, N. and Balkrishna, A. (2011) "Heart rate variability changes during high frequency yoga breathing and breath awareness." *BioPsychoSocial Medicine* doi: 10.1186/1751-0759-5-4; Hayano, J. and Yasuma, F. (2003) "Hypothesis: Respiratory sinus arrhythmia is an intrinsic resting function of cardiopulmonary system." *Cardiovascular Research 58*, 1, 1–9.

## CHAPTER 7

1 Lin, I. B., O'Sullivan, P. B., Coffin, J. A. *et al.* (2013) "Disabling chronic low back pain as an iatrogenic disorder: A qualitative study in Aboriginal Australians." *BMJ Open 3*, e002654.

2 Van Oosterwijck, J., Nijs, J., Meeus, M. *et al.* (2011) "Pain neurophysiology education improves cognitions, pain thresholds, and movement performance in people with chronic whiplash: A pilot study." *Journal of Rehabilitation Research and Development 48*, 1, 43–58; Lee, H., McAuley, J. H., Hübscher, M., Kamper, S. J., Traeger, A. C. and Moseley, G. L. (2016) "Does changing pain-related knowledge reduce pain and improve function through changes in catastrophizing?" *Pain 157*, 4, 922–930; Moseley, G. L. (2003) "Unravelling the barriers to reconceptualisation of the problem in chronic pain: The actual and perceived ability of patients and health professionals to understand the neurophysiology." *Journal of Pain 4*, 184–189; Moseley, G. L. (2002a) "Combined physiotherapy and education is effective for chronic low back pain. A randomised controlled trial." *Aus J Physiother 48*, 4, 297–302; Ryan, C. G., Gray, H. G., Newton, M. and Granat, M. H. (2010) "Pain biology education and exercise classes compared to pain biology education alone for individuals with chronic low back pain: A pilot randomised controlled trial." *Manual Therapy 15*, 4, 382–387.

3 Moseley (2002a); Ryan *et al.* (2010); Moseley, G. L. (2002b) "Combined physiotherapy and education is effective for chronic low back pain. A randomised controlled trial." *Aus J Physiother 48*, 4, 297–302.

4 Swami Satyananda Saraswati (1981) *A Systematic Course in the Ancient Tantric Techniques of Yoga and Kriya*. New Delhi: Yoga Publications Trust, Bihar School of Yoga, Thompson Press; Goswami

Kriyananda (1976) *The Spiritual Science of Kriya Yoga*. Chicago: The Temple of Kriya Yoga.

5 Swami Satyananda Saraswati (1981).

6 Swami Satyananda Saraswati (1981).

7 Goswami Kriyananda (1976).

8 Swami Satyananda Saraswati (1981).

9 Swami Satyananda Saraswati (1981); Goswami Kriyananda (1976).

10 Butler, D. S. and Moseley, G. L. (2003) *Explain Pain*. Adelaide: Noigroup Publications; Moseley, G. L. and Butler, D. S. (2015) Fifteen years of explaining pain: The past, present, and future. *Journal of Pain 16*, 9, 807–813.

11 Menezes, C., Maher, C., McAuley, J. *et al.* (2011) "Self-efficacy is more important than fear of movement in mediating the relationship between pain and disability in chronic low back pain." *European Journal of Pain 15*, 213–219.

12 Solberg Nes, L., Roach, A. and Segerstrom, S. (2009) "Executive functions, self-regulation, and chronic pain: A review. *Ann Behav Med 37*, 173–183.

13 Solberg Nes, Roach and Segerstrom (2009).

14 Lame, I. E., Peters, M. L., Vlaeyan, J. W., Kleef, M. V. and Patjin, J. (2005) "Quality of life in chronic pain is more associated with beliefs about pain, than with pain intensity." *European Journal of Pain 9*, 1, 15–24.

15 Tsay, A., Allen, T., Proske, M. and Giummarra, M. (2015) "Sensing the body in chronic pain: A review of psychophysical studies implicating altered body representation." *Neuroscience and Biobehavioral Reviews 52*, 221–232.

16 Lame *et al.* (2005).

17 Moseley, G. L. (2007a) "Reconceptualising pain according to modern pain science." *Physical Therapy Reviews 12*, 169–178.

18 Moseley (2007a).

19 Moseley (2002a).

20 Moseley (2003).

21 Van Oosterwijck (2011); Meeus, M., Nijs, J., Van Oosterwijck, J., Van Alsenoy, V. and Truijen, S. (2010) "Pain physiology education improves pain beliefs in patients with chronic fatigue syndrome compared with pacing and self-management education: A double-blind randomized controlled trial." *Archives of Physical Medicine and Rehabilitation 91*, 8, 1153–1159; Van Oosterwijck, J., Meeus, M., Paul, L., De Schryver, M. *et al.* (2013) "Pain physiology education improves health status and endogenous pain inhibition in fibromyalgia: A double-blind randomized controlled trial." *Clinical Journal of Pain 29*, 10, 873–882.

22 Wood, L. and Hendrick, P. A. (2018) "A systematic review and meta-analysis of pain neuroscience education for chronic low back pain: Short- and long-term outcomes of pain and disability." *European Journal of Pain 23*, 2, 234–249; Tegner, H., Frederiksen, P., Esbensen, B. A. and Juhl, C. (2018) "Neurophysiological pain education for patients with chronic low back pain: A systematic review and meta-analysis." *Clinical Journal of Pain 34*, 8, 778–786.

23 Louw, A., Zimney, K., Puentedura, E. J. and Diener, I. (2016) "The efficacy of pain neuroscience education on musculoskeletal pain: A systematic review of the literature." *Physiotherapy Theory and Practice 32*, 5, 332–355.

24 Butler and Moseley (2003); Moseley (2007a).

25 Curry, L. (1987) *Integrating Concepts of Cognitive Learning Style: A Review with Attention to Psychometric Standards*. Ontario: Canadian College of Health Service Executives.

26 Moseley, G. L. (2007b) *Painful Yarns: Metaphors and Stories to Help Understand the Biology of Pain*. Canberra: Dancing Giraffe Press.

27 Leung, A., Gregory, N. S., Allen, L. A. and Sluka, K. A. (2016) "Regular physical activity prevents chronic pain by altering resident muscle macrophage phenotype and increasing interleukin-10 in mice." *Pain 157*, 1, 70–79.

28 Youngstedt, S. D. (2005) "Effects of exercise on sleep." *Clinics in Sports Medicine 24*, 2, 355–365.

29 Bherer, L., Erickson, K. and Liu-Ambrose, T. Y. (2013) "A review of the effects of physical activity and exercise on cognitive and brain functions in older adults." *Journal of Aging Research 2013*, 657508.

30 Dum, R. P., Levinthal, D. and Strick, P. (2016) "Motor, cognitive, and affective areas of the cerebral cortex influence the adrenal medulla." *PNAS 113*, 35, 9922–9927.

31 Leung *et al.* (2016).

32 Dobson, J. L., McMillan, J. and Li, L. (2014) "Benefits of exercise intervention in reducing neuropathic pain." *Frontiers in Cellular Neuroscience 8*, 102.

33 Mehling, W., Wrubel, J., Daubenmier, J. *et al.* (2011) "Body awareness: A phenomenological inquiry into the common ground of mind-body therapies." *Philosophy, Ethics, and Humanities in Medicine 6*, 6.

34 Streeter, C., Whitfield, T., Owen, L. *et al.* (2010) "Effects of yoga versus walking on mood, anxiety, and brain GABA levels: A randomized controlled MRS study." *Journal of Alternative and Complementary Medicine 16*, 11, 1145–1152.

35 Uebelacker, L., Epstein-Lubow, G., Brandon, G. (2010) "Hatha yoga for depression: Critical review of the evidence for efficacy, plausible mechanisms of action, and directions for future research." *Journal of Psychiatric Practice 16*, 1, 22–33.

36 Nijs, J., Kosek, E., Van Oosterwicjk, J. and Meeus, M. (2012) "Dysfunctional endogenous analgesia during exercise in patients with chronic pain: To exercise or not to exercise?" *Pain Physician 15*, ES205–ES213.

37 Nijs *et al.* (2012).

38 Leung *et al.* (2016).

39 Clark, A. and Mach, N. (2016) "Exercise-induced stress behavior, gut-microbiota-brain axis and diet: A systematic review for athletes." *Journal of the International Society of Sports Nutrition 13*, 43.

40 McLean, S., Clauw, D., Abelson, J. and Liberzon, I. (2005) "The development of persistent pain and psychological morbidity after motor vehicle collision: Integrating the potential role of stress response systems into a biopsychosocial model." *Psychosomatic Medicine 67*, 5, 783–790.

41 Butler, D. and Moseley, L. (2017) *Explain Pain Supercharged*. Adelaide: Noigroup Publications.

42 Porges, S. (2009) "The polyvagal theory: New insights into adaptive reactions of the autonomic nervous system." *Cleve Clin J Med 76*, S2, S86–S90.

## Chapter 8

1 Borg-Olivier, S. and Machliss, B. (2011) *Applied Anatomy and Physiology of Yoga*. Waverley, NSW: YogaSynergy Pty Ltd., p.240.

2 Clifton-Smith, T. and Rowley, J. (2011) "Breathing pattern disorders and physiotherapy: Inspiration for our profession." *Physical Therapy Reviews 16*, 1, 75–86.

3 Clifton-Smith and Rowley (2011); Bordoni, B. and Zanier, E. (2013) "Anatomic connections of the diaphragm: Influence of respiration on the body system." *Journal of Multidisciplinary Healthcare 6*, 281–291.

4 Clifton-Smith and Rowley (2011); van Dixhoorn, J. (1997) "Hyperventilation and dysfunctional breathing." *Biological Psychology 46*, 90–91; Key, J. (2013) "'The core': Understanding it, and retraining its dysfunction." *Journal of Bodywork and Movement Therapies 17*, 541–559; Bordoni and Zanier (2013).

5 Craig, A. D. (2002) "How do you feel? Interoception: The sense of the physiological condition of the body." *Nat Rev Neurosci 3*, 8, 655–666; Paulus, M.

P. (2013) "The breathing conundrum: Interoceptive sensitivity and anxiety. *Depression and Anxiety 30*, 4, 315–320.

6   Strigo, I. R. and Craig, A. D. (2016) "Interoception, homeostatic emotions and sympathovagal balance." *Philosophical Transactions of the Royal Society B: Biological Sciences* doi: 10.1098/rstb.2016.0010; Philippot, P., Chapelle, G. and Blairy, S. (2010) "Respiratory feedback in the generation of emotion." *Cognition and Emotion 5*, 605–627; Brown, R. P. and Gerberg, P. L. (2005) "Sudarshan Kriya yogic breathing in the treatment of stress, anxiety and depression: Part I—Neurophysioloigc model." *Journal of Alternative and Complementary Medicine 11*, 1, 189–201; Rainville, P., Bechara, A., Naqvi, N. and Damasio, A. R. (2006) "Basic emotions are associated with distinct patterns of cardiorespiratory activity." *International Journal of Psychophysiology 61*, 5–18; Boiten, F. A., Frijda, N. H. and Wientjes, C. J. (1994) "Emotions and respiratory patterns: Review and critical analysis." *Int J Psychophysiol 17*, 103–128.

7   Telles, S., Singh, N. and Puthige, R. (2013) "Changes in P300 following alternate nostril yoga breathing and breath awareness." *Biopsychosocial Medicine 7*, 1, 11; Sharma, V. K., Manivel, R., Subramaniyam, V. *et al.* (2014) "Effect of fast and slow pranayama practice on cognitive functions in healthy volunteers." *Journal of Clinical and Diagnostic Research 8*, 1, 10–13; Schmalzl, L., Powers, C., Zanesco, A. P., Yetzb, N., Groessl, E. J. and Saron, C. D. (2018) "The effect of movement-focused and breath-focused yoga practice on stress parameters and sustained attention: A randomized controlled pilot study." *Consciousness and Cognition 65*, 109–125.

8   Strigo and Craig (2016); Sovik, R. (2000) "The science of breathing—The yogic view." *Prog Brain Res 122*, 491–505; Schmalzl, L., Powers, C. and Henje Blom, E. (2015) "Neurophysiological and neurocognitive mechanisms underlying the effects of yoga-based practices: Towards a comprehensive theoretical framework." *Front Hum Neurosci 9*, 235; Calabrese, P., Perrault, H., Dinh, T. P., Eberhard, A. and Benchetrit, G. (2000) "Cardiorespiratory interactions during resistive load breathing." *American Journal of Physiology: Regulatory, Integrative and Comparative Physiology 279*, 6, 2208–2213.

9   van Dixhoorn (1997), p.90.

10  Jafari, H., Courtois, I., Van den Bergh, O., Vlaeyen, J. W. S. and Van Diest, I. (2017) "Pain and respiration: A systematic review." *Pain 158*, 6, 995–1006.

11  van Dixhoorn (1997), p.90.

12  Clifton-Smith and Rowley (2011), p.76.

13  Clifton-Smith and Rowley (2011); Chaitow, L. (2012) "Breathing pattern disorders and lumbopelvic pain and dysfunction: An update." Accessed on 14/12/18 at http://leonchaitow.com/2012/01/23/breathing-pattern-disorders-and-lumbopelvic-pain-and-dysfunction-an-update; Schleifer, L. M., Ley, R.

and Spalding, T. W. (2002) "A hyperventilation theory of job stress and musculoskeletal disorders." *American Journal of Industrial Medicine 41*, 5, 420–432; Clausen, T., Scharf, A., Menzel, M. *et al.* (2004) "Influence of moderate and profound hyperventilation on cerebral blood flow, oxygenation and metabolism." *Brain Research 1019*, 1–2, 113–123.

14  Clifton-Smith and Rowley (2011).

15  Gardner, W. N. (2004) "Hyperventilation." *American Journal of Respiratory and Critical Care Medicine 170*, 2, 105–106.

16  Clifton-Smith and Rowley (2011).

17  van Dixhoorn, J. and Folgering, H. (2015) "The Nijmegen Questionnaire and dysfunctional breathing." *ERJ Open Research 1*, 1, 00001-2015.

18  van Dixhoorn and Folgering (2015), p.2.

19  Swami Jnaneshvara Bharati (n.d.) Traditional Yoga and Meditation of the Himalayan Masters, Self Realization through the Yoga Sutras, Vedanta, Samaya Sri Vidya Tantra. Accessed on 14/12/18 at http://swamij.com/yoga-sutras-13339.htm.

20  Pearson, N. (2007) *Understand Pain, Live Well Again: Pain Education for Busy Clinicians and People with Persistent Pain*. Penticton: Life is Now, Inc.

21  Saoji, A. A., Raghavendra, B. R. and Manjunath, N. K. (2017) "Effects of yogic breath regulation: A narrative review of scientific evidence." *Journal of Ayurveda and Integrative Medicines* doi: 10.1016/j.jaim.2117.07.008.

22  Zautra, A. J., Fasman, R., Davis, M. C. and Craig, A. D. B. (2010) "The effects of slow breathing on affective responses to pain stimuli: An experimental study." *Pain 149*, 12–18.

23  Bernardi, L., Gabutti, A., Porta, C. and Spicuzza, L. (2001) "Slow breathing reduces chemoreflex response to hypoxia and hypercapnia, and increases baroreflex sensitivity." *Journal of Hypertension 19*, 2221–2229; Bernardi, L., Porta, C., Gabutti, A., Spicuzza, L. and Sleight, P. (2001) "Modulatory effects of respiration." *Autonomic Neuroscience 90*, 47–56; Strauss-Blasche, G., Moser, M., Voica, M., McLeod, D., Klammer, N. and Marktl, W. (2000) "Relative timing of inspiration and expiration affects respiratory sinus arrhythmia." *Clinical and Experimental Pharmacology and Physiology 27*, 601–606; Esposito, P., Mereu, R., De Barbieri, G. *et al.* (2016) "Trained breathing-induced oxygenation acutely reverses cardiovascular autonomic dysfunction in patients with type 2 diabetes and renal disease." *Acta Diabetologica 53*, 2, 217–226.

24  Spicuzza, L., Gabutti, A., Porta, C., Montano, N. and Bernardi, L. (2000) "Yoga and chemoreflex response to hypoxia and hypercapnia." *Lancet 356*, 1495–1496.

25  Brown and Gerberg (2005).

26  Calabrese *et al.* (2000).

27  Sovik (2000).

28  Porges, S. W. (2001) "The polyvagal theory: Phylogenetic substrates of a social nervous system." *Int J Psychophysiol 42*, 2, 123–146; Schmalzl, L.,

Streeter, C. C. and Khalsa, S. B. S. (2016) "Research on the Psychophysiology of Yoga." In: S. B. S. Khalsa, L. Cohen, T. McCall and S. Telles (eds) *The Principles and Practice of Yoga in Healthcare.* Edinburgh: Handspring Publishing. 49–68.

29  Schmalzl, Powers and Henje Blom (2015); Thayer, J. F. and Sternberg, E. (2006) "Beyond heart rate variability: Vagal regulation of allostatic systems." *Annals of the New York Academy of Sciences 1088,* 1, 361–372.

30  Sharma *et al.* (2014).

31  Saoji, Raghavendra and Manjunath (2017).

32  Brown and Gerbarg (2005).

33  Saoji, Raghavendra and Manjunath (2017).

34  Schmalzl, Powers and Henje Blom (2015); Chang, C. and Glover, G. H. (2009) "Relationship between respiration, end-tidal $CO_2$ and BOLD signals in resting-state fMRI." *Neuroimage 47,* 4, 1381–1393.

35  Schmalzl, Powers and Henje Blom (2015); Borsook, D., Upadhyay, J., Chudler, E. H. and Becerra, L. (2010) "A key role of the basal ganglia in pain and analgesia: Insights gained through human functional imaging." *Mol Pain 6,* 27.

36  Telles, S., Sharma, S. K. and Balkrishna, A. (2014) "Blood pressure and heart rate variability during yoga-based alternate nostril breathing practice and breath awareness." *Medical Science Montiro Basic Research 20,* 1, 184–193; Sinha, A. N., Deepak, D. and Gusain, V. S. (2013) "Assessment of the effects of pranayama/alternate nostril breathing on the parasympathetic nervous system in young adults." *Journal of Clinical and Diagnostic Research 7,* 5, 821–823.

37  Telles, Singh and Puthige (2013).

38  Schmalzl *et al.* (2018).

39  Schmalzl, Streeter and Khalsa (2016).

40  Saoji, Raghavendra and Manjunath (2017).

41  Brown and Gerbarg (2005).

42  Brown and Gerbarg (2005), p.190.

43  Saoji, Raghavendra and Manjunath (2017), p.8.

44  Jafari, H., Courtois, I., Van den Bergh, O., Vlaeyen, J. W. S. and Van Diest, I. (2017) "Pain and respiration: A systematic review." *Pain 158,* 6, 995–1006.

45  Glynn, C. J., Lloyd, J. W. and Folkhard, S. (1981) "Ventilatory response to intractable pain." *Pain 11,* 201–211.

46  Suess, W. M., Alexander, A. B., Smith, D. D., Sweeney, H. W. and Marion, R. J. (1980) "The effects of psychological stress on respiration: A preliminary study of anxiety and hyperventilation." *Psychophysiology 17,* 535–540.

47  Jafari *et al.* (2017), p.998.

48  Jafari *et al.* (2017).

49  Perri, M. and Halford, E. (2008) "Pain and faulty breathing: A pilot study." *J Bodyw Mov Ther 4,* 297–306; McLaughlin, L., Goldsmith, C. H. and Coleman, K. (2011) "Breathing evaluation and retraining as an adjunct to manual therapy." *Manual Therapy 16,* 1, 51–52.

50  Hruska, J. (1997) "Influences of dysfunctional respiratory mechanics on orofacial pain." *Dent Clin North Am 41,* 2, 211–227.

51  Haugstad, G., Haugstad, T. and Kirste, U. (2006) "Posture, movement patterns, and body awareness in women with chronic pelvic pain." *J Psychosom Res 61,* 5, 637–644.

52  McLaughlin, Goldsmith and Coleman (2011); O'Sullivan, P. and Beale, D. (2007) "Changes in pelvic floor and diaphragm kinematics and respiratory patterns in subjects with sacroiliac joint pain following a motor learning intervention." *Manual Therapy 12,* 209–218; Hodges, P. W. and Moseley, G. L. (2003) "Pain and motor control of the lumbopelvic region: Effect and possible mechanisms." *Journal of Electromyography and Kinesiology 13,* 361–370; Janssens, L., Brumagne, S., Polspoel, K., Troosters, T. and McConnell, A. (2010) "The effect of inspiratory muscles fatigue on postural control in people with and without recurrent low back pain." *Spine 35,* 10, 1088–1094; Smith, M. D., Russell, A. and Hodges, P. W. (2006) "Disorders of breathing and continence have a stronger association with back pain than obesity and physical activity." *Australian Journal of Physiotherapy 52,* 11–16; Beekmans, N., Vermeersch, A., Lysens, R., *et al.* (2016) "The presence of respiratory disorders in individuals with low back pain: A systematic review." *Manual Therapy 26,* 77–86.

53  Smith, Russell and Hodges (2006).

54  Van Ryswyk, E. and Antic, N. A. (2016) "Opioids and sleep-disordered breathing." *Chest 150,* 4, 934–944.

55  Van Ryswyk and Antic (2016).

56  Key (2013); Bordoni and Zanier (2013).

57  Martin, S. L., Kerr, K. L., Bartley, E. J., Kuhn, B. L. *et al.* (2012) "Respiration-induced hypoalgesia: Exploration of potential mechanisms." *Journal of Pain 13,* 755–763.

58  Jafari *et al.* (2017).

59  Kapitza, K. P., Passie, T., Bernateck, M. and Karst, M. (2010) "First non-contingent respiratory biofeedback placebo versus contingent biofeedback in patients with chronic low back pain: A randomized, controlled, double-blind trial." *Appl Psychophysiol Biofeedback 35,* 207–217.

60  Elkreem, H. M. A. (2014) "Effect of breathing exercise on respiratory efficiency and pain intensity among children receiving chemotherapy." *Journal of Education and Practice 5,* 18–32.

61  Park, E., Oh, H. and Kim, T. (2013) "The effects of relaxation breathing on procedural pain and anxiety during burn care." *Burns 39,* 1101–1106.

62  Busch, V., Magerl, W., Kern, U., Haas, J., Hajak, G. and Eichhammer, P. (2012) "The effect of deep and slow breathing on pain perception, autonomic activity, and mood processing: An experimental study." *Pain Med 13,* 215–228.

63  Zautra *et al.* (2010).

64  Arsenault, M., Ladouceur, A., Lehmann, A., Rainville, P. and Piché, M. (2013) "Pain modulation

induced by respiration: Phase and frequency effects." *Neuroscience 252*, 501–511.

65 Iwabe, T., Ozaki, I. and Hashizume, A. (2014) "The respiratory cycle modulates brain potentials, sympathetic activity, and subjective pain sensation induced by noxious stimulation." *Neuroscience Research 84*, 47–59.

66 Martin *et al.* (2012).

67 Duschek, S., Werner, N. S. and Reyes del Paso, G. A. (2013) "The behavioral impact of baroreflex function: A review." *Psychophysiology 50*, 1183–1193.

68 Duschek, Werner and Reyes del Paso (2013).

69 Bernardi *et al.* (2001).

70 Strauss-Blasche *et al.* (2000).

71 Jafari *et al.* (2017).

72 Jafari *et al.* (2017).

73 Martin *et al.* (2012).

74 Busch *et al.* (2012).

75 Chalaye, P., Goffaux, P., Lafrenaye, S. and Marchand, S. (2009) "Respiratory effects on experimental heat pain and cardiac activity." *Pain Med 10*, 1334–1340.

76 Zautra (2010).

77 Jafari *et al.* (2017).

78 Jafari *et al.* (2017).

79 Jafari *et al.* (2017), p.1004.

80 van Dixhoorn (1997).

## CHAPTER 9

1 Bhavanani, A. B. (2011) *Understanding the Yoga Darshan*. 1st edition. Puducherr: Dhivyananda Creations.

2 Herbert, M. S., Goodin, B. R., Pero, S. T. *et al.* (2014) "Pain hypervigilance is associated with greater clinical pain severity and enhanced experimental pain sensitivity among adults with symptomatic knee osteoarthritis." *Ann Behav Med 48*, 1, 50–60.

3 Chapple, C. K. (2008) *Yoga and the Luminous: Patanjali's Spiritual Path to Freedom*. Albany, NY: State University of New York Press; Chapple, C. K., Sternlieb, B. and Antunes, C. (2015) *Sacred Thread: Patanjali's Yoga Sutras*. Pondicherry: Prisma Press.

4 Bharati, S. J. (n.d.) "Yoga Sutras 4.18–4.21 Illumination of the Mind." Accessed on 14/12/18 at http://swamij.com/yoga-sutras-41821.htm.

5 Mehling, W. E., Gopisetty, V., Daubenmier, J., Price, C. J., Hecht, F. M. and Stewart, A. (2009) "Body awareness: Construct and self–report measures." *PLoS One 4*, 5, e5614, p.2.

6 Chesler, A. T., Szczot, M., Bharucha-Goebel, D. *et al.* (2016) "The role of PIEZO2 in human mechanosensation." *New England Journal of Medicine 375*, 14, 1355–1364.

7 Lutz, A., Brefczynski-Lewis, J., Johnstone, T. and Davidson, R. J. (2008) "Regulation of the neural circuitry of emotion by compassion meditation: Effects of meditative expertise." *PLoS One 3*, 3, e1897.

8 Ly, M., Motzkin, J. C., Philippi, C. L. *et al.* (2012) "Cortical thinning in psychopathy." *American Journal of Psychiatry 169*, 7, 743–749.

9 Lazar, S. W., Kerr, C. E., Wasserman, R. H. *et al.* (2005) "Meditation experience is associated with increased cortical thickness." *Neuroreport 16*, 17, 1893–1897; Holzel, B. K., Carmody, J., Vangel, M. *et al.* (2011a) "Mindfulness practice leads to increases in regional brain gray matter density." *Psychiatry Research 191*, 1, 36–43.

10 Holzel, B. K., Lazar, S. W., Gard, T., Schuman-Olivier, Z., Vago, D. R. and Ott, U. (2011b) "How does mindfulness meditation work? Proposing mechanisms of action from a conceptual and neural perspective." *Perspectives on Psychological Science 6*, 6, 537–559.

11 Lazar *et al.* (2005); Holzel *et al.* (2011a); Holzel *et al.* (2011b).

12 Valenzuela-Moguillansky, C., Reyes-Reyes, A. and Gaete, M. I. (2017) "Exteroceptive and interoceptive body-self awareness in fibromyalgia patients." *Front Hum Neurosci 11*, 117.

13 Valenzuela-Moguillansky, Reyes-Reyes and Gaete (2017).

14 Herbert *et al.* (2014).

15 Holzel *et al.* (2011b); Cramer, H., Lauche, R., Daubenmier, J. *et al.* (2018) "Being aware of the painful body: Validation of the German Body Awareness Questionnaire and Body Responsiveness Questionnaire in patients with chronic pain." *PLoS One 13*, 2, e0193000; Gard, G. (2005) "Body awareness therapy for patients with fibromyalgia and chronic pain." *Disability and Rehabilitation 27*, 12, 725–728.

16 Mehling *et al.* (2009).

17 Bergström, M., Ejelöv, M., Mattsson, M. and Stålnacke, B.-M. (2014) "One-year follow-up of body awareness and perceived health after participating in a multimodal pain rehabilitation programme: A pilot study." *European Journal of Physiotherapy 16*, 4, 246–254.

18 Cohen, L. and M.D. Anderson Cancer Center (2014) "Effects of Meditation on Cognitive Function and Quality of Life." Accessed on 14/12/18 at https://clinicaltrials.gov/ct2/show/NCT02162329.

19 Holzel *et al.* (2011b); Benson, H. (1993) "The Relaxation Response." In: D. Goleman and J. Gurin (eds) *Mind Body Medicine How to Use Your Mind for Better Health*. New York, NY: Consumer Reports Book. 125–257; Kabat-Zinn, J. (1984) "The clinical use of mindfulness meditation for the self-regulation of chronic pain." *Journal of Behavioral Medicine 8*, 2, 163–190; Morone, N. E. and Greco, C. M. (2007) "Mind-body interventions for chronic pain in older adults: A structured review." *Pain Med 8*, 4, 359–375; Rosenzweig, S., Greeson, J. M., Reibel, D. K., Green, J. S., Jasser, S. A. and Beasley, D. (2010) "Mindfulness-based stress reduction for chronic pain conditions: Variation in treatment outcomes and role of home meditation practice." *J Psychosom*

*Res 68*, 1, 29–36; Vallath, N. (2010) "Perspectives on yoga inputs in the management of chronic pain." *Indian Journal of Palliative Care 16*, 1, 1–7; Schaffer, S. and Yucha, C. V. (2004) "Relaxation and pain management: The relaxation response can play a role in managing chronic and acute pain." *American Journal of Nursing 104*, 8, 75–82; Tilbrook, H., Cox, H., Hewitt, C. *et al.* (2011) "Yoga for chronic low back pain: A randomized trial." *Annals of Internal Medicine 155*, 9, 569–578; Astin, J. (2004) "Mind-body therapies for the management of pain." *Clinical Journal of Pain 20*, 1, 27–32; Baird, C. and Sands, L. (2004) "A pilot study of the effectiveness of guided imagery with progressive muscle relaxation to reduce chronic pain and mobility difficulties of osteoarthritis." *Pain Management Nursing 5*, 3, 97–104; Saper, R., Lemaster, C., Delitto, A. *et al.* (2017) "Yoga, physical therapy, or education for chronic low back pain: A randomized noninferiority trial." *Annals of Internal Medicine 167*, 2, 85–94; Cramer, H. (2017) "Effects of yoga on chronic neck pain: A systematic review and meta-analysis." *Clinical Rehabilitation 31*, 11, 1457–1465; Sutar, R., Yadav, S. and Desai, G. (2016) "Yoga intervention and functional pain syndromes: A selective review." *Int Rev Psychiatry 28*, 3, 316–322; Hilton, L., Hempel, S., Ewing, B. A. *et al.* (2017) "Mindfulness meditation for chronic pain: Systematic review and meta-analysis." *Ann Behav Med 51*, 2, 199–213.

20    Bhavanani (2011).

21    Giri, S. G. (1999) *The Ashtanga Yoga of Patanjali.* Tami Nadu: Satya Press, p.88.

22    Holzel *et al.* (2011a).

23    Lee, M., Silverman, S., Hansen, H., Patel, V. and Manchikanti, L. (2011) "A comprehensive review of opioid-induced hyperalgesia." *Pain Physician 14*, 145–161; Portenoy, R. K. (1996) "Opioid therapy for chronic nonmalignant pain." *Pain Research and Management 1*, 1, 17–28; Martell, B. A., O'Connor, P. G., Kerns, R. D. *et al.* (2007) "Systematic review: Opioid treatment for chronic back pain: Prevalence, efficacy, and association with addiction." *Annals of Internal Medicine 146*, 2, 116–127; Bogduk, N. and Andersson, G. (2009) "Is spinal surgery effective for back pain?" *F1000 Medical Reports* doi: 10.3410/M1-60.

24    Bogduk and Andersson (2009); Nystrom, B. (2012) "Spinal fusion in the treatment of chronic low back pain: Rationale for improvement." *Open Orthopaedics Journal 6*, 478–481; Thorlund, J. B., Juhl, C. B., Roos, E. M. and Lohmander, L. S. (2015) "Arthroscopic surgery for degenerative knee: Systematic review and meta-analysis of benefits and harms." *BMJ 350*, h2747; Brinjikji, W., Luetmer, P. H., Comstock, B. *et al.* (2015) "Systematic literature review of imaging features of spinal degeneration in asymptomatic populations." *American Journal of Neuroradiology 36*, 4, 811–816; Beard, D. J, Rees, J. L., Cook, J. A. *et al.* (2018) "Arthroscopic subacromial decompression for subacromial shoulder pain (CSAW): A multicentre, pragmatic,

parallel group, placebo-controlled, three-group, randomised surgical trial." *Lancet 391*, 10118, 329–338; Teunis, T. L. B., Reilly, B. T. and Ring, D. (2014) "A systematic review and pooled analysis of the prevalence of rotator cuff disease with increasing age." *Journal of Shoulder and Elbow Surgery 23*, 12, 1913–1921.

25    Chapple (2008); Chapple, Sternlieb and Antunes (2015).

26    Bharati, S. J. (n.d.) "Clearing the Clouded Mind Through Yoga." Accessed on 14/12/18 at www.swamij.com/cloudedmind.htm.

27    Ramachandran, V. and Blakeslee, S. (1998) *Phantoms in the Brain: Probing the Mysteries of the Human Mind.* 1st edition. New York, NY: HarperCollins, p.54.

28    Colmenero, L. H., Marmol, J. M. P., Marti-Garcia, C. *et al.* (2018) "Effectiveness of mirror therapy, motor imagery, and virtual feedback on phantom limb pain following amputation: A systematic review." *Prosthetics and Orthotics International 42*, 3, 288–298.

29    Vingerhoets, G., de Lange, F. P., Vandemaele, P., Deblaere, K. and Achten, E. (2002) "Motor imagery in mental rotation: An fMRI study." *NeuroImage 17*, 3, 1623–1633.

30    Ramachandran and Blakeslee (1998).

31    Moseley, L. (2011) "Why Things Hurt." [Video] *TEDxAdelaide*. Accessed on 14/12/18 at www.youtube.com/watch?v=gwd-wLdIHjs.

32    Moseley (2011).

33    Herbert *et al.* (2014); Cramer *et al.* (2018); Cramer, H., Mehling, W. E., Saha, F. J., Dobos, G. and Lauche, R. (2018) "Postural awareness and its relation to pain: Validation of an innovative instrument measuring awareness of body posture in patients with chronic pain." *BMC Musculoskeletal Disorders 19*, 1, 109.

34    Lazar *et al.* (2005); Holzel *et al.* (2011a); Holzel *et al.* (2011b); Hilton *et al.* (2017); Schmalzl, L. and Kerr, C. E. (2016) "Editorial: Neural mechanisms underlying movement-based embodied contemplative practices. *Front Hum Neurosci 10*, 169.

35    Gard (2005); Maglione, M. A., Hempel, S., Maher, A. R. *et al.* (2016) *Mindfulness Meditation for Chronic Pain.* Santa Monica, CA: Rand Corporation.

36    Gendlin, E. T. (2007) *Focusing.* 3rd edition. New York, NY: Bantam Books.

37    Rome, D. I. (2014) *Your Body Knows the Answer.* Boulder, CO: Shambala Publications.

38    Siegel, D. J. (2011) *Mindsight.* New York, NY: Bantam Books.

39    Levine, P. A. (1997) *Waking the Tiger.* Berkeley, CA: North Atlantic Books; Payne, P., Levine, P. A. and Crane-Godreau, M. A. (2015) "Somatic experiencing: Using interoception and proprioception as core elements of trauma therapy." *Front Psychol 6*, 93.

40    Chimenti, R., Frey-Law, L. and Sluka, K. (2018) "A mechanism-based approach to physical therapist

management of pain." *Phys Ther* 98, 5, 302–314, p.305.

41 Bharati, S. J. (n.d.) "Yoga Sutras 1.12–1.16, Practice and Non-Attachment." Accessed on 14/12/18 at www.swamij.com/yoga-sutras-11216.htm.

42 Valenzuela-Moguillansky, Reyes-Reyes and Gaete (2017); Bray, H. and Moseley, G. L. (2011) "Disrupted working body schema of the trunk in people with back pain." *British Journal of Sports Medicine* 45, 3, 168–173; Martinez, E., Aira, Z., Buesa, I., Aizpurua, I., Rada, D. and Azkue, J. J. (2018) "Embodied pain in fibromyalgia: Disturbed somatorepresentations and increased plasticity of the body schema." *PLoS One* 13, 4, e0194534; Valenzuela Moguillansky, C., O'Regan, J. K. and Petitmengin, C. (2013) "Exploring the subjective experience of the 'rubber hand' illusion." *Front Hum Neurosci* 7, 659; Trojan, J., Diers, M., Valenzuela-Moguillansky, C. and Torta, D. M. (2014) "Body, space, and pain." *Front Hum Neurosci* 8, 369; Schwoebel, J., Friedman, R., Duda, N. and Coslett, H. B. (2001) "Pain and the body schema: Evidence for peripheral effects on mental representations of movement." *Brain* 124, 10, 2096–2104; Martinez, E., Aira, Z., Buesa, I., Aizpurua, I., Rada, D. and Azkue, J. (2018) "Embodied pain in fibromyalgia: Disturbed somatorepresentations and increased plasticity of the body schema." *PLoS One* 13, 4, e0194534.

43 Moseley, G. L., Olthof, N., Venema, A. *et al.* (2008) "Psychologically induced cooling of a specific body part caused by the illusory ownership of an artificial counterpart." *Proc Natl Acad Sci* 105, 35, 13169–13173; Botvinick, M. and Cohen, J. (1998) "Rubber hands 'feel' touch that eyes see. *Nature* 391, 756; Ehrsson, H., Holmes, N. and Passingham, R. (2005) "Touching a rubber hand: Feeling of body ownership is associated with activity in multisensory brain areas." *Journal of Neuroscience* 25, 45, 10564–10573; Ehrsson, H., Spence, C. and Passingham, R. (2004) "That's my hand! Activity in premotor reflects feeling of ownership of a limb." *Science* 305, 875–877; Ehrsson, H., Wiech, K., Weiskopf, N., Dolan, R. and Passingham, R. (2007) "Threatening a rubber hand that you feel is yours elicits a cortical anxiety response." *Proc Natl Acad Sci* 104, 9828–9833; Longo, M., Schuur, F., Kammers, M., Tsakiris, M. and Haggard, P. (2008) "What is embodiment? A psychometric approach." *Cognition* 107, 978–998; Tsakiris, M. (2010) "My body in the brain: A neurocognitive model of body ownership." *Neuropsychologia* 48, 703–712; Tsakiris, M. and Haggard, P. (2005) "The rubber hand illusion revisited: Visuotactile integration and self-attribution." *Journal of Experimental*

*Psychology: Human Perception and Performance 31*, 80–91; Tsakiris, M., Hesse, M., Boy, C., Haggard, P. and Fink, G. (2007) "Neural signatures of body ownership: A sensory network for bodily self-consciousness." *Cerebral Cortex* 16, 645–660; Costantini, M. and Haggard, P. (2007) "The rubber hand illusion: Sensitivity and reference frame for body ownership." *Conscious Cognition* 16, 229–240; Capelari, E. and Brasil-Neto, J. (2009) "Feeling pain in the rubber hand: Integration of visual, proprioceptive, and painful stimuli." *Perception* 38, 92–99; Kammers, M., de Vignemont, F., Verhagen, L. and Dijkerman, H. (2009) "The rubber hand illusion in action." *Neuropsychologia* 47, 204–211; Schutz-Bosbach, S., Tausche, P. and Weiss, C. (2009) "Roughness perception during the rubber hand illusion." *Brain Cognition* 70, 136–144; Lewis, E. and Lloyd, D. (2010) "Embodied experience: A first-person investigation of the rubber hand illusion." *Phenomenology and the Cognitive Sciences* 9, 317–339; Barnsley, N., McAuley, J. H., Mohan, R., Dey, A., Thomas, P. and Moseley, G. L. (2011) "The rubber hand illusion increases histamine reactivity in the real arm." *Current Biology* 21, 23, R945–946; Moguillansky, C., O'Regan, J. and Petitmengin, C. (2013) "Exploring the subjective experience of the 'rubber hand' illusion." *Front Hum Neurosci* 7, 659.

44 Steptoe, W., Steed, A. and Slater, M. (2013) "Human tails: Ownership and control of extended humanoid avatars." *IEEE Transactions on Visualization and Computer Graphics* 19, 4, 583–590.

45 Chapple (2008).

46 Flor, H. (2002) "Painful memories: Can we train chronic pain patients to 'forget' their pain?" *EMBO Reports* 3, 4, 288–291.

47 Grossan, M. (2011) *Stressed? Anxiety? Your Cure is in the Mirror.* Charleston, SC: Murray Grossan, MD.

48 Fazzio, L. R. and Langer, E. (2013) *Improving Memory and Function in Chronic Pain Sufferers Through a Mindfulness Intervention.* Los Angeles, CA and Cambridge, MA: Loyola Marymount University and Harvard University.

49 Bray and Moseley (2011); Schwoebel *et al.* (2001); Valenzuela-Moguillansky, C. (2013) "Pain and body awareness: An exploration of the bodily experience of persons suffering from fibromyalgia." *Psychological Experiments in First-Person Research 8*, 3, 339–350; Gilpin, H. R., Moseley, G. L., Stanton, T. R. and Newport, R. (2015) "Evidence for distorted mental representation of the hand in osteoarthritis." *Rheumatology (Oxford)* 54, 4, 678–682.

50 Martinez *et al.* (2018).

51 Bhavanani (2011).

52 Fazzio and Langer (2013).

## Chapter 10

1 Cohen, S., Janicki-Deverts, D., Doyle, W. J. *et al.* (2012) "Chronic stress, glucocorticoid receptor resistance, inflammation, and disease risk." *PNAS* 109, 16, 5995–5999.

2 Zhang, J. M. and An, J. (2007) "Cytokines, inflammation and pain." *International Anesthesiology Clinics* 45, 2, 27–37.

3   Watkins, L. R., Milligan, E. D. and Maier, S. F. (2003) "Glial proinflammatory cytokines mediate exaggerated pain states: Implications for clinical pain." *Adv Exp Med Biol 521*, 1–21.

4   Ren, K. and Dubner, R. (2010) "Interactions between the immune and nervous systems in pain." *Nature Medicine 16*, 11, 1267–1276.

5   Okifuji, A. and Hare, B. D. (2015) "The association between chronic pain and obesity." *Journal of Pain Research 8*, 399–408.

6   James, M. J. and Cleland, L. G. (1997) "Dietary n-3 fatty acids and therapy for rheumatoid arthritis." *Semin Arthritis Rheum 27*, 2, 85–97; James, M., Proudman, S. and Cleland, L. (2010) "Fish oil and rheumatoid arthritis: Past, present and future." *Proceedings of the Nutrition Society 69*, 3, 316–323; Hurst, S., Zainal, Z., Caterson, B., Hughes, C. E. and Harwood, J. L. (2010) "Dietary fatty acids and arthritis." *Prostaglandins, Leukotrienes, and Essential Fatty Acids 82*, 4–6, 315–318.

7   Maroon, J. C. and Bost, J. W. (2006) "Omega-3 fatty acids (fish oil) as an anti-inflammatory: An alternative to nonsteroidal anti-inflammatory drugs for discogenic pain. *Surgical Neurology 65*, 4, 326–331.

8   Altman, R. D. and Marcussen, K. C. (2001) "Effects of a ginger extract on knee pain in patients with osteoarthritis." *Arthritis and Rheumatism 44*, 11, 2531–2538; Srivastava, K. C. and Mustafa, T. (1992) "Ginger (Zingiber officinale) in rheumatism and musculoskeletal disorders. *Medical Hypotheses 39*, 4, 342–348.

9   Stoner, G. and Wang, L. S. (2013) "Natural Products as Anti-inflammatory Agents." In: *Obesity, Inflammation and Cancer*. Springer New York. 341–361.

10  Richard, D. M., Dawes, M. A., Mathias, C. W., Acheson, A., Hill-Kapturczak, N. and Dougherty, D. M. (2009) "L-tryptophan: Basic metabolic functions, behavioral research and therapeutic indications." *International Journal of Tryptophan Research: IJTR 2*, 45–60; Martin, S. L., Power, A., Boyle, Y., Anderson, I. M., Silverdale, M. A. and Jones, A. K. P. (2017) "5-HT modulation of pain perception in humans." *Psychopharmacology 234*, 19, 2929–2939; Young, S. N. (1996) "Behavioral effects of dietary neurotransmitter precursors: Basic and clinical aspects." *Neurosci Biobehav Rev 20*, 2, 313–323; Sidransky, H. (2002) *Tryptophan: Biochemical and Health Implications*. Boca Raton, FL: CRC Press.

11  Katz, D. L. and Meller, S. (2014 "Can we say what diet is best for health?" *Annual Review of Public Health 35*, 83–103.

12  Pollan, M. (2009) *Food Rules: An Eater's Manual*. New York: Penguin Books.

13  Serra-Majem, L., Roman, B. and Estruch, R. (2006) "Scientific evidence of interventions using the Mediterranean diet: A systematic review." *Nutrition Reviews 64*, S1, S27–S47; Tortosa, A., Bes-Rastrollo, M., Sanchez-Villega, A., Basterra-Gortari, F. J., Nuñez-Cordoba, J. M. and Martinez-Gonzalez, M. A. (2007) "Mediterranean diet inversely associated with the incidence of metabolic syndrome: The SUN prospective cohort." *Diabetes Care 30*, 11, 2957–2959; Sköldstam, L., Hagfors, L. and Johannson, G. (2003) "An experimental study of a Mediterranean diet intervention for patients with rheumatoid arthritis." *Annals of Rheumatic Diseases 62*, 3; Sánchez-Villegas, A., Pérez-Comago, A., Zazpe, I., Santiago, S., Lahortiga, F. and Martinez-González, M. A. (2017) "Micronutrient intake adequacy and depression risk in the SUN cohort study." *European Journal of Nutrition* doi: 10.1007/s00394-017-1514-z.

14  Adam, T. C. and Epel, E. S. (2007) "Stress, eating and the reward system." *Physiology and Behavior 91*, 449–458.

15  Steptoe, A., Hamer, M. and Chida, Y. (2007) "The effects of acute psychological stress on circulating inflammatory factors in humans: A review and meta-analysis." *Brain, Behavior, and Immunity 21*, 901–912; Björntorp, B. (2001) "Do stress reactions cause abdominal obesity and comorbidities?" *Obesity Reviews 2*, 73–86; Epel, E., Lapidus, R., McEwen, B. and Brownell, K. (2001) "Stress may add bite to appetite in women: A laboratory study of stress-induced cortisol and eating behavior." *Psychoneuroendocrinology 26*, 37–49.

16  Garg, N. and Lerne, J. S. (2013) "Sadness and consumption." *Journal of Consumer Psychology 23*, 1, 106–113; Alba, J. W. and Williams, E. F. (2013) "Pleasure principles: A review of research on hedonic consumption." *Journal of Consumer Psychology 23*, 1, 2–18.

17  Black, P. H. (2006) "The inflammatory consequences of psychologic stress: Relationship to insulin resistance, obesity, atherosclerosis and diabetes mellitus, type II." *Medical Hypotheses 67*, 4, 879–891; Alberti, K., Zimmet, P. and Shaw, J. (2005) "The metabolic syndrome: A new worldwide definition." *Lancet 366*, 9491, 1059–1062.

18  Streeter, C. C., Gerberg, P. L., Saper, R. B., Ciraulo, D. A. and Brown, R. P. (2012) "Effects of yoga on the autonomic nervous system, gamma-aminobutyric-acid, and allostasis in epilepsy, depression, and post-traumatic stress disorder." *Medical Hypotheses 78*, 5, 571–579; Ross, A. and Thomas, S. (2010) "The health benefit of yoga and exercise: A review of comparison studies." *Journal of Alternative and Complementary Medicine 16*, 10, 3–12.

19  Ervin, R. B. and Ogden, C. L. (2013) "Consumption of added sugars among US adults, 2005–2010." *NCHS Data Brief, 122*, 1–8; United States Department of Agriculture, Economic Research Service (2012) *USDA Sugar Supply: Tables 51–53: US Consumption of Caloric Sweeteners*. Washington, DC: United States Department of Agriculture.

20  Johnson, R. K., Appel, L., Brands, M., *et al.* (2009) "Dietary sugars intake and cardiovascular health: A scientific statement from the American Heart Association." *Circulation 120*, 11, 1011–1020.

21  Lustig, R. (2013) "Fructose: It's 'alcohol without the buzz.'" *Advances in Nutrition 4*, 2, 226–235.

22 Volkow, N. D. and Li, T.-K. (2004) "Drug addiction: The neurobiology of behavior gone awry." *Nature Reviews Neuroscience 5*, 12, 963–970; Brownell, K. D. and Gold, M. S. (2012) *Food and Addiction: A Comprehensive Handbook.* New York, NY: Oxford University Press; Avena, N., Rada, P. and Hoebel, B. (2008) "Evidence for sugar addiction: Behavioral and neurochemical effects of intermittent, excessive sugar intake." *Neuroscience Behavior Review 52*, 1, 20–39.

23 National Institutes of Health (2012) *NIH Human Microbiome Project defines normal bacterial makeup of the body.* Accessed on 16/12/18 at www.nih.gov/news-events/news-releases/nih-human-microbiome-project-defines-normal-bacterial-makeup-body.

24 Guarner, F. and Malagelada, J. R. (2003) "Gut flora in health and disease." *Lancet 361*, 512–519; Falk, P. G., Hooper, L. V., Midtvedt, T. and Gordon, J. I. (1998) "Creating and maintaining the gastrointestinal ecosystem: What we know and need to know from gnotobiology." *Microbiology and Molecular Biology Reviews 62*, 1157–1170; Furness, J. B., Kunze, W. A. and Clerc, N. (1999) "Nutrient tasting and signaling mechanisms in the gut. II. The intestine as a sensory organ: neural, endocrine, and immune responses." *American Journal of Physiology 277*, 5.1, G922–G928.

25 Moschen, A. R., Wieser, V. and Tilg, H. (2012) "Dietary factors: Major regulators of the gut's microbiota." *Gut and Liver 6*, 4, 411–416; Foster, J. A., Rinaman, L. and Cryan, J. F. (2017) "Stress and the gut-brain axis: Regulation by the microbiome." *Neurobiology of Stress 7*, 124–136.

26 Brown, K., DeCoffe, D., Molcan, E. and Gibson, D. L. (2012) "Diet-induced dybiosis of the intestinal microbiota and the effects on immunity and disease." *Nutrients 4*, 8, 1095–1119.

27 Vangay, P., Ward, T., Gerber, J. S. and Knights, D. (2015) "Antibiotics, pediatric dysbiosis, and disease." *Cell Host and Microbe 17*, 5, 553–564; Langdon, A., Crook, N. and Dantas, G. (2016) "The effects of antibiotics on the microbiome throughout development and alternative approaches for therapeutic modulation." *Genome Medicine 8*, 39; Zaura, E., Brandt, B. W., Teixeira de Mattos, M. J. *et al.* (2015) "Same exposure but two radically different responses to antibiotics: Resilience of the salivary microbiome versus long-term microbial shifts in feces." *mBio 6*, 6, e01693-15.

28 Kang, M., Mischel, R. A., Bhave, S. *et al.* (2017) "The effect of gut microbiome on tolerance to morphine mediated antinociception in mice." *Scientific Reports 7*, 42658; Rogers, M. A. M. and Aronoff, D. M. (2016) "The influence of non-steroidal anti-inflammatory drugs on the gut microbiome." *Clinical Microbiology and Infection 22*, 2, 178.e1–178.e9; Liang, X., Bittinger, K., Li, X., Abernethy, D. R., Bushman, F. D. and FitzGerald, G. A. (2015) "Bidirectional interactions between indomethacin and the murine intestinal microbiota." *eLife 4*, e08973; Babrowski,

T., Holbrook, C., Moss, J. and Gottlieb, L. (2012) "Pseudomonas aeruginosa virulence expression is directly activated by morphine and is capable of causing lethal gut-derived sepsis in mice during chronic morphine administration." *Annals of Surgery 255*, 2, 386–393.

29 Langdon, Crook, and Dantas (2016).

30 Othman, M., Agüero, R. and Lin, H. C. (2008) "Alterations in intestinal microbial flora and human disease." *Current Opinion in Gastroenterology 24*, 1, 11–16; Pimentel, M., Wallace, D., Hallegua, D. *et al.* (2004) "A link between irritable bowel syndrome and fibromyalgia may be related to findings on lactulose breath testing." *Annals of Rheumatic Diseases 63*, 4, 450–452.

31 Goebel, A., Buhner, S., Schedel, R., Lochs, H. and Sprotte, G. (2008) "Altered intestinal permeability in patients with primary fibromyalgia and in patients with complex regional pain syndrome." *Rheumatology (Oxford) 47*, 8, 1223–1227.

32 Kamiya, T., Wang, L., Forsythe, P. *et al.* (2006) "Inhibitory effects of *Lactobacillus reuteri* on visceral pain induced by colorectal distension in Sprague-Dawley rats." *Gut 55*, 2, 191–196.

33 Kunze, W. A., Mao, Y. K., Wang, B. *et al.* (2009) "Lactobacillus reuteri enhances excitability of colonic AH neurons by inhibiting calcium-dependent potassium channel opening." *Journal of Cellular and Molecular Medicine 13*, 2261–2270.

34 Arora, H. C., Eng, C. and Shoskes, D. A. (2017) "Gut microbiome and chronic prostatitis/chronic pelvic pain syndrome." *Annals of Translational Medicine 5*, 2, 30.

35 Yano, J. M., Yu, K., Donaldson, G. P. *et al.* (2015) "Indigenous bacteria from the gut microbiota regulate host serotonin biosynthesis." *Cell 161*, 264–276.

36 Foster, Rinaman and Cryan (2017); Lima-Ojeda, J. M., Rupprecht, R. and Baghai, T. C. (2017) "I am I and my bacterial circumstances: Linking gut microbiome, neurodevelopment, and depression." *Frontiers in Psychiatry 8*, 153; Moloney, R. D., Johnson, A. C., O'Mahony, S. M., Dinan, T. G., Greenwood-Van Meerveld, B. and Cryan, J. F. (2016) "Stress and the microbiota-gut-brain axis in visceral pain: Relevance to irritable bowel syndrome." *CNS Neuroscience and Therapeutics 22*, 102–117.

37 Wang, Y. and Kasper, L. H. (2014) "The role of microbiome in central nervous system disorders." *Brain, Behavior, and Immunity 38*, 1–12.

38 Chiu, I. M., Heesters, B. A., Ghasemlou, N. *et al.* (2013) "Bacteria activate sensory neurons that modulate pain and inflammation." *Nature 501*, 7465, 52–57.

39 Rousseaux, C., Thuru, X., Gelot, A. *et al.* (2007) "Lactobacillus acidophilus modulates intestinal pain and induces opioid and cannabinoid receptors." *Nature Medicine 13*, 1, 35–37.

40 Goldenberg, J. Z., Ma, S. S., Saxton, J. D. *et al.* (2013) "Probiotics for the prevention of Clostridium

difficile-associated diarrhea in adults and children." *Cochrane Database Syst Rev 5*, CD006095.

41  Vitetta, L., Coulson, S., Linnane, A. W. and Butt, H. (2013) "The gastrointestinal microbiome and musculoskeletal diseases: A beneficial role for probiotics and prebiotics." *Pathogens 2*, 4, 606–626.

42  Średnicka-Tober, D., Barański, M., Seal, C. J. *et al.* (2016) "Higher PUFA and n-3 PUFA, conjugated linoleic acid, α-tocopherol and iron, but lower iodine and selenium concentrations in organic milk: A systematic literature review and meta- and redundancy analyses." *British Journal of Nutrition 115*, 6, 1043–1060.

43  Barański, M., Średnicka-Tober, D., Volakakis, N. *et al.* (2014) "Higher antioxidant and lower cadmium concentrations and lower incidence of pesticide residues in organically grown crops: A systematic literature review and meta-analyses." *British Journal of Nutrition 112*, 5, 794–811.

44  Alavanja, M. C. R., Ross, M. K. and Bonner, M. R. (2013) "Increased cancer burden among pesticide applicators and others due to pesticide exposure." *CA: A Cancer Journal for Clinicians 63*, 120–142; Silva, J. F., Mattos, I. E., Luz, L. L., Carmo, C. N. and Abydos, R. D. (2016) "Exposure to pesticides and prostate cancer: Systematic review of the literature." *Reviews on Environmental Health 31*, 3, 311–327; Gangemi, S., Miozzi, E., Teodoro, M. *et al.* (2016) "Occupational exposure to pesticides as a possible risk factor for the development of chronic disease in humans (Review)." *Molecular Medicine Reports 14*, 5, 4475–4488; Samel, A. and Seneff, S. (2013) "Glyphosate, pathways to modern diseases II: Celiac sprue and gluten intolerance." *Interdisciplinary Toxicology 6*, 4, 159–184.

45  Baudry, J., Assmann, K. E., Touvier, M. *et al.* (2018) "Association of frequency of organic food consumption with cancer risk: Findings from the NutriNet-Santé Prospective Cohort Study." *JAMA Internal Medicine* doi:10.1001/jamainternmed.2018.4357.

46  Gardner, Z. E., McGuffin, M. and American Herbal Products Association (eds) (2013) *American Herbal Products Association's Botanical Safety Handbook.* 2nd edition. Boca Raton, FL: American Herbal Products Association, CRC Press.

47  Altman, R. D. and Barthel, H. R. (2011) "Topical therapies for osteoarthritis." *Drugs 71*, 10, 1259–1279.

48  Palma, C. and Manzini, S. (1998) "Substance P induces secretion of immunomodulatory cytokines by human astrocytoma cells." *Journal of Neuroimmunology 81*, 1–2, 127–137.

49  Mason, L., Moore, R. A., Derry, S., Edwards, J. E. and McQuay, H. J. (2004) "Systematic review of topical capsaicin for the treatment of chronic pain." *BMJ 328*, 7446, 991; Derry, S., Lloyd, R., Moore, R. A. and McQuay, H. J. (2009) "Topical capsaicin for chronic neuropathic pain in adults." *Cochrane Database Syst Rev 4*, CD007393; Pittler, M. H. and Ernst, E. (2008) "Complementary therapies for neuropathic and neuralgic pain: Systematic review." *Clinical Journal of Pain 24*, 8, 731–733; Peppin, J. F. and Pappagallo, M. (2014) "Capsaicinoids in the treatment of neuropathic pain: A review." *Therapeutic Advances in Neurological Disorders 7*, 1, 22–32.

50  Knuesel, O., Weber, M. and Suter, A. (2002) "Arnica montana gel in osteoarthritis of the knee: An open multicenter clinical trial." *Advances in Therapy 19*, 5, 209–218.

51  Terry, R., Posadzki, P., Watson, L. K. and Ernst, E. (2011) "The use of ginger (Zingiber officinale) for the treatment of pain: A systematic review of clinical trials." *Pain Med 12*, 1808–1818.

52  Henrotin, Y., Clutterbuck, A. L., Allaway, D. *et al.* (2010) "Biological actions of curcumin on articular chondrocytes." *Osteoarthritis and Cartilage 18*, 2, 141–149.

53  Efthimiou, P. and Kukar, M. (2010) "Complementary and alternative medicine use in rheumatoid arthritis: Proposed mechanism of action and efficacy of commonly used modalities." *Rheumatology International 30*, 5, 571–586; Chandran, B. and Goel, A. (2012) "A randomized, pilot study to assess the efficacy and safety of curcumin in patients with active rheumatoid arthritis." *Phytotherapy Research 26*, 11, 1719–1725; Panahi, Y., Rahimnia, A. R., Sharafi, M., Alishiri, G., Saburi, A. and Sahebkar, A. (2014) "Curcuminoid treatment for knee osteoarthritis: A randomized double-blind placebo-controlled trial." *Phytotherapy Research 28*, 11, 1625–1631; Belcaro, G., Cesarone, M. R., Dugall, M. *et al.* (2010) "Efficacy and safety of Meriva, a curcumin-phosphatidylcholine complex, during extended administration in osteoarthritis patients." *Alternative Medicine Review 15*, 4, 337–344; Kuptniratsaikul, V., Thanakhumtorn, S., Chinswangwatanakul, P., Wattanamongkonsil, L. and Thamlikitkul, V. (2009) "Efficacy and safety of Curcuma domestica extracts in patients with knee osteoarthritis." *J Altern Complement Med 15*, 8, 891–897.

54  Cameron, M., Gagnier, J. J., Little, C. V., Parsons, T. J., Blümle, A. and Chrubasik, S. (2009) "Evidence of effectiveness of herbal medicinal products in the treatment of arthritis: Part I: Osteoarthritis." *Phytotherapy Research 23*, 11, 1497–4515; Siddiqui, M. Z. (2011) "Boswellia serrata, a potential anti-inflammatory agent: An overview." *Indian Journal of Pharmaceutical Sciences 73*, 3, 255–261; Sengupta, K., Alluri, K. V., Satish, A. R. *et al.* (2008) "A double blind, randomized, placebo controlled study of the efficacy and safety of 5-Loxin for treatment of osteoarthritis of the knee." *Arthritis Research and Therapy 10*, 4, R85; Vishal, A. A., Mishra, A. and Raychaudhuri, S. P. (2011) "A double blind, randomized, placebo controlled clinical study evaluates the early efficacy of aflapin in subjects with osteoarthritis of knee." *International Journal of Medical Sciences 8*, 7, 615–622.

55  Fetrow, C. W. and Avila, J. R. (2001) "Efficacy of the dietary supplement S-adenosyl-L-methionine."

*Annals of Pharmacotherapy 35*, 11, 1414–1425; Soeken, K. L., Lee, W. L., Bausell, R. B., Agelli, M. and Berman, B. M. (2002) "Safety and efficacy of S-adenosylmethionine (SAMe) for osteoarthritis." *Journal of Family Practice 51*, 5, 425–430; De Silva, V., El-Metwally, A., Ernst, E. *et al.* (2011) "Evidence for the efficacy of complementary and alternative medicines in the management of osteoarthritis: A systematic review." *Rheumatology 50*, 5, 911–920; Rutjes, A. W. S., Nüesch, E., Reichenbach, S. *et al.* (2009) "S-Adenosylmethionine for osteoarthritis of the knee or hip." *Cochrane Database of Systematic Reviews 4*, CD007321.

56  Chrubasik, S., Eisenberg, E., Balan, E., Weinberger, T., Luzzati, R. and Conradt, C. (2000) "Treatment of low back pain exacerbations with willow bark extract: A randomized double-blind study." *American Journal of Medicine 109*, 1, 9–14; Fuster, V. and Sweeny, J. M. (2011) "Aspirin: A historical and contemporary therapeutic overview." *Circulation 123*, 7, 768–778; Ernst, E. and Chrubasik, S. (2000) "Phyto-anti-inflammatories. A systematic review of randomized, placebo-controlled, double-blind trials." *Rheumatic Diseases Clinics of North America 26*, 1, 13–27; Gagnier, J. J., van Tulder, M., Berman, B. and Bombardier, C. (2006) "Herbal medicine for low back pain." *Cochrane Database Syst Rev 2*, CD004504; Biegert, C., Wagner, I., Lüdtke, R. *et al.* (2004) "Efficacy and safety of willow bark extract in the treatment of osteoarthritis and rheumatoid arthritis: Results of 2 randomized double-blind controlled trials." *Journal of Rheumatology 31*, 11, 2121–2130.

57  Levy, R. M., Saikovsky, R., Shmidt, E., Khokhlov, A. and Burnett, B. P. (2009) "Flavocoxid is as effective as naproxen for managing the signs and symptoms of osteoarthritis of the knee in humans: A short-term randomized, double-blind pilot study." *Nutrition Research 29*, 5, 298–304.

58  Setty, A. R. and Sigal, L. H. (2005) "Herbal medications commonly used in the practice of rheumatology: Mechanisms of action, efficacy, and side effects." *Seminars in Arthritis and Rheumatism 34*, 6, 773–784; Chrubasik, J. E., Roufogalis, B. D. and Chrubasik, S. (2007) "Evidence of effectiveness of herbal antiinflammatory drugs in the treatment of painful osteoarthritis and chronic low back pain." *Phytotherapy Research: PTR 21*, 7, 675–683; Ernst, E. (2011) "Herbal medicine in the treatment of rheumatic diseases." *Rheumatic Disease Clinics of North America 37*, 1, 95–102; Sanders, M. and Grundmann, O. (2011) "The use of glucosamine, devil's claw (Harpagophytum procumbens), and acupuncture as complementary and alternative treatments for osteoarthritis." *Alternative Medicine Review: A Journal of Clinical Therapeutic 16*, 3, 228–238.

59  Piscoya, J., Rodriguez, Z., Bustamante, S. A., Okuhama, N. N., Miller, M. J. and Sandoval, M. (2001) "Efficacy and safety of freeze-dried cat's claw in osteoarthritis of the knee: Mechanisms of action of the species Uncaria guianensis." *Inflammation Research 50*, 9, 442–428; Mur, E., Hartig, F., Eibl, G. and Schirmer, M. (2002) "Randomized double blind trial of an extract from the pentacyclic alkaloid-chemotype of uncaria tomentosa for the treatment of rheumatoid arthritis." *J Rheumatol 29*, 4, 678–681; Erowele, G. I. and Kalejaiye, A. O. (2009) "Pharmacology and therapeutic uses of cat's claw." *American Journal of Health-System Pharmacy: AJHP: Official Journal of the American Society of Health-System Pharmacists 66*, 11, 992–995.

60  Sarzi Puttini, P. and Caruso, I. (1992) "Primary fibromyalgia syndrome and 5-hydroxy-L-tryptophan: A 90-day open study." *Journal of International Medical Research 20*, 2, 182–189; Turner, E. H., Loftis, J. M. and Blackwell, A. D. (2006) "Serotonin a la carte: Supplementation with the serotonin precursor 5-hydroxytryptophan." *Pharmacology and Therapeutics 109*, 3, 325–338.

61  Diener, H. C., Rahlfs, V. W. and Danesch, U. (2004) "The first placebo-controlled trial of a special butterbur root extract for the prevention of migraine: Reanalysis of efficacy criteria." *European Neurology 51*, 2, 89–97; Lipton, R. B., Göbel, H., Einhäupl, K. M., Wilks, K. and Mauskop, A. (2004) "Petasites hybridus root (butterbur) is an effective preventive treatment for migraine." *Neurology 63*, 12, 2240–2244; Sutherland, A. and Sweet, B. V. (2010) "Butterbur: An alternative therapy for migraine prevention." *American Journal of Health-System Pharmacy: AJHP: Official Journal of the American Society of Health-System Pharmacists 67*, 9, 705–711.

62  Vogler, B. K., Pittler, M. H. and Ernst, E. (1998) "Feverfew as a preventive treatment for migraine: A systematic review." *Cephalalgia 18*, 10, 704–708; Pittler, M. H. and Ernst, E. (2004) "Feverfew for preventing migraine." *Cochrane Database of Systematic Reviews*, CD002286; Schiapparelli, P., Allais, G., Castagnoli Gabellari, I., Rolando, S., Terzi, M. G. and Benedetto, C. (2010) "Non-pharmacological approach to migraine prophylaxis: Part II." *Neurological Sciences: Official Journal of the Italian Neurological Society and of the Italian Society of Clinical Neurophysiology 31*, S1, S137–139; Diener, H. C., Pfaffenrath, V., Schnitker, J., Friede, M. and Henneicke-von Zepelin, H. H. (2005) "Efficacy and safety of 6.25 mg t.i.d. feverfew CO2-extract (MIG-99) in migraine prevention: A randomized, double-blind, multicentre, placebo-controlled study." *Cephalalgia: An International Journal of Headache 25*, 11, 1031–1041.

63  Mauskop, A. and Altura, B. M. (1998) "Role of magnesium in the pathogenesis and treatment of migraines." *Clinical Neuroscience 5*, 1, 24–27; Peikert, A., Wilimzig, C. and Köhne-Volland, R. (1996) "Prophylaxis of migraine with oral magnesium: Results from a prospective, multi-center, placebo-controlled and double-blind randomized study." *Cephalalgia: An International Journal of Headache 16*, 4, 257–263; Pfaffenrath, V., Wessely, P., Meyer,

C. *et al.* (1996) "Magnesium in the prophylaxis of migraine—a double-blind placebo-controlled study." *Cephalalgia: An International Journal of Headache 16*, 6, 436–440; Mauskop, A., Altura, B. T. and Altura, B. M. (2002) "Serum ionized magnesium levels and serum ionized calcium/ ionized magnesium ratios in women with menstrual migraine." *Headache 42*, 4, 242–248; Facchinetti, F., Sances, G., Borella, P., Genazzani, A. R. and Nappi, G. (1991) "Magnesium prophylaxis of menstrual migraine: Effects on intracellular magnesium." *Headache 31*, 5, 298–301.

## CHAPTER 11

1   Feuerstein, G. (1989) *The Yoga-Sutra of Patañjali: A New Translation and Commentary.* New edition. Rochester, VT: Inner Traditions.

2   The University of California, San Francisco, School of Nursing Symptom Management Faculty Group (1994) "A Model for Symptom Management." *Journal of Nursing Scholarship 26*, 4, 272–276.

3   Ecker, B., Ticic, R. and Hulley, L. (2012) *Unlocking the Emotional Brain: Eliminating Symptoms at Their Roots Using Memory Reconsolidation.* New York: Routledge.

4   Amrita Aromatherapy (n.d.) "Holistic vs. Reductionist Paradigm." Accessed on 14/12/18 at www.amrita.net/holistic-paradigm.

5   Sarbacker, S. R. and Kimple, K. (2015) *The Eight Limbs of Yoga: A Handbook for Living Yoga Philosophy.* New York, NY: North Point Press, p.3.

6   Lee, M. (2000) *Phoenix Rising Yoga: Bridge from Body to Soul.* Deerfield Beach, FL: Health Communications.

7   Feuerstein (1989), p.3.

8   Feuerstein (1989).

9   Gass, R. (2010) *What is Transformational Change?* Accessed on 14/1/19 at http://hiddenleaf. electricembers.net/wp-content/uploads/2010/06/ What-is-Transformational-Change.pdf.

10  Mythical Realm (n.d.) "Rise of the Phoenix." Accessed on 14/12/18 at http://mythicalrealm.com/ creatures/phoenix.html.

11  Fronsdal, G. (2008) *The Dhammapada: A New Translation of the Buddhist Classic with Annotations.* Boston, MA: Shambhala.

12  Farb, N. A. S., Segal, Z. V., Mayberg, H. *et al.* (2007) "Attending to the present: Mindfulness meditation reveals distinct neural modes of self-reference." *Social Cognitive and Affective Neuroscience 2*, 4, 313–322.

13  Cooper, M. (2013) *The Handbook of Person-Centred Psychotherapy and Counselling* New York, NY: Palgrave Macmillan.

14  Knowles, M. S. (1990) *Andragogy in Action:* San Francisco, CA: Jossey-Bass Publishers.

15  Lee, M. (2000) *Phoenix Rising Yoga: Bridge from Body to Soul.* Deerfield Beach, FL: Health Communications.

16  Fromm, E., Funk, R. and Fromm, E. (2010) *The Pathology of Normalcy.* Riverdale, NY: American Mental Health Foundation Books.

17  Khalsa, S. B., Cohen, L., McCall, T. and Telles, S. (2006) *The Principles and Practice of Yoga in Health Care.* Edinburgh: Handspring Publishing.

18  Belluz, J. (2015) *I read more than 50 scientific studies about yoga. Here's what I learned.* Accessed on 24/4/19 at https://www.vox.com/2015/7/22/9012075/yoga-health-benefits-exercise-science.

19  Bhavanani, Y. (2015) *Are We Practicing Yoga Therapy or Yogopathy?* [LinkedIn SlideShare] Accessed on 14/12/18 at www.slideshare.net/anandabhavanani/ are-we-practicing-yoga-therapy-or-yogopathy.

20  Fronsdal (2008); Gethin, R. M. L. (1998) *The Foundations of Buddhism.* Oxford: Oxford University Press.

21  Travis, J. W. (2004) *Wellness Inventory.* Asheville, NC: Wellness Associates.

22  Travis (2004).

23  White, F. (1998) *The Overview Effect: Space Exploration and Human Evolution.* Reston, VA: American Institute of Aeronautics and Astronautics.

24  Ecker, Ticic and Hulley (2012).

25  Lee (2000).

26  Perls, F. S. (1973) *The Gestalt Approach and Eyewitness to Therapy: Fritz Perls.* Palo Alto, CA: Science and Behaviour Books; Beck, J. S. (2011) *Cognitive Behavior Therapy: Basics and Beyond.* New York, NY: The Guilford Press.

27  Sneed, J. and Hammer, T. (2018) "Phenomenological inquiry into Phoenix Rising yoga therapy." *International Journal of Yoga Therapy 28*, 1, 87–95.

## CHAPTER 12

1   National Institute on Drug Abuse (2015) "Drugs of Abuse: Opioids." Bethesda, MD: National Institute on Drug Abuse. Accessed on 14/12/18 at www. drugabuse.gov/drugs-abuse/opioids.

2   National Institute on Drug Abuse (2015).

3   National Institute on Drug Abuse (2015).

4   National Institute on Drug Abuse (2018) *Principles of Drug Addiction Treatment: A Research-Based Guide.* 3rd edition. Bethesda, MD: National Institute on Drug Abuse. Accessed on 14/12/18 at www.drugabuse.gov/publications/principles-drug-addiction-treatment-research-based-guide-third-edition.

5   National Institute on Drug Abuse (2015).

6   Monnat, S. (2016) *Communities and Banking. Drugs, Death, and Despair in New England.* Boston, MA: Federal Reserve Bank of Boston. Accessed on 14/12/18 at www.bostonfed.org/publications/

communities-and-banking/2016/fall/drugs-death-and-despair-in-new-england.aspx.

7  National Institute on Drug Abuse (2015).

8  The Joint Commission (2017) *The Joint Commission's Pain Standards: Origin and Evolution*. Oakbrook Terrace, IL: The Joint Commission. Accessed on 14/12/18 at www.jointcommission.org/assets/1/6/Pain_Std_History_Web_Version_05122017.pdf.

9  National Institute on Drug Abuse (2015).

10  National Institute on Drug Abuse (2018); Substance Abuse and Mental Health Services Administration (2016) *Office of the Surgeon General (US). Facing Addiction in America: The Surgeon General's Report on Alcohol, Drugs, and Health.* "Chapter 5, Recovery: The Many Paths to Wellness." Accessed on 14/12/18 at www.ncbi.nlm.nih.gov/books/NBK424846.

11  National Institute on Drug Abuse (2015).

12  National Institute on Drug Abuse (2015); National Institute on Drug Abuse (2018); Substance Abuse and Mental Health Services Administration (2016); Center for Disease Control Prevention (2017) "Opioid Overdose: Data." Atlanta, GA: Center for Disease Control Prevention. Accessed on 14/12/18 at www.cdc.gov/drugoverdose/data/overdose.html.

13  National Institute on Drug Abuse (2015).

14  Center for Disease Control Prevention (2016) "Opioid Overdose: Guideline Resources." Atlanta, GA: Center for Disease Control Prevention. Accessed on 14/12/18 at www.cdc.gov/drugoverdose/prescribing/resources.html.

15  Qaseem, A., Wilt, T. J., McLean, R. M. and Forciea, M. A. (2017) "Noninvasive treatment for acute, subacute, and chronic low back pain: A clinical practice guideline from the American College of Physicians." *Annals of Internal Medicine 166*, 7, 514–530.

16  Barnes, P. M., Bloom, B. and Nahin, R. (2017) *CDC National Health Statistics Report #12. Complementary and Alternative Medicine Use Among Adults and Children: United States.* Accessed on 14/12/18 at https://nccih.nih.gov/research/statistics/2007/camsurvey_fs1.htm.

17  Clarke, T.C., Barnes, P.M., Black, L.I., Stussman, B.J. and Nahin, R.L. (2018) "Use of Yoga, Meditation, and Chiropractors Among U.S. Adults Aged 18 and over." *NCHS Data Brief, no 325*. Hyattsville, MD: National Center for Health Statistics.

18  American Society of Addiction Medicine (2011) "Definition of Addiction." Accessed on 14/12/18 at www.asam.org/resources/definition-of-addiction.

19  American Psychiatric Association (2013) *Diagnostic and Statistical Manual of Mental Disorders.* 5th edition. Washington, DC: American Psychiatric Association Publishing.

20  American Psychiatric Association (2013).

21  American Society of Addiction Medicine (2011).

22  Khantzian, E. J. (1997) "The self-medication hypothesis of substance use disorders: A reconsideration and recent applications." *Harvard Review of Psychiatry 4*, 5, 231–244.

23  National Institute on Drug Abuse (2015).

24  Felitti, V., Anda, R., Nordenberg, D. *et al.* (1998) "Relationship of childhood abuse and household dysfunction to many of the leading causes of death in adults: The Adverse Childhood Experiences (ACE) study." *American Journal of Preventative Medicine 14*, 245–258.

25  Dube, S., Felitti, V., Dong, M., Chapman, D., Giles, W. and Anda, R. (2003) "Childhood abuse, neglect, and household dysfunction and risk for illicit drug use: The Adverse Childhood Experiences study." *Pediatrics 3*, 3, 564–572.

26  Douglas, K., Chan, G., Gelernter, J. *et al.* (2010) "Adverse childhood events as risk factors for substance dependence: Partial mediation by mood and anxiety disorders." *Addictive Behaviors 35*, 7–13.

27  Felitti *et al.* (1998); Dube *et al.* (2003); Douglas *et al.* (2010).

28  Chiesa, A. and Serretti, A. (2014) "Are mindfulness-based interventions effective for substance use disorders? A systematic review of the evidence." *Substance Use and Misuse 49*, 492–512.

29  Del Vecchio, P. (2012) "SAMHSA's Working Definition of Recovery, Updated." Accessed on 14/12/18 at https://blog.samhsa.gov/2012/03/23/samhsas-working-definition-of-recovery-updated.

30  Department of Behavioral Health and Intellectual Disability Services (2012) *Recovery/Remission from Substance Use Disorders: An Analysis of Reported Outcomes in 415 Scientific Reports, 1868–2011.* Philadelphia, PA. Accessed on 14/12/18 at www.naadac.org/assets/2416/whitewl2012_recoveryremission_from_substance_abuse_disorders.pdf; Grant, B. F., Goldstein, R. B., Saha, T. D. *et al.* (2015) "Epidemiology of DSM-5 alcohol use disorder: Results from the national epidemiologic survey on alcohol and related conditions III." *JAMA Psychiatry 72*, 8, 757–766.

31  National Institute on Drug Abuse (2018).

32  National Institute on Drug Abuse (2018).

33  National Institute on Drug Abuse (2018).

34  Posadzki, P., Choi, J., Soo Lee, M. and Ernst, E. (2014) "Yoga for addictions: A systematic review of randomized clinical trials." *Focus on Alternative and Complementary Therapies 19*, 1, 1–8.

35  Posadzki *et al.* (2014); Bowen, S., Chawla, N., Collins, S. *et al.* (2009) "Mindfulness-based relapse prevention for substance use disorders: A pilot efficacy trial." *Substance Abuse 30*, 4, 295–305; Hallgren, M., Romberg, K., Bakshi, A. and Andreasson, S. (2014) "Yoga as an adjunct treatment for alcohol dependence: A pilot study." *Complementary Therapies in Medicine 22*, 3, 441–445; Khalsa, S., Khalsa, G., Khalsa, H. and Khalsa, M. (2008) "Evaluation of a residential kundalini yoga lifestyle pilot program for addiction in India." *Journal of Ethnicity in Substance Abuse 7*, 67–69; Kochupillai, V., Kumar P., Sing, D. *et al.* (2005) "Effect of rhythmic breathing (sudarshan kriya and pranayam) on immune functions and tobacco addiction." *Annals of the New York Academy of Sciences 1056*, 242–252; Marefat, M.,

Peymanzad, H. and Alikhajeh, Y. (2011) "The study of the effects of yoga exercise on addicts' depression and anxiety in rehabilitation period." *Procedia Social and Behavioral Sciences 30*, 1494–1498; Vedamurthachar, A., Janakiramaiah, N., Hegde, J. *et al.* (2006) "Antidepressant efficacy and hormonal effects of Sudarshana Kriya yoga (SKY) in alcohol dependent individuals." *Journal of Affective Disorder 94*, 240–253.

36   Khanna, S. and Greeson, J. (2013) "A narrative review of yoga and mindfulness as complementary therapies for addiction." *Complementary Therapies in Medicine 21*, 3, 244–252.

37   Posadzki *et al.* (2014); McIver, S., O'Halloran, P. and McGartland, M. (2009) "Yoga as a treatment for binge eating disorder: A preliminary study." *Complementary Therapies in Medicine 17*, 196–202; Shaffer, H., LaSalvia, T. and Stein, J. (1997) "Comparing Hatha yoga with dynamic group psychotherapy for enhancing methadone maintenance treatment: A randomized clinical trial." *Alternative Therapies 3*, 4, 57–66.

38   Bowen *et al.* (2009).

39   Sarkar, S. and Varshney, M. (2017) "Yoga and substance use disorders: A narrative review." *Asian Journal of Psychiatry 25*, 191–196.

40   Marefat, Peymanzad and Alikhajeh (2011).

41   Center for Disease Control Prevention (2017); Vedamurthachar *et al.* (2006).

42   Vallejo, Z. and Amaro, H. (2009) "Adaptation of mindfulness-based stress reduction program for addiction relapse prevention." *The Humanistic Psychologist 37*, 192–206; Witkiewitz, K. and Marlatt, G. (2004) "Relapse prevention for alcohol and drug problem: That was Zen, this is Tao." *American Psychologist 59*, 4, 224–235.

43   Vallejo and Amaro (2009).

44   Satchidananda, S. (2012) *The Yoga Sutras of Pantajali*. Buckingham, VA: Integral Yoga Publications.

45   Sargeant, W. (2009) *The Bhagavad Gita*. New York, NY: Excelsior Editions.

46   Alcoholics Anonymous (2001) *Alcoholics Anonymous*. 4th edition. New York, NY: A. A. World Services; Plantania, J. (2005) *The 12-Step Restorative Yoga Workbook*. Scotts Valley, CA: Createspace Independent Publishing Platform.

47   Plantania (2005).

48   Plantania (2005).

49   Hallgren *et al.* (2014); Khalsa *et al.* (2008); Shaffer, LaSalvia and Stein (1997); Bock, B., Fava, J., Gaskins, R. *et al.* (2012) "Yoga as a complementary treatment for smoking cessation in women." *Journal of Women's Health 21*, 2, 240–248; Sarkar and Varshney (2017).

50   Sarkar and Varshney (2017).

51   Marefat, Peymanzad and Alikhajeh (2011); Sarkar and Varshney (2017); Bharshankar, J., Mandape, A., Phatak, M. and Bharshankar, R. (2015) "Autonomic functions in raja-yoga meditators." *Indian Journal of Physiological Pharmacology 59*, 396–401.

52   Chiesa and Serretti (2014).

53   Kabat-Zinn, J. (2003) "Mindfulness-based interventions in context: Past, present and future." *Clinical Psychology: Science and Practice 10*, 2, 144–156. See also Black, D. (2014) "Mindfulness-based interventions: An antidote to suffering in the context of substance use, misuse, and addiction." *Substance Use and Misuse 49*, 487–491; Carlson, B. and Larkin, H. (2009) "Meditation as coping intervention for treatment of addiction." *Journal of Religion and Spirituality in Social Work: Social Thought 28*, 379–392.

54   Carlson and Larkin (2009).

55   Carlson and Larkin (2009).

56   Carlson and Larkin (2009).

57   Carlson and Larkin (2009); Larimer, M., Palmer, R. and Marlatt, A. (1999) "Relapse prevention: An overview of Marlatt's cognitive-behavioral model." *Alcohol, Research and Health 23*, 151–160; Witkiewitz, K., Marlatt, G. and Walker, D. (2005) "Mindfulness-based relapse prevention for alcohol and substance use disorders." *Journal of Cognitive Psychotherapy: An International Quarterly 19*, 3, 211–228.

58   Sarkar and Varshney (2017).

59   Witkiewitz, Marlatt and Walker (2005); Vallejo and Amaro (2009); Witkiewitz and Marlatt (2004).

60   Garland, E. (2013) *Mindfulness-Oriented Recovery Enhancement for Addiction, Stress, and Pain*. Washington, DC: NASW Press.

61   Tovio by Advocacy Unlimited (n.d.) "Cultivate Mind, Body, Spirit." Accessed on 14/12/18 at http://toivocenter.org.

## Chapter 13

1   Sausys, A. (2014) *Yoga for Grief Relief: Simple Practices for Transforming Your Grieving Mind and Body*. Oakland, CA: New Harbinger Publications.

2   IASP (2017) "IASP Terminology." Accessed on 14/1/19 at www.iasp-pain.org/terminology?navItemNumber=576.

3   Boss, P. (1999) *Ambiguous Loss: Learning to Live with Unresolved Grief*. Cambridge, MA: Harvard University Press.

4   Lunche, H. J. (1999) *Understanding Grief: A Guide for the Bereaved*. Berkeley, CA: SVL Press.

5   Worden, J. W. (2009) *Grief Counseling and Grief Therapy: A Handbook for the Mental Health Practitioner*. 4th edition. New York, NY: Springer Publishing Co.

6   Cardoso, A., Arias-Carrion, O., Paes, F. *et al.* (2014) "Neurological aspects of grief." *CNS & Neurological Disorders: Drug Targets (Formerly Current Drug Targets: CNS & Neurological Disorders) 13*, 930–936.

7   Erickson, K. I., Gildengers, A. G. and Butters, M. A. (2013) "Physical activity and brain plasticity in late

adulthood." *Dialogues in Clinical Neuroscience 15*, 1, 99–108.

8   Davidson, R. (2012) *The Emotional Life of Your Brain: How Its Unique Patterns Affect the Way You Think, Feel, and Live—and How You Can Change Them.* New York, NY: Hudson Street Press.

9   Sausys (2014).

10  Worden (2009).

11  Worden (2009), p.44.

12  Tennant, F. (2013) "The physiologic effects of pain on the endocrine system." *Pain and Therapy 2*, 2, 75–86.

13  Satyananda, Swami (2008) *Asana Pranayama Mudra Bandha.* Munger: Bihar School of Yoga.

14  Sausys (2014).

15  Satyananda, Swami (1976) *Four Chapters on Freedom.* Bihar: Yoga Publications Trust.

16  Sausys (2014).

17  Worden (2009).

## Chapter 14

1   Arman, M. and Hok, J. (2016) "Self-care follows from compassionate care: Chronic pain patients' experience of integrative rehabilitation." *Scandinavian Journal of Caring Sciences 30*, 374–381; Frampton, S. B., Guastello, S. and Lepore, M. (2013) "Compassion at the foundation of patient-centered care: The importance of compassion in action." *Journal of Comparative Effectiveness Research 2*, 5, 443–455; Sirois, F. M. and Rowse, G. (2016) "The role of self-compassion in chronic illness care." *Journal of Clinical Outcome Management 23*, 11, 521–527.

2   Goetz, J. L., Keltner, D. and Simon-Thomas, E. (2010) "Compassion: An evolutionary analysis and empirical review." *Psychological Bulletin 136*, 3, 351–374; Gilbert, P. and Mascaro, J. (2017) "Compassion Fears, Blocks and Resistances: An Evolutionary Investigation." In: E. M. Seppala, E. Simon-Thomas, S. L. Brown, M. C. Worline, C. D. Cameron and J. R. Doty (eds) *The Oxford Handbook of Compassion Science.* New York, NY: Oxford University Press. 399–418; Goetz, J. L. and Simon-Thomas, E. (2017) "The Landscape of Compassion: Definitions and Scientific Approaches." In: E. M. Seppala, E. Simon-Thomas, S. L. Brown, M. C. Worline, C. D. Cameron and J. R. Doty (eds) *The Oxford Handbook of Compassion Science.* New York, NY: Oxford University Press. 3–15; Brown, S. L. and Brown, R. M. (2017) "Compassionate Neurobiology and Health." In: E. M. Seppala, E. Simon-Thomas, S. L. Brown, M. C. Worline, C. D. Cameron and J. R. Doty (eds) *The Oxford Handbook of Compassion Science.* New York, NY: Oxford University Press. 159–172; Carter, C. S., Bartal, I. B. and Porges, E. C. (2017) "The Roots of Compassion: An Evolutionary and Neurobiological Perspective." In: E. M. Seppala, E. Simon-Thomas, S. L. Brown, M. C. Worline, C. D. Cameron and J. R. Doty (eds) *The Oxford Handbook of Compassion Science.* New York, NY: Oxford University Press. 173–187; Seppala, E. M., Hutcherson, C. A., Nguyen, D. T. H., Doty, J. R. and Gross, J. J. (2014) "Loving-kindness meditation: A tool to improve healthcare provider compassion, resilience, and patient care." *Journal of Compassionate Health Care 1*, 5; Neumann, M., Edelhauser, F., Tauschel, D. *et al.* (2011) "Empathy decline and its reasons: A systematic review of studies with medical students and residents." *Academic Medicine 86*, 996–1009;

Nunes, P., Williams, S., Sa, B. and Stevenson, K. (2011) "A study of empathy decline in students from five health disciplines during their first year of training." *International Journal of Medical Education 2*, 12–17; Piff, P. K. and Moskowitz, J. P. (2017) "The Class-Compassion Gap: How Socioeconomic Factors Influence Compassion." In: E. M. Seppala, E. Simon-Thomas, S. L. Brown, M. C. Worline, C. D. Cameron and J. R. Doty (eds) *The Oxford Handbook of Compassion Science.* New York, NY: Oxford University Press. 317–330; Conway, C. C. and Slavich, G. M. (2017) "Behavior Genetics of Prosocial Behavior." In: P. Gilbert (ed.) *Compassion: Concepts, Research and Applications.* London: Routledge. 151–170; Vitaliano, P. P., Zhang, J. and Scanlan, J. M. (2003) "Is care-giving hazardous to one's health? A meta-analysis." *Psychological Bulletin 129*, 946–972; Plante, T. G. (ed.) (2015) *The Psychology of Compassion and Cruelty: Understanding the Emotional, Spiritual, and Religious Influences.* Santa Barbara, CA: Praeger; Shea, S. and Lionis, C. (2017) "The Call for Compassion In Health Care." In: E. M. Seppala, E. Simon-Thomas, S. L. Brown, M. C. Worline, C. D. Cameron and J. R. Doty (eds) *The Oxford Handbook of Compassion Science.* New York, NY: Oxford University Press. 457–473; Porges, S. W. (2017) "Vagal Pathways: Portals to Compassion." In: E. M. Seppala, E. Simon-Thomas, S. L. Brown, M. C. Worline, C. D. Cameron and J. R. Doty (eds) *The Oxford Handbook of Compassion Science.* New York, NY: Oxford University Press. 189–202.

3   Shea, S., Wynyard, R., West, E. and Lionis, C. (2011) "Reaching a consensus in defining and moving forward with the science and art of compassion in healthcare." *Journal of Holistic Health Care 8*, 58–60; Keogh, B. (2013) *Review into the Quality of Care and Treatment Provided by 14 Hospital Trusts in England: Overview Report.* London: NHS; NHS Confederation (2008) *Futures Debate: Compassion in Healthcare: The Missing Dimension of Healthcare Reform?* Accessed on 14/12/18 at www.nhsconfed.org/~/media/Confederation/Files/Publications/Documents/compassion_healthcare_future08.pdf; Nauert, R. (2015) "Compassion missing in American health care." *Psych Central.* Accessed on 14/12/18 at https://psychcentral.com/news/2011/09/09/compassion-missing-in-american-health-care/29295.html; Crowther, J.,

Wilson, K. C. M., Horton, S. and Lloyd-Williams, M. (2013) "Compassion in healthcare: Lessons from a qualitative study of the end of life care of people with dementia." *Journal of the Royal Society of Medicine 106*, 12, 492–497; Lown, B. A., Rosen, J. and Marttila, J. (2011) "An agenda for improving compassionate care: A survey shows about half of patients say such care is missing." *Health Affairs (Millwood) 9*, 1772–1778; Twenge, J. M., Campbell, W. K. and Freeman, E. C. (2012) "Generational differences in young adults' life goals, concern for others, and civic orientation, 1966–2009." *Journal of Personality and Social Psychology 102*, 5, 1045–1062; Zarins, S. and Konrath, S. (2017) "Changes over Time in Compassion-Related Variables in the United States." In: E. M. Seppala, E. Simon-Thomas, S. L. Brown, M. C. Worline, C. D. Cameron and J. R. Doty (eds) *The Oxford Handbook of Compassion Science*. New York, NY: Oxford University Press. 331–352.

4   Seppala, E. M., Simon-Thomas, E., Brown, S. L., Worline, M. C., Cameron, C. D. and Doty, J. R. (eds) (2017) *The Oxford Handbook of Compassion Science*. New York, NY: Oxford University Press.

5   Goetz, Keltner and Simon-Thomas (2010).

6   Gilbert, P. (2017) "Compassion: Definitions and Controversies." In: P. Gilbert (ed.) *Compassion, Concepts, Research and Applications*. London: Routledge. 3–15; Gilbert, P. and Choden, P. (2014) *Mindful Compassion*. Oakland, CA: New Harbinger.

7   Neff, K. and Germer, C. (2017) "Self-Compassion and Psychological Well-Being." In: E. M. Seppala, E. Simon-Thomas, S. L. Brown, M. C. Worline, C. D. Cameron and J. R. Doty (eds) *The Oxford Handbook of Compassion Science*. New York, NY: Oxford University Press. 371–385.

8   Neff, K. D. (2003) "Self-compassion: An alternative conceptualization of a healthy attitude toward oneself." *Self and Identity 2*, 85–102.

9   Neff, K. and Brown, B. (2017) *Module 2: Self-Compassion with Kristin Neff and Brene Brown*. Courageworks online course. Accessed on 14/12/18 at https://catalog.pesi.com/sales/bh_001195_brenebrown_organic-15321.

10  Breines, J. G. and Chen, S. (2012) "Self-compassion increases self-improvement motivation." *Personality and Social Psychology Bulletin 38*, 9, 1133–1143; Neff, K. D., Hsieh, Y. and Dejitterat, K. (2005) "Self-compassion, achievement goals, and coping with academic failure. *Self and Identity 4*, 3, 263–287; Neely, M. E., Schallert, D. L., Mohammed, S. S., Roberts, R. M. and Chen, Y. (2009) "Self-kindness when facing stress: The role of self-compassion, goal regulation, and support in college students' well-being." *Motivation and Emotion 33*, 88–97; Williams, J. G., Stark, S. K. and Foster, E. E. (2008) "Start today or the very last day? The relationships among self-compassion, motivation, and procrastination." *American Journal of Psychological Research 4*, 37–44; Sirois, F. M. (2014) "Procrastination and stress: Exploring the role of self-compassion." *Self Identity 13*, 128–145.

11  Neff and Germer (2017).

12  Strauss, C., Lever Taylor, B., Gu, J., Kuyken, W., Baer, R., Jones, F. and Cavanagh, K. (2016) "What is compassion and how can we measure it? A review of definitions and measures." *Clinical Psychology Review 47*, 15–27.

13  Strauss *et al.* (2016).

14  Frampton, Guastello and Lepore (2013); Seppala *et al.* (2014); Shea and Lionis (2017); Hojat, M. (2009) "Ten approaches for enhancing empathy in health and human services cultures." *Journal of the Health and Human Services Administration 31*, 4, 412–450; Fotaki, M. (2015) "Why and how is compassion necessary to provide good quality healthcare?" *International Journal of Health Policy Management 4*, 4, 199–201; Fogarty, L. A., Curbow, B. A., Wingard, J. R., McDonnell, K. and Somerfield, M. R. (1999) "Can 40 seconds of compassion reduce patient anxiety?" *Journal of Clinical Oncology 17*, 1, 371–379; Shaltout, H. A., Tooze, J. A., Rosenberger, M. A. and Kemper, K. J. (2012) "Time, touch, and compassion: Effects on autonomic nervous system and well-being." *Explore 8*, 3, 177–184; Ackerman, S. J. and Hilsenroth, M. J. (2003) "A review of psychotherapist characteristics and techniques positively impacting on the therapeutic alliance." *Clinical Psychology Review 23*, 1, 1–33; Hardy, G., Cahill, J. and Barkham, M. (2007) "Active Ingredients of the Therapeutic Relationship That Promote Client Change: A Research Perspective." In: P. Gilbert and R. L. Leahy (eds) *The Therapeutic Relationship in the Cognitive and Behavioral Psychotherapies*. Hove: Routledge. 24–42; Klimecki, O. and Singer, T. (2011) "Empathic Distress Rather Than Compassion Fatigue? Integrating Findings from Empathy Research in Psychology and Social Neuroscience." In: B. Oakley. A. Knafo, G. Madhavan and D. S. Wilson (eds) *Pathological Altruism*. New York, NY: Oxford University Press. 368–383; Boellinghaus, I., Jones, F. W. and Hutton, J. (2014) "The role of mindfulness and loving-kindness meditation in cultivating self-compassion and other-focused concern in health care professionals." *Mindfulness 5*, 2, 129–138.

15  Seppala, E., Rossomando, T. and Doty, J. R. (2013) "Social connection and compassion: Important predictors of health and well-being." *Social Research 80*, 2, 411; Konrath, S. and Brown, S. (2013) "The Effects of Giving on Givers." In: N. Roberts and M. Newman (eds) *Handbook of Health and Social Relationships*. Washington, DC: American Psychological Association; Brown, S. L., Nesse, R. M., Vinokur, A. D. and Smith, D. M. (2003) "Providing social support may be more beneficial than receiving it: Results from a prospective study of mortality." *Psychological Science 14*, 320–327; Cosley, B. J., McCoy, S. K., Saslow, L. R. and Epel, E. S. (2010) "Is compassion for others stress buffering? Consequences of compassion and social support

for physiological reactivity to stress." *Journal of Experimental Social Psychology 46*, 816–823; Raposa, E. B., Laws, H. B. and Ansell, E. B. (2016) "Prosocial behavior mitigates the negative effects of stress in everyday life." *Clinical Psychological Science 4*, 4, 691–698.

16 Goetz, Keltner and Simon-Thomas (2010); Gilbert and Mascaro (2017); Goetz and Simon-Thomas (2017); Brown and Brown (2017); Carter, Bartal and Porges (2017); Neumann *et al.* (2011); Nunes *et al.* (2011); Piff and Moskowitz (2017); Conway and Slavich (2017); Vitaliano, Zhang and Scanlan (2003); Plante (2015); Shea and Lionis (2017); Porges (2017).

17 Gilbert and Mascaro (2017).

18 Shea and Lionis (2017); Keogh (2013); Nauert (2015); Crowther *et al.* (2013); Crawford, P., Brown, B., Kvangarsnes, M. and Gilbert, P. (2014) "The design of compassionate care." *Journal of Clinical Nursing 23*, 23–24, 3587–3599.

19 Institute of Medicine (2001) *Crossing the Quality Chasm: A New Health System for the 21st Century.* Washington, DC: National Academy Press.

20 Frampton, Guastello and Lepore (2013); Shea and Lionis (2017).

21 Arman and Hok (2016), p.380.

22 Shea and Lionis (2017); Crawford *et al.* (2014); Brown, B., Crawford, P., Gilbert, P., Gilbert, J. and Gale, C. (2014) "Practical compassions: Repertoires of practice and compassion talk in acute mental healthcare." *Sociology of Health and Illness 36*, 383–399.

23 Seppala *et al.* (2014); Boellinghaus, Jones and Hutton (2014); Klimecki, O. M., Leiberg, S., Ricard, M. and Singer, T. (2014) "Differential pattern of functional brain plasticity after compassion and empathy training." *Social Cognitive and Affective Neuroscience 9*, 6, 873–879; Condon, P. and DeSteno, D. (2017) "Enhancing Compassion: Social Psychological Perspectives." In: E. M. Seppala, E. Simon-Thomas, S. L. Brown, M. C. Worline, C. D. Cameron and J. R. Doty (eds) *The Oxford Handbook of Compassion Science.* New York, NY: Oxford University Press. 287–298; Condon, P., Desbordes, G., Miller, W. B. and DeSteno, D. (2013) "Meditation increases compassionate responses to suffering." *Psychological Science 24*, 2125–2127; Lutz, A., Brefczynski-Lewis, J., Johnstone, T. and Davidson, R. J. (2008) "Regulation of the neural circuitry of emotion by compassion meditation: Effects of meditative expertise." *PLoS One 3*, 3, e1897; Mascaro, J. S., Rilling, J. K., Tenzin Negi, L. and Raison, C. L. (2013) "Compassion meditation enhances empathic accuracy and related neural activity." *Social Cognitive and Affective Neuroscience 8*, 48–55.

24 Klimecki, O. M., Leigberg, S., Lamm, C. and Singer, T. (2013) "Functional neural plasticity and associated changes in positive affect after compassion training." *Cerebral Cortex 23*, 7, 1552–1561; Weng, H. Y., Fox, A. S., Shackman, A. J. *et al.*

(2013) "Compassion training alters altruism and neural responses to suffering." *Psychological Science 24*, 7, 1171–1180; Jazaieri, H., McGonigal, K., Jinpa, T., Doty, J. R., Gross, J. J. and Goldin, P. R. (2014) "A randomized controlled trial of compassion cultivation training: Effects on mindfulness, affect, and emotion regulation." *Motivation and Emotion 38*, 1, 23–25.

25 Singer, T. and Bolz, M. (eds) (2013) *Compassion: Bridging Practice and Science.* Munich: Max Planck Society. Accessed on 14/12/18 at www.compassion-training.org.

26 Seppala *et al.* (2017).

27 Salzberg, S. (1995) *Loving-Kindness: The Revolutionary Art of Happiness.* Boston, MA: Shambhala Publications.

28 Seppala *et al.* (2014), p.1.

29 Halifax, J. (2012) "A heuristic model of enactive compassion." *Current Opinion in Supportive and Palliative Care 6*, 228–235.

30 Halifax (2012).

31 Halifax (2012); Halifax, J. (2013) "Understanding and Cultivating Compassion in Clinical Settings." In: T. Singer and M. Bolz (eds) *Compassion: Bridging Practice and Science.* Munich: Max Planck Society. 208–226; 467–478.

32 Ortner, C. N. M., Kilner, S. J. and Zelazo, P. D. (2007) "Mindfulness meditation and reduced emotional interference on a cognitive task." *Motivation and Emotion 31*, 4, 271–283.

33 Zeidan, F., Johnson, S. K., Diamond, B. J., David, Z. and Goolkasian, P. (2010) "Mindfulness meditation improves cognition: Evidence of brief mental training." *Consciousness and Cognition 19*, 2, 597–605; MacLean, K. A., Ferrer, E., Aichele, S. R. *et al.* (2010) "Intensive meditation training improves perceptual discrimination and sustained attention." *Psychological Science 21*, 6, 829–839.

34 Halifax (2012).

35 Fredrickson, B. L. and Branigan, C. (2003) "Positive emotions broaden the scope of attention and thought-action repertoires." *Cognition and Emotion 19*, 3, 313–332.

36 Seppala *et al.* (2014); Boellinghaus, Jones and Hutton (2014).

37 Singer, T., Critchley, H. D. and Preuschoff, K. (2009) "A common role of insula in feelings, empathy and uncertainty." *Trends in Cognitive Science 13*, 334–340; Fukushima, H., Terasawa, Y. and Umeda, S. (2011) "Association between interoception and empathy: Evidence from heartbeat-evoked brain potential." *Int J Psychophysiol 79*, 259–265; Panksepp, J. (2006) "The Core Emotional Systems of the Mammalian Brain: The Fundamental Substrates of Human Emotions." In: J. Corrigall, H. Payne and H. Wilkinson (eds) *About a Body: Working with the Embodied Mind in Psychotherapy.* Hove and New York, NY: Routledge; Singer, T. (2012) "The past, present and future of social neuroscience: A European perspective." *NeuroImage 61*, 2, 437–449; Bornemann, B. and Singer, T. (2013) "A Cognitive

Neuroscience Perspective: The ReSource Model of Compassion." In: T. Singer and M. Bolz (eds) *Compassion: Bridging Practice and Science*. Munich: Max Planck Society. 178–191; Craig, A. D. (2003) "Interoception: The sense of the physiological condition of the body." *Current Opinion in Neurobiology 13*, 4, 500–505.

38  Jha, A. P., Stanley, E. A., Kiyonaga, A., Wong, L. M. and Gelfand, L. (2010) "Examining the protective effects of mindfulness training on working memory capacity and affective experience." *Emotion 10*, 54–64.

39  Goetz, Keltner and Simon-Thomas (2010).

40  Halifax (2013); Schmidt, S. (2004) "Mindfulness and healing intention: Concepts, practice, and research evaluation." *J Alternat Complement Med 10*, 7–14.

41  Halifax (2012).

42  Taylor, M. J. (2016) *Yoga Therapy as a Creative Inquiry into Suffering*. Keynote presentation at Symposium on Yoga Therapy and Research, June 10.

43  Halifax (2012); Lamm, C., Batson, C. D. and Decety, J. (2007) "The neural substrate of human empathy: Effects of perspective-taking and cognitive appraisal." *Journal of Cognitive Neuroscience 19*, 42–58; Silvia, P. J. (2002) "Self-awareness and emotional intensity." *Cognition and Emotion 16*, 195–216.

44  Gilbert and Mascaro (2017), p.403; Gilbert and Choden (2014); Singer and Bolz (2013).

45  Taylor (2018).

46  Singer, Critchley and Preuschoff (2009); Fukushima, Terasawa and Umeda (2011); Panksepp (2006); Singer (2012); Bornemann and Singer (2013); Craig (2003).

47  Devi, N.J. (2007) *The Secret Power of Yoga; A Woman's Guide to the Heart and Spirit of the Yoga Sutras*. New York: Three Rivers Press, p.180.

48  Mate, G. (2017) *Compassionate Inquiry*. Lecture, Scotia Bank Theatre, Edmonton, AB.

49  Porges (2017), p.190.

50  Porges (2017), p.191.

51  Gilbert and Mascaro (2017), p.403.

52  Halifax (2013).

53  Halifax (2012).

54  Pearson, N. (n.d.) *Breathing Techniques for People in Pain*. [Audio CD] Accessed on 14/12/18 at https://paincareu.com/shop/page/2.

55  Seppala *et al.* (2014).

56  Taylor (2016).

57  Taylor (2018).

58  Halifax (2013).

59  Sargeant, W. and Chapple, C. K. (eds) (1984) *The Bhagavad Gita*. Revised edition. Albany, NY: State University of New York Press.

60  Satchidananda, Sri Swami (1990) *The Yoga Sutras of Patanjali*. Buckingham, VA: Integral Yoga Publications.

61  Easwaran, E. (2007) *The Upanishads*. 2nd edition. Berkeley, CA: Nilgiri Press.

62  Satchidananda (1990).

63  Satchidananda (1990).

64  Satchidananda (1990).

65  Satchidananda (1990).

66  Stryker, R. (2011) *The Four Desires: Creating a Life of Purpose, Happiness, Prosperity, and Freedom*. New York, NY: Delacorte Press.

67  Busia, K. (2010) *The Yoga Sutras of Patanjali*. Accessed on 14/12/18 at www.kofibusia.com/yogasutras/yogasutras3.php.

68  Sargeant and Chapple (1984).

69  Purdie, F. and Morley, S. (2016) "Compassion and chronic pain." *Pain 157*, 12, 2625–2627; Chapin, H. L., Darnall, B. D., Seppala, E. M., Doty, J. R., Hah, J. M. and Mackey, S. C. (2014) "Pilot study of a compassion meditation intervention in chronic pain." *Journal of Compassionate Health Care 1*, 4, 1–12; Okifuji, A., Turk, D. C. and Curran, S. L. (1999) "Anger in chronic pain: Investigations of anger targets and intensity." *Journal of Psychosomatic Research 47*, 1–12; Dow, C. M., Roche, P. A. and Ziebland, S. (2012) "Talk of frustration in the narratives of people with chronic pain." *Chronic Illness 8*, 3, 176–191; Rudich, Z., Lerman, S. F., Gurevich, B., Weksler, N. and Shahar, G. (2008) "Patients' self-criticism is a stronger predictor of physician's evaluation of prognosis than pain diagnosis or severity in chronic pain patients." *Journal of Pain 9*, 3, 210–216; Lumley, M. A., Cohen, J. L., Borszcz, G. S. *et al.* (2011) "Pain and emotion: A biopsychosocial review of recent research." *Journal of Clinical Psychology 67*, 9, 942–968; Neff, K. D. (2003) "The development and validation of a scale to measure self-compassion." *Self Identity 2*, 3, 223–250.

70  Neff and Germer (2017); Neff, Hsieh and Dejitterat (2005); Sirois (2014); Neff (2003); Neff, K. D., Rude, S. S. and Kirkpatrick, K. L. (2007) "An examination of self-compassion in relation to positive psychology functioning and personality traits." *Journal of Research in Personality 41*, 4, 908–916. Breines, J. G., Thoma, M. V., Gianferante, D., Hanlin, L., Chen, X. and Rohleder, N. (2014) "Self-compassion as a predictor of interleukin-6 response to acute psychosocial stress." *Brain, Behavior, and Immunity 37*, 109–114.

71  Wren, A. A., Somers, T. J., Wright, M. A. *et al.* (2012) "Self-compassion in patients with persistent musculoskeletal pain: Relationship of self-compassion to adjustment to persistent pain." *Journal of Pain and Symptom Management 43*, 4, 759–770.

72  Purdie, F. and Morley, S. (2015) "Self-compassion, pain and breaking a social contract." *Pain 156*, 11, 2354–2363, p.2354.

73  Costa, J. and Pinto-Gouveia, J. (2011) "Acceptance of pain, self-compassion and psychopathology: Using the chronic pain acceptance questionnaire to identify patients' subgroups." *Clinical Psychology and Psychotherapy 18*, 4, 292–302.

74  Costa and Pinto-Gouveia (2011); Vowles, K., McNeil, D., Gross, R., McDaniel, M. and Mouse, A. (2007) "Effects of pain acceptance and pain control strategies on physical impairment in individuals

with chronic low back pain." *Behavior Therapy 38*, 412–425. McCracken, L. (1998) "Learning to live with pain: Acceptance of pain predicts adjustments in persons with chronic pain." *Pain 74*, 21–27. McCracken, L. (1999) "Behavioral constituents of chronic pain acceptance: Results from factor analysis of the Chronic Pain Acceptance Questionnaire." *Journal of Back Musculoskeletal Rehabilitation 13*, 93–100; McCracken, L. and Eccleston, C. (2005) "A prospective study of acceptance of pain and patient functioning with chronic pain." *Pain 118*, 164–169; Viane, I., Crombez, G., Eccleston, C. *et al.* (2003) "Acceptance of pain in an independent predictor of mental well-being in patients with chronic pain: Empirical evidence and reappraisal." *Pain 106*, 65–72.

75 Zeidan, F., Martucci, K. T., Kraft, R. A., Gordon, N. S., McHaffie, J. G. and Coghill, R. C. (2011) "Brain mechanisms supporting the modulation of pain by mindfulness meditation." *Journal of Neuroscience 31*, 14, 5540–5548; Zeidan, F., Emerson, N. M., Farris, S. R. *et al.* (2015) "Mindfulness meditation-based pain relief employs different neural mechanisms than placebo and sham mindfulness meditation-induced analgesia." *Journal of Neuroscience 35*, 46, 15307–15325; Zeidan, F., Adler-Neal, A. L., Wells, R. E. *et al.* (2016) "Mindfulness-meditation-based pain relief is not mediated by endogenous opioids." *Journal of Neuroscience 36*, 11, 3391–3397.

76 Chapin *et al.* (2014).

77 Carson, J. W., Keefe, F. J., Lynch, T. R. *et al.* (2005) "Loving-kindness meditation for chronic low back pain: Results from a pilot trial." *J Holist Nurs 23*, 287–304.

78 Lutz *et al.* (2008); Klimecki, O. M., Leigberg, S., Lamm, C. and Singer, T. (2013) "Functional neural plasticity and associated changes in positive affect after compassion training." *Cerebral Cortex 23*, 7, 1552–1561; Grant, J. A. (2013) "Being with Pain: A Discussion of Meditation-Based Analgesia." In: T. Singer and M. Bolz (eds) *Compassion: Bridging Practice and Science.* Munich: Max Planck Society. 252–269.

79 Klimecki *et al.* (2014); Klimecki *et al.* (2013); Klimecki, O. M. and Singer, T. (2017) "The Compassionate Brain." In: E. M. Seppala, E. Simon-Thomas, S. L. Brown, M. C. Worline, C. D. Cameron and J. R. Doty (eds) *The Oxford Handbook of Compassion Science.* New York, NY: Oxford University Press. 109–120; Engen, H. G. and Singer, T. (2015) "Compassion-based emotion regulation up-regulates experienced positive affect and associated neural networks." *Social Cognitive and Affective Neuroscience 10*, 9, 1291–1301.

80 Sirois and Rowse (2016); Purdie and Morley (2016); Fosam, H. (2016) "Compassion and chronic pain." Accessed on 14/12/18 at www.clinicalpainadvisor. com/chronic-pain/compassionchronic-painempathy/article/579587.

81 Belton, J. (2019) Email correspondence.

82 Belton (2019).

83 Neff (2003).

84 Pearson (n.d.).

85 Kriyananda, G. (1997–2009) *Oral Teachings 1997–2009.*

86 Le Page, J. and Le Page, L. (2013) *Mudras for Healing and Transformation.* Pennsauken, NJ: BookBaby.

87 Seppala *et al.* (2014); Boellinghaus, Jones and Hutton (2014).

88 Boellinghaus, Jones and Hutton (2014); Neff, K. D. and Pommier, E. (2013) "The relationship between self-compassion and other-focused concern among college undergraduates, community adults, and practicing meditators." *Self and Identity 12*, 2, 160–176.

89 Seppala *et al.* (2014); Neff and Brown (2017).

90 Shea and Lionis (2017).

91 Porges (2017).

92 Neff and Germer (2017), p.379, p.381.

93 Hutton (2014).

94 Seppala *et al.* (2014).

95 Shapiro, S. L., Astin, J. A., Bishop, S. R. and Cordova, M. (2005) "Mindfulness-based stress reduction for health care professionals: Results from a randomized trial." *International Journal of Stress Management 12*, 164–176.

96 Neff, K. D. and Germer, C. K. (2013) "A pilot study and randomized controlled trial of the mindful self-compassion program." *Journal of Clinical Psychology 69*, 1, 28–44.

97 Neff (2003).

98 Pearson, L. (2016) "The Resurrection Breath. Advanced Pain Care Yoga Training." In: *Oral Teachings of Goswami Kriyananda 1997–2009.*

99 Pearson (2016).

100 Salzberg (1995).

101 Figley, C. R. and Figley, K. R. (2017) "Compassion Fatigue Resilience." In: E. M. Seppala, E. Simon-Thomas, S. L. Brown, M. C. Worline, C. D. Cameron and J. R. Doty (eds) *The Oxford Handbook of Compassion Science.* New York, NY: Oxford University Press. 387–397.

102 Klimecki and Singer (2011).

103 Klimecki and Singer (2011); Brown *et al.* (2014); Klimecki *et al.* (2014); Klimecki and Singer (2017); Singer, T. and Klimecki, O. M. (2014) "Empathy and compassion." *Current Biology 24*, 18, R875–R878.

104 Singer and Klimecki (2014) "Empathy and compassion." *Current Biology 24*, 18, R875–R878; Klimecki, O. M. and Singer, T. (2013) "Empathy from the Perspective of Social Neuroscience." In: J. Armony and P. Vuilleumier (eds) *Handbook of Human Affective Neuroscience.* New York, NY: Cambridge University Press. 533–549; Davis, M. H. (1983) "Measuring individual differences in empathy: Evidence for a multidimensional approach." *Journal of Personality and Social Psychology 44*, 1, 113–126.

105 Davis (1983).

106 Gilbert and Mascaro (2017).

107 Goetz, Keltner and Simon-Thomas (2010).

108 Zaki, J. and Cikara, M. (2015) "Addressing empathic failures." *Current Direction in Psychological Science* 24, 6, 471–476.

109 Goetz and Simon-Thomas (2017); Loewenstein, G. and Small, D. A. (2007) "The scarecrow and the tin man: The vicissitudes of human sympathy and caring." *Review of General Psychology 11*, 2, 112–126.

110 Klimecki *et al.* (2014); Klimecki *et al.* (2013); Engen and Singer (2015); Corradi-Dell'Acqua, C., Hofstetter, C. and Vuilleumeir, P. (2011) "Felt and seen pain evoke the same local patterns of cortical activity in insular and cingulate cortex." *Journal of Neuroscience: The Official Journal of the Society for Neuroscience 31*, 49; Lamm, C., Decety, J. and Singer, T. (2011) "Meta-analysis evidence for common and distinct neural networks associated with directly experienced pain and empathy for pain." *NeuroImage 54*, 3, 2492–2505; Klimecki, O., Ricard, M. and Singer, T. (2013) "Empathy vs Compassion: Lessons from 1st and 3rd Persons Methods." In: T. Singer and M. Bolz (eds) *Compassion: Bridging*

*Practice and Science.* Munich: Max Planck Society. 272–278.

111 Klimecki and Singer (2017), p.116.

112 Klimecki, Ricard and Singer (2013), p.272.

113 Seppala *et al.* (2014).

114 Klimecki and Singer (2011).

115 Gilbert, P., Catarino, F., Duarte, C. *et al.* (2017) "The development of compassionate engagement and action scales for self and others." *Journal of Compassionate Health Care 4*, 4.

116 Shea and Lionis (2017).

117 Maturana, H. (2013) In: P. Senge (2013) *Systems Thinking and the Gap Between Aspirations and Performance.* Keynote Presentation at Garrison Institute October 13. Accessed on 14/12/18 at www.youtube.com/watch?v=_PFo7zdiw34.

118 Belton, J. (2015) "Permission to Exit the Holding Pattern of Pain and Uncertainty." Accessed on 14/1/19 at www.mycuppajo.com/pain-and-uncertainty.

## Chapter 15

1 Edwards, I., Jones, M., Thacker, M. and Swisher, L. L. (2014) "The moral experience of the patient with chronic pain: Bridging the gap between first and third person ethics." *Pain Med 15*, 3, 364–378; Dezutter, J., Luyckx, K. and Wachholtz, A. (2015) "Meaning in life in chronic pain patients over time: Associations with pain experience and psychological well-being." *Journal of Behavioral Medicine 38*, 2, 384–396; Dezutter, J., Casalin, S., Wachholtz, A., Luyckx, K., Hekking, J. and Vandewiele, W. (2013) "Meaning in life: An important factor for the psychological well-being of chronically ill patients?" *Rehabilitation Psychology 58*, 4, 334–341.

2 Edwards *et al.* (2014).

3 Edwards *et al.* (2014).

4 Edwards *et al.* (2014).

5 Edwards *et al.* (2014).

6 Edwards *et al.* (2014).

7 Edwards *et al.* (2014).

8 Edwards *et al.* (2014).

9 Cacioppo, J. T. and Cacioppo, S. (2014) "Social relationships and health: The toxic effects of perceived social isolation: social relationships and health." *Social Personal Psychology Compass 8, 2,* 58–72; Cacioppo, J. T., Hawkley, L. C., Norman, G. J. and Berntson, G. G. (2011) "Social isolation." *Annals of the New York Academy of Science 1231*, 1, 17–22; Ong, A. D., Uchino, B. N. and Wethington, E. (2016) "Loneliness and health in older adults: A mini-review and synthesis." *Gerontology 62*, 4, 443–449.

10 Cacioppo and Cacioppo (2014); Cacioppo *et al.* (2011); Ong, Uchino and Wethington (2016).

11 Cacioppo and Cacioppo (2014); Ong, Uchino and Wethington (2016).

12 Cacioppo *et al.* (2011); Ryan, R. M. and Deci, E. L. (2001) "On happiness and human potentials: A

review of research on hedonic and eudaimonic well-being." *Annual Review of Psychology 52*, 1, 141–166.

13 Cacioppo and Cacioppo (2014); Cacioppo *et al.* (2011); Ong, Uchino and Wethington (2016).

14 Cacioppo and Cacioppo (2014).

15 Cole, S. W. (2013) "Social regulation of human gene expression: Mechanisms and implications for public health." *Am J Public Health 103*, S1, S84–S92.

16 Norman, G. J., Hawkley, L., Ball, A., Berntson, G. G. and Cacioppo, J. T. (2013) "Perceived social isolation moderates the relationship between early childhood trauma and pulse pressure in older adults." *Int J Psychophysiol 88*, 3, 334–338.

17 Karayannis, N. V., Baumann, I., Sturgeon, J. A., Melloh, M. and Mackey, S. C. (2018) "The impact of social isolation on pain interference: A longitudinal study." *Ann Behav Med 53*, 1, 65–74; Oliveira, V. C., Ferreira, M. L., Morso, L., Albert, H. B., Refshauge, K. M. and Ferreira, P. H. (2015) "Patients' perceived level of social isolation affects the prognosis of low back pain: Social isolation and low back pain." *European Journal of Pain 19*, 4, 538–545; Evers, A. W., Kraaimaat, F. W., Geenen, R., Jacobs, J. W. and Bijlsma, J. W. (2003) "Pain coping and social support as predictors of long-term functional disability and pain in early rheumatoid arthritis." *Behaviour Research and Therapy 41*, 11, 1295–1310.

18 Karayannis *et al.* (2018).

19 López-Martínez, A. E., Esteve-Zarazaga, R. and Ramírez-Maestre, C. (2008) "Perceived social support and coping responses are independent variables explaining pain adjustment among chronic pain patients." *Journal of Pain 9*, 4, 373–379.

20 Koenig, H. G., McCullough, M. E. and Larson, D. B. (2001) *Handbook of Religion and Health.* Oxford and New York, NY: Oxford University Press.

21 Eisenberger, N. I., Jarcho, J. M., Lieberman, M. D. and Naliboff, B. D. (2006) "An experimental study

of shared sensitivity to physical pain and social rejection." *Pain 126*, 1, 132–138.

22 Eisenberger *et al.* (2006).

23 Frankl, V. E. (2006) *Man's Search for Meaning.* Mini book edition. Boston, MA: Beacon Press.

24 Dezutter, Luyckx and Wachholtz (2015).

25 Dezutter, Luyckx and Wachholtz (2015).

26 Boyle, P. A., Barnes, L. L., Buchman, A. S. and Bennett, D. A. (2009) "Purpose in life is associated with mortality among community-dwelling older persons." *Psychosom Med 71*, 5, 574–579; Krause, N. (2009) "Meaning in life and mortality." *J Gerontol B Psychol Sci Soc Sci 64*, 4, 517–527; Sone, T., Nakaya, N., Ohmori, K. *et al.* (2008) "Sense of life worth living (Ikigai) and mortality in Japan: Ohsaki study." *Psychosom Med 70*, 6, 709–715; Ryff, C. D. (2014) "Psychological well-being revisited: Advances in the science and practice of eudaimonia." *Psychother Psychosom 83*, 1, 10–28.

27 Ryff (2014).

28 Ryff (2014).

29 Vaillant, G. (2008) "Positive emotions, spirituality and the practice of psychiatry." *Mens Sana Monographs 6*, 1, 48.

30 Cole, S. W., Levine, M. E., Arevalo, J. M. G., Ma, J., Weir, D. R. and Crimmins, E. M. (2015) "Loneliness, eudaimonia, and the human conserved transcriptional response to adversity." *Psychoneuroendocrinology 62*, 11–17.

31 Cole *et al.* (2015).

32 Dezutter *et al.* (2013).

33 Dezutter *et al.* (2013).

34 Dezutter, Luyckx and Wachholtz (2015).

35 Edwards *et al.* (2014).

36 Vaillant, G. (2008); Koenig, H. G. (2012) "Religion, spirituality, and health: The research and clinical implications." *ISRN Psychiatry*, 1–33; King, M. B. and Koenig, H. G. (2009) "Conceptualising spirituality for medical research and health service provision." *BMC Health Services Research 9*, 1; Monod, S., Brennan, M., Rochat, E., Martin, E., Rochat, S. and Büla, C. J. (2011) "Instruments measuring spirituality in clinical research: A systematic review." *Journal of General Internal Medicine 26*, 11, 1345–1357.

37 Vaillant (2008); Koenig (2012); King and Koenig (2009); Wachholtz, A. B. and Pearce, M. J. (2009) "Does spirituality as a coping mechanism help or hinder coping with chronic pain?" *Current Pain and Headache Reports 13*, 2, 127–132.

38 Koenig, McCullough and Larson (2001); Koenig (2012); King and Koenig (2009); Monod *et al.* (2011); Wachholtz and Pearce (2009); Büssing, A., Michalsen, A., Balzat, H.-J. *et al.* (2009) "Are spirituality and religiosity resources for patients with chronic pain conditions?" *Pain Med 10*, 2, 327–339.

39 Koenig, McCullough and Larson (2001); Wachholtz and Pearce (2009).

40 Koenig (2012); Monod *et al.* (2011).

41 Wachholtz and Pearce (2009).

42 Wachholtz and Pearce (2009).

43 Koenig, McCullough and Larson (2001); Wachholtz and Pearce (2009).

44 Koenig (2012); Wachholtz and Pearce (2009).

45 Koenig (2012); Wachholtz and Pearce (2009).

46 Wachholtz and Pearce (2009).

47 Thomson, J. A. K. and Tredennick, H. (2004) *The Nicomachean Ethics.* Further revised edition. London and New York, NY: Penguin Books.

48 Ryan and Deci (2001).

49 Ryan and Deci (2001).

50 Ryan and Deci (2001); Ryff, C. D., Singer, B. H. and Dienberg Love, G. (2004) "Positive health: Connecting well-being with biology." *Philos Trans R Soc B Biol Sci 359*, 1449, 1383–1394.

51 Ryan and Deci (2001); Thomson and Tredennick (2004).

52 Thomson and Tredennick (2004); Blackburn, S. (2003) *Ethics: A Very Short Introduction.* New York, NY: Oxford University Press.

53 Ryff *et al.* (2004).

54 Ryan and Deci (2001); Ryff *et al.* (2004); Keyes, C. L. and Simoes, E. J. (2012) "To flourish or not: Positive mental health and all-cause mortality." *Am J Public Health 102*, 11, 2164–2172.

55 Ryan and Deci (2001); Ryff (2014); Ryff *et al.* (2004); Keyes and Simoes (2012).

56 Ryff (2014); Ryff *et al.* (2004); Ryff, C. D. and Keyes, C. L. (1995) "The structure of psychological well-being revisited." *J Pers Soc Psychol 69*, 4, 719–727.

57 Ryff *et al.* (2004); Ryff and Keyes (1995).

58 Ryff and Keyes (1995).

59 Ryff and Keyes (1995).

60 Ryff and Keyes (1995).

61 Ryff and Keyes (1995).

62 Ryan and Deci (2001).

63 Ryff and Keyes (1995).

64 Cole (2013); Cole *et al.* (2015); Fredrickson, B. L., Grewen, K. M., Algoe, S. B. *et al.* (2015) "Psychological well-being and the human conserved transcriptional response to adversity." *PLoS One 10*, 3, e0121839; Fredrickson, B. L., Grewen, K. M., Coffey, K. A. *et al.* (2013) "A functional genomic perspective on human well-being." *Proc Natl Acad Sci 110*, 33, 13684–13689.

65 Cole *et al.* (2015).

66 Fredrickson *et al.* (2015).

67 Fredrickson *et al.* (2013).

68 Ryff *et al.* (2004).

69 Ryff (2014)

70 Keyes and Simoes (2012).

71 Schleicher, H., Alonso, C., Shirtcliff, E. A., Muller, D., Loevinger, B. L. and Coe, C. L. (2005) "In the face of pain: The relationship between psychological well-being and disability in women with fibromyalgia." *Psychother Psychosom 74*, 4, 231–239.

72 Schleicher *et al.* (2005).

73 Schleicher *et al.* (2005).

74 Dezutter, Luyckx and Wachholtz (2015); Dezutter *et al.* (2013).

75 Schleicher *et al.* (2005).

76  Ross, A., Bevans, M., Friedmann, E., Williams, L. and Thomas, S. (2014) "'I am a nice person when i do yoga!!!': A qualitative analysis of how yoga affects relationships." *J Holist Nurs 32*, 2, 67–77; Fiori, F., Aglioti, S. M. and David, N. (2017) "Interactions between body and social awareness in yoga." *J Altern Complement Med 23*, 3, 227–233.

77  Ross *et al.* (2014); Ivtzan, I. and Papantoniou, A. (2014) "Yoga meets positive psychology: Examining the integration of hedonic (gratitude) and eudaimonic (meaning) wellbeing in relation to the extent of yoga practice." *J Bodyw Mov Ther 18*, 2, 183–189.

78  Stoler-Miller, B. (2004) *The Bhagavad-Gita*. New York, NY: Bantam Classics.

79  Stoler-Miller (2004); Miller, R. (2012) *The Samkhya Karika*. San Rafael, CA: Integrative Restoration Institute; Stoler-Miller, B. (1998) *Yoga: Discipline of Freedom*. New York, NY: Bantam Books; Sullivan, M., Moonaz, S., Weber., K., Taylor, J. N. and Schmalzl, L. (2017) "Towards an explanatory framework for yoga therapy informed by philosphical and ethical perspectives." *Altern Ther Health Med 24*, 1, 38–47.

80  Sullivan *et al.* (2017).

81  Easwaran, E. (2007) *The Upanishads*. Tomales, CA: The Blue Mountain Center of Meditation.

82  Easwaran (2007).

83  Easwaran (2007).

84  Stoler-Miller (2004); Miller (2012); Stoler-Miller (1998).

85  Ross *et al.* (2014).

86  Easwaran (2007).

87  Stoler-Miller (2004).

88  Easwaran (2007).

89  Ross *et al.* (2014).

90  Ross *et al.* (2014); Stoler-Miller (2004).

91  Ross *et al.* (2014).

92  Black, D. S., Cole, S. W., Irwin, M. R. *et al.* (2013) "Yogic meditation reverses NF-κB and IRF-related transcriptome dynamics in leukocytes of family dementia caregivers in a randomized controlled trial." *Psychoneuroendocrinology 38*, 3, 348–355;

Bower, J. E., Greendale, G., Crosswell, A. D. *et al.* (2014) "Yoga reduces inflammatory signaling in fatigued breast cancer survivors: A randomized controlled trial." *Psychoneuroendocrinology 43*, 20–29.

93  Stoler-Miller (2004).

94  Stoler-Miller (2004).

95  Ross *et al.* (2014).

96  Edwards *et al.* (2014).

97  Fiori, Aglioti and David (2017); Rani, J. N. and Rao, K. P. (1994) "Body awareness and yoga training." *Perceptual and Motor Skills 79*, 1103–1106; Fiori, F., David, N. and Aglioti, S. M. (2014) "Processing of proprioceptive and vestibular body signals and self-transcendence in Ashtanga yoga practitioners." *Front Hum Neurosci* doi: 10.3389/fnhum.2014.00734.

98  Stoler-Miller (2004).

99  Doniger, W. (2010) *The Hindus: An Alternative History*. New York, NY: Penguin Books; Raveh, D. (2016) *Sutras, Stories and Yoga Philosophy: Narrative and Transfiguration*. London and New York, NY: Routledge, Taylor and Francis Group; Sullivan, M. and Robertson, L. (in press) "Understanding yoga therapy: Applied philosophy and science for health and well-being."

100  Embree, A. T., Hay, S. N. and De Bary, W. T. (eds) (1988) *Sources of Indian Tradition*. 2nd edition. New York, NY: Columbia University Press.

101  Ross *et al.* (2014).

102  Thomson and Tredennick (2004); Smith, J. D. (ed.) (2009) *Mahābhārata*. London: Penguin.

103  Gupta, B. (2006) "'Bhagavad Gītā' as duty and virtue ethics: Some reflections." *Journal of Religious Ethics 34*, 3, 373–395.

104  Cole *et al.* (2015); Keyes and Simoes (2012); Fredrickson *et al.* (2015).

105  Edwards *et al.* (2014).

106  Edwards *et al.* (2014).

107  Smith, J. A., Greer, T., Sheets, T. and Watson, S. (2011) "Is there more to yoga than exercise? *Altern Ther Health Med 17*, 3, 22.

108  Fiori, Aglioti and David (2017).

# Index

abdominal pain 47–8
acceptance
  of change 30
  niyama of 76
  self- 265
accuracy/inaccuracy of senses 133, 165
addiction
  12-step recovery model 214–6
  biological vulnerabilities to 210
  components of treatments 212
  definitions 208–10
  integrative models 216–9
  mindfulness-based interventions for 217–8
  opioid crisis 206–8
  recovery models 210–3
  remission from 211
  "substance use disorder" 209–10
  Toivo Center 218–9
  yoga lifestyle approach 213–9
Adverse Childhood Experiences (ACE) study 210
affective domain of compassion 239–40, 243, 245
allodynia 87
alternate nostril breathing 147, 149
American College of Physicians 16, 42, 208
American Medical Association 16
American Pain Society 42
American Psychiatric Association 209
ambiguous loss 222
amygdala 97
anterior cingulate cortex 96
appropriation of yoga 53
Aristotle 56, 263, 271, 276
Arman, M. 238
arthritis 42–5
attention domain of compassion 239, 242, 245
attitude towards pain 232–3
autonomic nervous system
  dysregulation-pain relationship 106–7
  integration within 107–8
  overview 100–1
  parasympathetic nervous system 104–5
  and self-regulation 105–6
  sympathetic nervous system 104–5
  yoga and regulation of 113–5
  see also polyvagal theory
Avicenna 56
awareness
  bodily dissociation 166
  body awareness 160–8

Body Awareness Questionnaire 162
Body Awareness Scale 162
body schema 168–72
  equanimity and 114, 116–7
  internal 77–8
  Multidimensional Assessment of Interoceptive
    Awareness 162
  non-judgemental 162
  obstacles to 159
  overview 159

back pain 40–2, 130
Barron, F. 63
belief systems 55, 62
Belton, J. 256
Bhakti yoga 73
Bhavanani, A. B. 163, 199
bodily dissociation 166
body, rejection of 258
body awareness 160–8
Body Awareness Questionnaire 162
Body Awareness Scale 162
body schema 168–72
body-self neuromatrix 102
Bolz, M. 238
Bosch, P. R. 43
Boss, P. 222
brain see physiological processes
breathing (pranayama)
  alternate nostril breathing 147, 149
  breath awareness 144–5
  breath regulation 145–8
  breath visualization 147
  breathing pattern disorders 143–4
  clinical relevance 155–7
  deep slow breathing 146–7, 148
  definitions 142
  faster paced breathing 149
  grounding effect of 32–3
  hyperventilation 143–4, 151
  influence of pain on 150–1
  longer-smoother-softer breath 146–8
  Nijmegen Questionnaire 144
  opioids effects on 151
  overview 77, 141–3
  research 148–51, 152–5
  respiratory alkalosis 143
  Resurrection Breath 253

315